Specialty Care in the Era of Managed Care

Specialty Care in the Era of Managed Care

Cleveland Clinic versus
University Hospitals of Cleveland

John A. Kastor, M.D.
Professor of Medicine
University of Maryland School of Medicine
Baltimore, Maryland

The Johns Hopkins University Press
Baltimore

The Johns Hopkins University Press
2715 North Charles Street
Baltimore, Maryland 21218-4363
www.press.jhu.edu

Library of Congress Cataloging-in-Publication Data

Kastor, John A.
  Specialty care in the era of managed care : Cleveland Clinic
versus University Hospitals of Cleveland / John A. Kastor.
    p. ; cm.
  Includes bibliographical references and index.
  ISBN 0-8018-8174-9 (hardcover : alk. paper)
  1. Cleveland Clinic Foundation. 2. University Hospitals of
Cleveland (Ohio). 3. Academic medical centers—Effect of
managed care on—Ohio—Cleveland. 4. Hospitals—Ohio—
Cleveland—Administration. 5. Managed care plans (Medical
care)—Ohio—Cleveland.
  [DNLM: 1. Cleveland Clinic Foundation. 2. University
Hospitals of Cleveland (Ohio). 3. Hospitals, Private—trends—
Ohio. 4. Hospitals, Teaching—trends—Ohio. 5. Managed Care
Programs—Ohio. 6. Specialties, Medical—trends—Ohio.
WX 27 AO3 K19s 2005] I. Title.
  RA982.C62C555 2005
  362.11'068'0977132—dc22   2004028271

A catalog record for this book is available from the British Library.

To the memory of my mother and stepfather,

Ellen Voigt Bentley and Julius Long Stern

Contents

Photographs appear following pages 83 and 185

Preface

Limiting the care of patients by specialists forms one of the fundamental tenets of managed care. The mantra dictates that patients should first see their primary care physicians, who will evaluate and treat most of the patients' ills and refer them to specialists only when absolutely necessary. This approach will reduce the cost of care by limiting the ministrations of highly paid specialists and avoiding the expensive tests they love to order and the procedures they can't wait to perform. The generalist will also, as a participant in a health *maintenance* organization, or HMO—or so the theory goes—render preventive medicine and thereby avoid or at least delay the need for expensive specialty care. Where, then, does this leave those providers who specialize in being specialists?[1]

To learn more about this conflict, I studied the two leading centers for specialty care in Cleveland: the Cleveland Clinic, one of America's most successful group practices, and University Hospitals of Cleveland, the primary teaching hospital of the Case Western Reserve University School of Medicine. I learned what I learned by using the same technique employed in two previous studies:[2,3] interviewing as many people as possible who could add to the story.

I'm a cardiologist and have long wondered how the Cleveland Clinic reached its eminence in our field. I knew of the fundamental discoveries made by members of its staff in the 1950s and 1960s, which introduced contemporary methods of diagnosing and treating coronary disease. But to have continued to lead as the decades passed required some accomplishments about which I was ignorant. As someone who has always worked in academic medical centers, I wondered how this institution, located in an old rust-belt city with more than its share of urban difficulties and without a medical school, had prospered and, in the judgment of *U.S. News & World Report*, surpassed, at least in cardiac care, the most famous and respected of our medical school-related teaching hospitals.

In the process of talking to people at the Clinic, I constantly heard about the rivalry for the Clinic's patients by its principal competitor, University Hospitals of Cleveland, located only one mile away at University Circle. Accordingly, I decided to sweep University Hospitals and its associated university into the study.

I interviewed 248 people, often in their offices, less frequently by telephone or e-mail. Ninety-five were from the Cleveland Clinic Foundation and 153 from University Hospitals of Cleveland and Case Western Reserve University (see appendix 1). The first interview was conducted in July 2002, and I sent the manuscript to the publisher twenty-four months later. A few facts of particular interest were added in subsequent months.

To enhance accuracy, I sent drafts of the material that I had written about our conversations to each person interviewed. With few exceptions, each interviewee responded promptly with useful comments and revisions, which saved me from making more mistakes than the manuscript may still contain. I then rewrote the text to include all their corrections and most of their revisions and added, often as footnotes, comments that conflicted from what I had learned from others. A few people with whom I spoke did not wish to be directly associated with particular quotations or identified in the appendix as having been interviewed.

I thank those who read and, in some cases, commented on one or more of the chapters: at the Cleveland Clinic—John Clough, Floyd Loop, and Eric Topol; at University Hospitals of Cleveland and Case Western Reserve University—Malvin Bank, Richard Baznik, Robert Daroff, Edward Hundert, John Lewis, Adel Mahmoud, Roger Meyer, Richard Pogue, Agnar Pytte, and Farah Walters. Diane Solov, who has covered the medical scene in Cleveland for a decade as a medical reporter for *The Plain Dealer,* provided much useful information through her articles in the newspaper. She helped further by answering several questions I put to her directly. The suggestions of each of these people assisted me in improving the accuracy and clarity of the text. Problems that remain must be assigned to the author.

At the Johns Hopkins University Press, I thank my editor Wendy Harris for her continuing advice and support. Maria denBoer expertly edited the copy and Becky Hornyak prepared the index, as they did for one of my previous books. The ever-faithful Phyllis Farrell at the University of Maryland checked my review of the proofs and, as usual, found some problems I had overlooked. Only I can be blamed for those that remain.

Specialty Care in the Era of Managed Care

CHAPTER ONE

Cleveland and Its Medical Centers

In the fall of 1996, the two dominant hospital systems in the city of Cleveland, Ohio, contended to acquire the Meridia Health System, itself a merger of four community hospitals on Cleveland's East Side. After an intense and, at times, bitter competition, the Meridia board of trustees, by a majority of one vote, awarded itself to the Cleveland Clinic Foundation, leaving the University Hospital Health System to lick its wounds. The rivalry for the Meridia prize involved not only the winning and losing institutions but also their trustees and CEOs, Farah Walters at University and Dr. Fred Loop at the Clinic, who competed repeatedly to control the region's medical specialty business.

To tell the story of this rivalry, one must start by looking at the site of the battle. About 500,000 people live in the city in which the Cleveland Clinic and University Hospitals of Cleveland are located, half as many as at the end of World War II.[1]* The median income is $26,840, and the level of poverty about 13 percent, both similar to most cities with more than 200,000

*The current population of the Cleveland metropolitan area is about 2.2 million.

residents.[2] Cleveland citizens are older, with 15 percent over age fifty-four, compared with 11 percent elsewhere. Fewer under age sixty-five lack insurance for health care, 8.6 percent compared with an average of 15 percent elsewhere, which is said to reflect the tight labor market and the relatively generous benefits companies find it necessary to provide.[2]

The city has become a "small employer town," according to Jon Christianson, a health care economist who has studied the region. "Cleveland has only three Fortune 500 companies now. There were thirty a few decades ago, I've been told."[3] Many of the leaders of the larger corporations in Cleveland tend to live there because of their jobs.[4] "They can be moved tomorrow," observed a former department chairman at Case Western Reserve University (CASE)* School of Medicine, who is now a senior executive at a large pharmaceutical house.[5]

The city, many claim, likes to call itself a big city but actually has many of the qualities of a small town.[6] One observer described it as having "big city problems with a small city mentality."[7] From the vantage point of New York City, to which he moved, a former CASE medical professor observed, "For all its harrumphing about being a world-class city, the cultural reality is that Cleveland is a small Midwestern town that has cultural organizations left over from the gifts of wealthy donors that a city its current size might not otherwise have."[8] As one of the Clinic surgeons observed, "Cleveland has a lousy football team, a weak baseball team, a first-class orchestra, and it's hardly a business center anymore."[9]

Despite its current problems, Cleveland has a proud industrial history.[10] "Cleveland was once third in cities with Fortune 500 company headquarters, a leader in iron, steel, oil, refining, and chemicals," recalls Robert Eckardt of the Cleveland Foundation. "Charitable giving was enormous and service on nonprofit boards expected of its leaders. Once it was the country's fifth largest city; now it's fifteenth to seventeenth."[11]

Although much of the manufacturing that brought an older Cleveland its wealth has left, headquarters of many firms remain there because, according to one of the city's leading lawyers and former chairman of the board of University Hospitals of Cleveland, "they like living here."[1] Suburban living—Shaker Heights being probably the best-known community—

---

*In 2003, the leaders of Case Western Reserve University adopted the name and style CASE for informal reference to their institution.

can be very comfortable and convenient. Substantial houses, many built in the 1920s, face winding, tree-covered streets, only a short distance from both the Cleveland Clinic and University Hospitals.

Accordingly, much executive talent remains in Cleveland. A particular fan of the town is Dr. James Block, the CEO of University Hospitals from 1986 to 1992. Block left Cleveland to become CEO of the Johns Hopkins Hospital and consequently has worked for two different boards of trustees in two cities of relatively similar size. "Although each has a large population of poor people in the core of the city," Block said, "the economic underpinnings are quite different. Cleveland has a larger number of corporate headquarters: auto parts, corporations like Sherwin-Williams and Glidden paints and Stouffer foods, and publicly traded banks. And there's tremendous wealth. All this brings talent to boards."[12] Block found that his trustees had more depth and quantity of executive leadership in Cleveland than in Baltimore.[12]

"An unknown jewel in many respects," is how a leading banker and trustee of the Cleveland Clinic sees Cleveland. "I find the mixture of culture, education, basic manufacturing, ethnic diversity, and wealth fascinating. And there are few places with such a depth of affordable housing." He believes that "those of us not born and raised here are less hard on Cleveland."[13]

Nevertheless, economic growth in Cleveland and surrounding areas remains slow.[13] The departure of the former drivers of much of the local economy has left the two health care systems—the Clinic, the larger of the two, and University Hospitals—as the city's largest nongovernmental[14] employers.[3] With the economic future of Cleveland so tied to these centers, larger employers and insurance plans have refrained from squeezing the hospitals with debilitating lower rates as in other markets. Furthermore, Cleveland companies have not formed employer consortia, which elsewhere have forced providers to accept lower payments.[15]

Despite the somewhat less onerous environment of the Cleveland medical scene, the leaders of the Clinic and University Hospitals needed to respond to the challenges of managed care and used methods that have also been applied with varying success elsewhere. Two features, however, make the Cleveland scene unique. One is the method by which the Clinic governs itself, a system of conducting its business with few parallels among other large clinical centers. The other was the presence until recently of a mutually damaging conflict that afflicted University Hospitals and its affiliated medical school.

This book describes how these and other features of the competitive relationship between these two large medical centers affected how specialty care would be delivered in the community and how that effort would affect the future of each. Finally, this study describes the efforts by the Cleveland Clinic to create a medical school, a longstanding goal of the institution.

CHAPTER TWO

Cleveland Clinic
The Clinical Factory

Three surgeons and one internist, all practitioners in Cleveland, Ohio, founded in 1919 what would become, by the beginning of the twenty-first century, a medical institution in which a group practice of more than 1,300 doctors would care for more than 800 inpatients and 5,500 outpatients each day and train more than 750 residents and fellows each year. In addition to the 155-acre main campus in Cleveland, the organization would grow to contain an outpatient clinic and two hospitals in Florida and ten community hospitals in Ohio. The magazine *U.S. News & World Report* would rank the Cleveland Clinic fourth in its 2004 "Honor Roll" of the best hospitals in the country.[1] In 2004, the Clinic admitted the first class of thirty-two students to its new medical college "devoted," as described by Dr. Floyd ("Fred") Loop, the Clinic CEO, "to the education of physician-investigators."[2]

Although they created a for-profit entity to construct the first building,[3] the founders* soon donated their holdings to the Cleveland Clinic Founda-

*Surgeons Frank E. Bunts, George W. Crile, and William E. Lower and internist John Phillips. For a more complete history of the Clinic, see *To Act as a Unit: The Story of the Cleveland Clinic* by John Clough,[4] on which much of this section is based.

tion, a nonprofit corporation which, since being established by the state of Ohio on February 5, 1921,[5] has owned the institution. The greatest trial that the founders and their associates faced occurred only eight years after the creation of the Clinic, when a fire, fed by burning nitrocellulose x-ray films, produced toxic fumes that helped to kill 123 people, among them a founder, the internist John Phillips.[6] This personal and financial tragedy plus the economic effects of the Great Depression made the 1930s a particularly difficult time for the young Clinic. Founder George Crile's immense surgical practice—he brought many members of Cleveland's first families to the Clinic[7]—continued to support the Clinic throughout much of the decade. He retained in his salary much less than he collected for his services. For many years after its founding the organization was known, not surprisingly, as "The Crile Clinic,"* the place to go when complicated surgery was required.[7,8]

Eventually, each of founders left the scene—Crile died in 1943—and new men and the Foundation's board of trustees led the growing enterprise. Beginning in 1955, a board of governors of physicians elected by the group practice gradually took over the management of its professional and organizational activities. During the first thirteen years of the board of governors' existence, the business manager and hospital administrator limited its authority, since they had been appointed by, and reported to, the trustees. In those simpler and less expensive days, however, the trustees usually supported the governors' projects because surpluses from operations provided what was needed and financing by debt was unnecessary. The administrators and some of the trustees set the doctors' salaries.[9]

As the board of trustees evolved over the years, the character of its members changed and its numbers increased. Now there are more than eighty trustees, for the most part the usual worthies who fill such positions. Ten are physicians. The executive committee of eighteen includes three doctors, two of whom are the Clinic's CEO and chief of staff.[10] This is the group most intimately involved in overseeing the Clinic. "Its responsibilities have become increasingly broad, objective, and complex," Loop said.[2]

The board itself, like so many similar boards, is too large for the average member to participate actively in management. "Being on the board was a

---

*Changing the name of the Clinic to the "Crile Clinic," in imitation of the Mayo Clinic, was considered and rejected.[7]

rubber stamp," said one former chairman of the board[11]—"show and tell," according to another—"but you do get access to the Clinic and its doctors when you need them."[11] "Trustees love the place and the docs who take care of them," according to Malachai Mixon, the board chairman.[12]

The Board of Governors Takes Over

By 1968, the governors' desire for greater and more rapid expansion conflicted with the opinion of some of the trustees, who feared that "the prudence of businesslike standards could easily be cast aside," as the official historian of the Clinic describes their attitude, and particularly with that of the business manager of the Clinic who reported to them.[13] The controversy led to a secret meeting at a Cleveland club of a small group of the Clinic's leading doctors who resolved to carry through the reassignment of the administrative functions from the board of trustees and its appointees to the board of governors. The business manager was removed from his position, and a new chairman of the board of governors, Dr. Carl Wasmuth, a lawyer as well as a physician, was elected. Wasmuth put aside his clinical practice and leadership of the department of anesthesiology and devoted himself solely to his administrative responsibilities, thereby reinstituting the tradition of physician leadership initially exercised in the days of the founders when the Clinic was much smaller and less complex. A second physician, a urologist this time, also closed his practice and, after taking an advanced management course at Harvard, joined the administration as vice chairman of the board of governors and director of operations. From this time forward, in a spirit of shared governance, the board of trustees tended to emphasize fiscal considerations—its investment and finance committees providing significant advice—while the board of governors directed the Clinic's medical affairs.[14] "Businessmen should stick to business issues and never get involved in medical issues," says Mal Mixon.[12] As trustee Robert Lintz puts it, "We're more interested in guiding than managing."[15]

As the Clinic grew, it faced a decision familiar to many universities and hospitals. Although its first building, which opened in 1921, faced Euclid Avenue* in what was then a wealthy, although already deteriorating,[18] section of the city, the Clinic, like many other medical centers, eventually

---

*Euclid Avenue was once known as "Millionaire's Row."[16,17]

found itself surrounded by empty lots, a minority population, and poor schools.[17,19] The local population's income and the real estate values had fallen as the Clinic's wealthier, formerly local clientele moved to the suburbs.[16,19] Today two mansions[18,20]* and two large, architecturally impressive churches[22] near the Clinic attest to the magnificence of the institution's earlier surroundings. Despite the environment, however, the governors and trustees decided, in the mid-1960s, not to move to a more congenial site to the east;[7,17] purchased adjacent property, then available at depreciated prices,[7]† for future expansion; and built a hotel for patients and their families, a parking garage, and, thanks to a generous bequest, an education building.

By 1988, the Clinic, which was then operating more than a thousand beds and had recently completed a large capital program funded for the first time in its history with borrowed money, began to experience serious financial difficulties[23] that led to depletion of its reserves.[17] Changing methods of reimbursement with the end of cost-based payment, the rise of managed care, losses from the operation of a branch of the Cleveland Clinic in Florida,‡ and a floundering computer system prompted a comprehensive review of the Clinic's operation. Assisted by an independent consulting firm, the Clinic estimated that it could lose $175 million over the next three years unless drastic action was taken.[24] The administration, according to a longtime department director present then and now, found the Clinic's leaders "so imbued with the need for consensus, we missed doing things."[17]

The chairman of the board of governors at the time was Dr. William Kiser, a skilled urologist and charismatic leader who was highly respected by the medical staff.[7] The staff saw Kiser as "an open man, easy to communicate with,"[25] and "a very pleasant man who greeted everyone in the halls with a friendly 'hello' and looked for consensus." He had been elected to the board of governors in 1972, had become chief operating officer two years later, and, on the resignation of the CEO, succeeded to the top position in 1976. "The board of governors and board of trustees selected me to be CEO," he remembers, "without a search."[9] Kiser's personality contrasted

---

*One, now owned by the Clinic at Euclid Avenue and East Eighty-ninth Street, was built by Francis Drury, whose firm made burners for the lamps fueled by John D. Rockefeller's kerosene.[21]

†Shattuck Hartwell, a plastic surgeon who was chief of staff from 1974 to 1987, remembers that these purchases were conducted by third parties to prevent the values from inflating if the sellers knew that the Clinic was the buyer.[7]

‡See the discussion later in this chapter.

strongly with that of his predecessor, a "smart man with a good business sense"[7] but whom Kiser remembers as "autocratic."[9]

As financial problems grew at the end of the 1980s, some of the governors concluded that something more than Kiser's gentle and winning ways was needed to restore prosperity to the Clinic: a CEO who could reach decisions more quickly[17] and was willing to introduce changes thought necessary at this difficult time.[26] Kiser resigned in July 1989.

New Chief Executive and Governance

A search committee of governors and trustees[11] reviewed the suitability of thirty-three internal and external candidates, both doctors and administrators, to become the new CEO. The committee, as William MacDonald, then chairman of the board of trustees, remembers, "was leaning toward an outside guy who was not a Clinic veteran."[11] The doctors on the committee strongly favored choosing a doctor then at the Clinic.[11]

Cardiac surgeon Fred Loop describes what followed: "The board [of governors] said we needed a change of leadership and tabled everything. I was one of the bigger complainers among the governors and was really worried about the place."[24] Colleagues suggested that Loop should become a candidate. "It wasn't my ambition to be a CEO until it was put to me, but I thought I could do a better job than any of those who had applied for it."[24] So he entered the lists, made a presentation to the search committee, and was eventually chosen.*

It had been the governors, not the trustees, who brought about the change in leadership, and the board of trustees was not informed until Kiser had resigned, causing some irritation among the more involved trustees.[11] "I should have spoken up," says Art Modell, the senior trustee at the time. Modell admired Kiser and regretted changing the leadership. "I had no power to do anything," he said, reflecting the superior authority of the board of governors over the trustees in this critical decision.[28] Loop would make certain to inform the executive committee of the trustees about all important issues that the governors were considering.[11]

The choice of Loop supported the custom that the Clinic, three of whose

---

*See Diane Solov's "Dr. CEO," a comprehensive story about Loop and the Cleveland Clinic in the April 18, 2004 edition of *The Plain Dealer Sunday Magazine*.[27]

founders had been surgeons, would continue to be dominated by surgeons[29,30] with their "surgical personality,"[31] which says "we can get it done" and "don't take 'no' for an answer."[30] Observers of the events suggested that, due to the financial status of the Clinic, if a doctor with Loop's business sense and proactive attitude hadn't become available, the trustees "might have pushed for a layman."[32] On November 8, 1989, Loop began "the toughest year of my life."[24]

Chairman of the highly successful department of cardiothoracic surgery at the Clinic from 1975 until 1989, Loop was a widely respected and busy cardiac surgeon who had contributed important advances to his specialty. Now, although he continued to operate on four patients each week for several years,[17] Loop had become responsible for reversing the financial losses, responding to the rapidly changing medical environment, and, somehow, continuing to develop and expand the Clinic's operation. Trustees differed about whether Loop should continue to operate. William MacDonald told him that some trustees felt "that he couldn't operate and do the CEO job."[11] Loop said that he could run the place and still operate but would decrease the number of cases he would do. Modell agreed that Loop's continuing to operate was wise, "so he's in the trenches."[28]

Loop moved into the CEO's office lined with dark wood walls at the end of a large suite of offices where the senior administrative staff of the Clinic works. The visitor cannot help but notice that most of the secretaries call their physician and administrative supervisors, including Loop, by their first names. Some formality, however, persists. "Suits and ties are still the norm," explains chief operating officer Frank Lordeman.[33]

Loop quickly controlled expenses without compromising patient care or the academic mission of the institution.[32] He did not renew the one-year contracts—routine at the Clinic and a terrifying concept to tenured members of medical faculties—of five members of the staff whom the CEO had concluded were relatively unproductive. "Sent a message," he says,[24] and afterward there was little housecleaning among the doctors. He encouraged the less industrious to retire, or, if they had a penchant for research, created suitable positions for them. "It was a slow, deliberate process," according to Thomas Seals, the director of the department of protective services from 1984 to 2003, who has known Loop for nineteen years.[17]

Loop restructured the administration by reducing the number of people directly reporting to him, thinking his predecessor had had, in twenty-five direct reports, too many. He turned over fifty administrators in the first five years of his administration.[34] The project of converting the accounts receivable into cash was reassigned from the chief financial officer to the chief operating officer.[34]

As Loop embarked on changes, not each of which was universally popular, trustee William MacDonald advised that he needed to emulate his predecessor's congenial personality and familiar personal relationship with the staff and employees, which included "a lot of handshaking."[11] This is not the style of the CEO, essentially a shy man.[35] His predecessor was characteristically "nice, perhaps, too nice. Fred can be a bit rough,"[11] but "not rigid."[35] Compared with his predecessor, Loop is more authoritarian, "more closed,"[25] "a benevolent autocrat," according to one of his colleagues.[36] "He takes a position, and that's that," according to one of the department chairmen.[26] Despite some characteristics that might be seen as disadvantageous, all acknowledge that Loop is "a strong and effective leader."[25] Thus, the Clinic had chosen someone with more of the forceful characteristics of the CEO who preceded the benevolent Kiser, a man whose term as CEO ended in part because he had come to be seen as high-handed.

The sixteen-member board of governors remained the principal governing group, its nine physicians serving five-year terms.* The staff elects a nominating committee, which is chaired by the outgoing governors, to propose a slate of about ten doctors. The governors then choose one or two from the list to fill the seats of those who are retiring.[37,38] The system thus gives the staff the democratic opportunity of naming the members of the nominating committee, while the final choice is made by the governors and the CEO. The governors then ask the staff to ratify the choices, a pro forma process since the nominees are always confirmed.[38]

By convention, three governors each come from the divisions of medicine and surgery, the two largest divisions, and three come from the other divisions.† "Each must be clinically excellent, which underlies everything

---

*As of 2004, the Clinic no longer limited the duration of service of the governors.[14]

†Unlike the custom at most medical schools, where the largest administrative units such as medicine and surgery are called "departments," at the Cleveland Clinic they are "divisions." Consequently, the subordinate units, such as cardiology in the division of medicine and cardiothoracic surgery in the division of surgery are called "departments" rather than "divisions" or "units," their

that works here," says Dr. Melinda Estes, CEO of Cleveland Clinic Florida, who served as an elected member from 1990 to 1995 and participates ex officio.* When deciding whether a colleague should become a member of the board of governors or hold another administrative position, the doctors on the staff base their choice on the candidate's reputation as a physician or investigator. "We would not select someone solely for taking a career path that emphasizes administration over medicine or research," says Robert Kay, the chief of staff.[40]

The CEO also appoints to the board of governors several senior administrators, some of whom are not physicians, and these include the chief operating officer, chief financial officer, chief academic officer, CEO of Cleveland Clinic Florida,[41] and CEO of Kaiser Permanente of Ohio in recognition of the role that group plays in Clinic operations.† Loop is the chairman, and Kay, a pediatric urologist and the chief of staff, is the vice chairman.

As the leading level of governance at the Clinic, the governors, acting in response to the advice of search committees, nominate—in effect, select—the CEO and appoint all division and department chairmen.[42] Chairmen of divisions and departments are formally reviewed every five years, and the board has the power to relieve or reappoint them. When someone has to go, however, "it follows full review and discussion by the board of governors," says Andrew Fishleder, a pathologist who is chairman of the division of education and served as an elected member of the board of governors from 1995 to 2000.[43]

Loop or Kay also chairs the weekly[31] meetings of the medical executive committee, consisting of the chairmen of the divisions, institutes, and key departments,[44] who, although officially reporting to the chief of staff and

---

almost universal titles in most medical schools. Clinic historian John Clough wonders whether the founders chose the word *division* for the principal administrative units in the Clinic because of their experience as physician-officers in World War I.[16]

Familiar to faculty working in medical schools are the divisions of anesthesiology, cancer center, eye institute (ophthalmology), medicine, pediatrics, radiology, and surgery. In addition, the Clinic accords divisional status to certain administrative units, including education, finance, general counsel, health affairs, information technology, managed care, marketing, nursing, operations, regional medical practice, and the research institute. Emergency medicine, neurology, psychiatry, and rehabilitation medicine are departments, each within the division of medicine.[39] The directors of the clinical divisions and departments are all called chairmen.

*In 2003, Estes became president and CEO of Fletcher Allen Health Care, the principal teaching hospital for the University of Vermont College of Medicine.

† See the discussion later in this chapter.

not to the CEO, individually meet with Loop when necessary. Although some believe that chairmen should not be elected governors since they can influence Clinic-wide decisions through their membership on the medical executive committee, the governors now believe that the presence of some chairmen on the board can be useful.[43]

The directors of the administrative divisions report directly to Loop. He meets with them in his administrative council, or "Loop's cabinet" as it is called,[44] over lunch four days per week. Doctors and administrators in the areas being studied attend Loop's cabinet, give their suggestions, and receive their instructions. This close association with the administration allows the CEO to keep aware of, and develop policies for,[37] all important features of the Clinic's management. Because of the management structure he has created, an important feature of which is Loop's desire to converse frequently with his associates,[45] decisions can be made quickly,[45] much faster than in the more bureaucratic organization typical of most academic medical centers. The sessions of the administrative council can be contentious, with all members contributing to the agenda, sometimes at the same time. "Everyone is smarter than someone," explains Lordeman. "But when we walk out, the contention stops, and we get done what we've decided, item by item."[46] Kevin Roberts, former treasurer at the Clinic and now chief financial officer at University Hospitals Health System, describes the process: "note the problem, marshal the forces, take ownership of a solution, implement it, move on."[47] As one of the doctors, who had been recruited from a widely respected medical school, said, "Things do happen here."[37] No minutes are taken during the meetings of Loop's cabinet.[48]

Specific issues under recent discussion at the administrative council include how to reduce the cost of the operating rooms and the pharmacy, how to improve the emergency room, and the admission process for beds and outpatient visits. How to improve "customer service" is a constant theme[42] for which the Clinic and a consultant are engaged in "a major effort. Patients have a tolerance level here," says Shawn Ulreich, the chairman of the division of nursing from 1998 to 2003. "They think, 'I'm at the Cleveland Clinic to see a famous physician, so I'll wait,' but that's not good enough for us."[49] For example, Ulreich's nurses often have to calm families and postoperative patients waiting in the postanesthesia recovery unit for a bed—a problem familiar to executives at many hospitals. Although this difficulty has become less severe, clearing beds for these patients continues to vex the Clinic's leaders. With 70 percent of the patients now entering the hospital on the same day as their operations and invasive diagnostic procedures, the Clinic constructed an attractive area where they and their families can wait. When families complained about not knowing the status of their relatives during the operative experience, Ulreich hired nurses specifically to respond to this need.[49]

The Clinic shares with many other hospitals the bane of not having enough nurses.[35] To relieve the shortage, the hospital employs nurses who are not on the regular nursing staff. The staff nurses object to working beside these nurses whose salaries, set by the agencies that employ them, are often greater than the amount the Clinic pays its staff nurses.[35]

Because of the increasing size of the Clinic, the board of governors focuses on performance of divisions and departments rather than individuals.[43] "Loop has never delegated the strategic planning function to any one executive," says Robert Ivancic, the Clinic's executive director of the division of human resources. "He feels strongly that it is the collective responsibility of the entire management team. He believes in the saying, 'No one is as smart as everyone.' "[45]

Much admired for his organizational and interpersonal skills,[12,26,31,35] Loop would rather be told things than read them in a report and doesn't favor sending memos back and forth. An informal man, who talks and makes his points quietly, Loop is only occasionally "a shouter."[50] This cardiac surgeon and executive, is, one is not surprised to learn, an ambitious man—"an understatement," according to one of his former executive colleagues[47]—but his personal ambition translates into accomplishment for the Cleveland Clinic. And he can make decisions quickly in keeping with his specialty. "He listens, then he decides," according to Kenneth Ouriel, like Loop, a surgeon and chairman of the surgery division since 2003.[31]

"No detail's too small for him," says Gene Altus, administrator of the board of governors and a regular attendee at the council, "but he doesn't micromanage. He sets goals." Altus continues, "Dr. Loop believes in innovation in both medicine and business. Will the enterprise add value to patient care and improve our fiscal situation?"[42] "Nothing gets by him," according to Ivancic,[45] or, as Tom Seals says, "he consumes information."[17] The chairman of the trustees sees Loop as "an unusual leader, a doctor who really understands the economics of medicine."[12] Consequently, the board rarely opposes what Loop recommends.[12]

Loop travels much less than is typical of many people in his position. "He avoids the limelight and is the opposite of the flashy CEO," says Robert Ivancic.[45] "He's not in it for the personal glory."[45] Tom Seals, whose department is responsible for the Clinic's vehicles, offered Loop use of a limousine to transport him to work. "Wouldn't let me give him a driver," although the Clinic does retain a large car and driver to transport VIPs and guests.* "Thought it wouldn't look good, that the staff might oppose it."[17]†

Ivancic has found him to be "a regular guy, who also happens to be a world-renowned cardiac surgeon and an extraordinary CEO. He's very supportive if we occasionally err, so long as we don't make the same mistakes twice."[45] There has been little turnover among the senior administrators once Loop assembled his own team. Ivancic, for example, has worked at the Clinic since recruited by Loop in 1991.[45]

Seals, an executive with deep respect for the CEO, remembers that, when he arrived at the Clinic to take the job, Loop, as director of the department of cardiothoracic surgery, "was the first department chair to invite me to his staff meeting. He's one of those few people you'll go up the hill with," says the former army officer. Seals sees in his boss "command presence," and greatly admires Loop's intellect and commitment to the institution.[17]

Clinic veterans consider it important and characteristic that the leader of the Cleveland Clinic be a superb clinician—Loop, sixty-seven years old in 2004, stopped operating four years ago. Melinda Estes adds, "The CEO has to be someone from the inside although this doesn't preclude our choosing a strong-willed person,"[41] which, all agree, is an apt description. Considering the history of Clinic leaders, one isn't surprised to hear Loop, the son of a doctor,[51] say, "Respected doctors should run big medical centers, particularly ours."[24] His colleagues agree.[52] "He supports the doctors and group collectively and individually."[36] As Dr. Andrew Novick, chairman of the highly successful clinical and research programs of the urological institute, puts it, "He's one of us, an academic surgeon who understands research and education."[53]

James Blazar, director of the marketing division, describes his boss as

---

*The first time I visited the Clinic, Loop's office sent the driver to pick me up at, and return me to, the airport. The ride was very comfortable both ways. Thereafter, I thought it best, to maintain at least some degree of impartiality, to arrange my own transportation.

†Loop's reserve and his desire to confirm the importance of the governors extends to his office telephone. Rather than answering "Dr. Loop's office," his secretaries have been told to greet callers with "Board of Governors."

"tough when he needs to be tough. Here you're fully accountable, including Fred. He has wide knowledge and the respect of everyone here," a fact that this writer confirms. "He's a visionary [a characteristic many apply to him[17,54]] who does not want pushovers. He wants you to be a thinker, give him your best advice, and take action. He knows quality, wants only the best people here. I feel he listens to me and learns from me, but he's so smart that I do most of the learning."[44] Loop's "history of success"[17] explains part of the almost universal support that he enjoys. In the opinion of a colleague who has known Loop throughout the period he has been CEO, "He's been brilliant building Cleveland Clinic into a regional powerhouse and raising us on the national stage."[54]

Ivancic remembers Loop's eulogy at the funeral of one of the Clinic's most generous donors, where he said, " 'The good hockey player goes to where the puck is. The great player goes to what the puck will be.' This could apply to Dr. Loop just as well. He's always been way ahead of the curve."[45]

The Group Practice

Now, as when it was founded, the Cleveland Clinic is clearly a doctors' organization, not accountable to a medical school or a private company.[51] "We are a group practice that happens to own a hospital"[39] is the mantra of the institution, and the fundamental mission and staff model have not changed since the founding.[55] The doctors—each of whom is a full-time salaried employee of the practice[56]—run the place.[26] The top executive is a surgeon, an active practitioner at the Clinic both before and for many years after he became CEO, not a professional hospital administrator or a physician who had emphasized management rather than the practice of medicine during most of his career.[46,57] Leadership by physicians assures, many at the Clinic believe, better relations with the practicing doctors, the chief resource of the place.[58] Despite the resistance of organized medicine in Cleveland to group practices in the Clinic's early days,[9] the system survived, and the doctors at the Clinic continued operating in this manner from the founding.

"Our mission has always been very clear," says Dr. Douglas Moodie, who came to the Cleveland Clinic from the Mayo Clinic in 1978 and was chairman of the department of pediatrics from 1987 to 2002.[59] "Number 1, number 2, and number 3 was to take care of patients. Everything was organized to make this happen." Moodie was struck from the time he arrived in Cleveland about how hard the staff worked. "They were here at all hours."[59] Moodie emphasizes the importance of pressure from peers and an entrepreneurial spirit as the motivators for the excellence of clinical care.[59]

When Dr. Donald Vidt, who directed the department of nephrology and hypertension from 1985 to 1991, came to the Clinic in 1964, he found "a small, friendly little place with about a hundred physicians on the staff."[25] Vidt had trained at University Hospitals (UH) of Cleveland but did not consider practicing there. "I knew I didn't want a research career, and there were few clinical opportunities at UH." When asked why he chose the Clinic, Vidt describes an "environment to practice subspecialty medicine and work with a patient population with a broad array of pathology plus the opportunity to teach the house staff and fellows."[25] The Clinic encourages its members to participate in the work of national organizations, and, responding to this policy, Vidt became a member of the House of Delegates of the American Medical Association.

"One purpose of the board of governors," says Rob Kay, the chief of staff and vice chairman of the board of governors, "is to ensure the integrity of the group practice."[40] As much as anyone at the Clinic, Kay, as chief of staff, is charged to maintain that culture.[56] "Each member must respect the other and never act at the expense of the group."[40] As two senior members of the staff put it, "We like to hang our coats next to each other,"[39] and "we care for each other as well as for the patients."[7] The trustees sense this. Patrick McCartan, a former managing partner of one of the largest law firms in the country and a member of the board's executive committee, finds "more cooperation among the doctors here than elsewhere. They're wedded to the group practice model. One for all, and all for one."[14]

When doctors move to the Clinic from a typical academic medical center, they must adjust to the dominance of the group practice. Michael Levine, who was recruited from the Johns Hopkins Hospital to chair the division of pediatrics in 2003, observed, "When they call it 'the Clinic,' that's just what they mean. People refer to their fellow physicians as 'partners,' more often than 'colleagues.'" Unlike at Hopkins, where "clinicians are second-class citizens, here you're not much if you're not a superb clinician, and, consequently, clinicians don't feel marginalized, as they may at some medical schools."[60] Whereas clinicians may have difficulty being promoted at traditional academic medical centers, "at the Clinic this is not a problem. The high clinical achievers are recognized."[60]

"Group practice is a uniquely American phenomenon," says former CEO Bill Kiser, "and is based on the thesis that doctors can accomplish more working together than alone."[9] Since each doctor is an employee of the Clinic, which handles the administrative details of the practice, the leaders, but not most of the staff, are burdened with these responsibilities,[9] which many doctors find onerous and some perform rather poorly. "The most striking feature of the Clinic is that almost all the doctors are freed of the business and financial aspects of practicing medicine," says Dr. Robert Stewart, a cardiac surgeon who worked at the Clinic for many years before being recruited by University Hospitals. "You could stay there your whole career and never know about Medicare, etc. It all gets taken care of seamlessly."[61]

Cleveland Clinic founder George Crile once said, "Mediocrity, well organized, is better than brilliancy with strife and discord."[62]* Although the Cleveland Clinic certainly has its stars and, as much as possible, each doctor is encouraged to become well known outside the institution, most members of the staff, who constitute the backbone of the institution, do not have national reputations. They are able doctors content to work in a group practice so highly structured that cardiologist Roger Mills calls it "the epitome of medical bureaucracy."[65] Joseph Iannotti, the chairman of orthopedics, agrees. "Compared with Penn [the University of Pennsylvania, from which Iannotti was recruited] the Cleveland Clinic is a monolith, a centrally organized system of medical care affecting the daily actions of everybody. At Penn, there were rules, but everyone believed they didn't have to follow them. It's the reverse here."[66] Despite what many see as the extreme bureaucracy of the place, and perhaps because of it, decision making can be quite nimble.[32]

Mills, who trained at highly competitive institutions and worked for several years at medical school hospitals and in private practice, finds "peer group interaction is the big thing for me. I can find the world's expert on anything here. As a clinician, it's the most fantastic environment. Patients are not *my* patients, as in private practice. They're *the Clinic's* patients."[65]

---

*When the Clinic's hospital opened, Crile resigned as director of surgery at Lakeside Hospital, which would become the adult medical and surgical facility of University Hospitals of Cleveland after it moved to the Western Reserve University campus. Thus, an important department of the precursor of University Hospitals was once led by the creator of its greatest competitor.[63,64]

His fellow cardiologist Gary Francis adds, "Fantastic cases, and the quality of my colleagues and the cardiology fellows is superb, some of the best docs I've ever worked with. There's great pride being here."[51]

Clinic surgeons have no reason to do additional cases[7,67] and, as Robert Kay says, "I never think about how much money I will be paid for doing a case."[40] Urology department chairman Andrew Novick adds, "Since clinic physicians are salaried, there are no financial gains or incentives to do additional cases. We flourish because our doctors are salaried. No one is practicing and sending dollars into their pockets."[53]

Another source of satisfaction for many of the staff is that, as neurosurgeon Joseph Hahn, chairman of the division of surgery from 1987 to 2003, describes his early years at the Clinic, "Here, I just had to operate. We don't tell everyone to be a triple threat [equally capable as a clinician, researcher, and teacher]. Not having that pressure," which Hahn felt would have been his lot at one of the medical schools where he was offered faculty positions, "is a joy. I have always felt a great sense of freedom here, even when I was just a junior staff member."[68] Hahn emphasizes, however, that, even though many of his colleagues are not required to be academically productive, "we do expect everyone to be a world-class surgeon or physician and a good teacher."[68] As one of the cardiologists says, "for those staff physicians who are less clinically active, it is expected that extramural support is forthcoming."[51]

"Our model is different," explains Delos ("Toby") Cosgrove, chairman of the department of cardiothoracic surgery, one of the Clinic's most renowned and successful units. "Everyone's incentives are aligned. We're all in this together. What's good for Toby C. is good for the Clinic and vice versa."[69] Clinic veterans point to the name *Cleveland Clinic*, not *Cleveland University*. "We're a mugwump* between a university and private practice," Cosgrove explains, because the Clinic has traditionally emphasized clinical care and teaching of postgraduates, not research.[69] "Being doctor-driven lets us focus on patient care," adds Robert Kay. "In contrast to some universities that emphasize basic research, here, excellence in clinical medicine is

---

*A "mugwump," from the Algonquian word for chief, was originally a liberal Republican who, in 1884, deserted James G. Blaine, the party's nominee for president, and supported Grover Cleveland, the Democratic candidate who won the election.[70] A wag at the time reportedly said that a mugwump had his mug on one side of a fence and his wump on the other. The word is now used for an independent, particularly in politics.

critical to the advancement of our physicians while the basic scientists are rewarded for their research. However, we never sacrifice patient care for research."[71] Loop believes that the Clinic has prospered primarily "because of strong, innovative doctors."[55]

The biggest cause for complaint among the staff is the workload,[29,51,65,72] though few leave because of it.[51] "It's the bane of our existence and our virtue," says James Young, a cardiologist who became chairman of medicine in 2004.[72] Although many, probably most, Clinic physicians work more, the expected routine for a typical general physician involves seeing patients for thirty-eight hours per week, Monday through Friday, from 8:00 a.m. to 12 noon and 1:00 p.m. to 5:00 p.m. The doctor has a half day off per week but has patients one evening per week from 6:00 to 8:00 p.m. and a half Saturday once per month.[73] Nevertheless, this means "fewer patients per week than I saw when I was in private practice," says Michael Rabovsky, the medical director at the Beachwood regional practice site, a suburban outpatient facility that the Clinic owns. "And I have no worries about malpractice or contracting with the insurer that the patients have." Rabovsky remembers that "on the day I signed on, there was a computer on my desk with all kinds of useful information about the patients I would see plus specific medical information. The Clinic is supremely supportive."[73]

Every patient whose insurance includes the Cleveland Clinic can see any of the more than 1,300 physicians there, allowing the referring physician to avoid having to check whether the patient's insurance allows him or her to see a particular doctor so long as the doctor is content to refer within the Clinic, hardly a problem when one considers the depth and breadth of the medical competence there. "I can just pick up the phone and discuss any patient's problem with a world-renowned specialist."[73] Clinic staff appreciate being able to receive all their medical care at the Clinic without charge.[74]

Senior nephrologist Marc Pohl had a full schedule from the day he joined the staff[29] because the majority of patients are referred to the Clinic as an entity rather than to individual doctors. So long as the new physician practices well, no doctor need worry about personally attracting patients.[51] Compensation will not depend solely upon the staff member's personal ability to develop a practice. The clinical load means that, according to Pohl, "You get very good at clinical medicine, but there's little protected time in internal medicine."[29] This continuous call on the doctors' time in the Clinic "makes it difficult, except for the most ambitious and hardworking members of the staff, to conduct unfunded research or write papers."[29]

The Clinic is not a place for doctors who don't want to do clinical work. "All except Fred [Loop]* see patients," says neurosurgeon Joe Hahn. "If a doc needs to see me, he can find me in the changing room and talk to me there about whatever is on his mind. Our stars, like Toby Cosgrove, have been here all along," adds Hahn. "They don't leave."[68]

Efficiency helps to compensate for the high volume.[37] All agree that the technical support is excellent. Procedures are performed swiftly and capably, and the professional and technical expertise is excellent.[29] Salary also helps. Although Clinic policy prohibits the staff from discussing specifics, cardiologist Mills acknowledges earning more than he was paid at the medical schools at which he previously worked and almost as much as he was making in private practice.[65] Then there's the liberal vacation policy. When they start, staff physicians receive twenty vacation days, which increase to thirty-five for more senior doctors. Physicians can attend professional meetings for as many as twenty-six days each year; the Clinic will pay expenses for ten days.[29]

Throughout much of its history, "a significant number of the staff had trained here, and the chairmen frequently were Clinic veterans, familiar with its customs and culture," says Robert Coulton, the director of professional staff affairs.[56] Recently, however, the need for a larger staff—meaning annual growth of more than 8 percent[56]—required recruiting physicians who had not previously worked at the Clinic, so much so that the training program has become "less of a feeder," says Coulton.† Recruits from medical schools are often alarmed by the prospect of holding only one-year appointments, but they are disabused of this anxiety quickly when they learn that all but those who commit the most egregious offenses are annually reappointed.[37]

The specialists, who constitute most of the staff, are not required to sign a noncompete clause when they join the staff. "We take the risk," says Coulton, that they will not leave and enter a competitive practice in the community.[56] The Clinic, however, does require that those staff members,

---

*Loop, who became CEO in 1989, continued to operate until 1999.[2]

†"In this respect," says Coulton, "we're different from Mayo's [the Mayo Clinic in Rochester, Minnesota], where more of the staff come from the inside."[56]

mostly primary care physicians who work in the community health centers and leave after one year of employment, not practice within a ten-mile radius from where they worked for one year. "We would enforce it," says Coulton, "but it seldom happens."[56]

Loop and the governors have recruited highly visible academic physicians and surgeons from outside the Clinic to fill vacancies in some of the divisions and departments.[53] "We have to be sure that mediocre people don't fill these positions," says Loop.[55] Coulton has heard the senior leadership ask, "Does this appointment elevate the mean, or is this a 'convenient hire'?"[56]

"The culture at the Clinic," according to biochemist George Stark, chairman of the Lerner Research Institute from 1992 to 2002, "prizes excellence above everything else. The people here really care about what it takes to be the best. We have the unashamed ambition to be number one in everything."[30] As Hilel Lewis, the chairman of ophthalmology, says, "The culture supports excellence and is good at implementing dreams. What's important is making contributions."[57] Loop certainly agrees, insisting that "the organization is a meritocracy."[2]

John Clough, a rheumatologist who is the executive director of the Cleveland Clinic Foundation Press and editor of the official history of the Clinic,[4] has heard colleagues at the Clinic question whether "these superstars will necessarily fit into our egalitarian organization."[16] "I don't like outside recruiting so much," says Robert Hermann, former chairman of the department of general surgery. When he joined the Clinic in 1962, there were only three other general surgeons and the entire staff of the Clinic numbered only ninety physicians and surgeons, less than 10 percent of the number now.[75] "We should give an edge to inside candidates. Better the devil, you know."[75] Hermann warns that excessive recruiting of leaders from the outside could cause the Clinic to lose some of its most valuable doctors.[75]

Former surgery chief Joseph Hahn finds that preferential promoting of local candidates still prevails at the Clinic. "If the qualifications of the candidates are equal, we'll go with the insider, particularly if the department or division's okay. If a shakeup is needed, we usually go outside."[68] When three division chairmanships changed in 2003, Clinic veterans were chosen for medicine and surgery while an outside candidate, Michael Levine from the Johns Hopkins University, was recruited for pediatrics. The chairman of the search committee remembers that Loop and the governors wanted to build the division and favored an outside person with experience at a first-class academic medical center.[76]

The board of governors does not use headhunters to find physicians for their staff but does employ them to locate some administrators,[56] usually those to fill what human resources director Robert Ivancic calls "one-of-a-kind jobs where we have no search expertise." When hiring hospital directors and most executives, "we do the searching ourselves." Many of those hired are local. "Since Cleveland's a unique market, we hire people who know the market," Ivancic says.[77]

Contracts, Reviews, Compensation

The contracts that bind the physicians to the Clinic are reviewed annually. The doctors have no tenure in the university sense or contracts longer than one year, as is characteristic of the employment of most faculty in academic medical centers. The performance of each doctor is reviewed yearly in a formal process known as the "annual professional review" (APR), a procedure that the Clinic leadership proudly describes.[9,37,39,40,55] Education, research, contributions to the literature, leadership of national professional societies, and service to the group all figure in the evaluation of staff members' performance during the past year. However, the most important standard applied to most of the staff is the quality of the clinical care delivered.[9]

One-fourth of the staff is evaluated each quarter. The mechanics of the system include a "pre-APR" performed by the chairman of the doctor's specialty, who then sends his recommendation to his division chairman who is joined by one of the governors for the official APR with the doctor. At the review, the doctor has the opportunity to suggest changes and improvements and to plan how his career will progress.[37] As a result of this final review, the Clinic offers a contract and salary for the next year.[39] "Time-wise, the system is inefficient," acknowledges former CEO Kiser, "but it's the glue that holds the group together."[9]

The Clinic pays no bonuses, a point that many of the interviewees emphasize.[39,56] Robert Coulton explains, "It's very tough to establish a basis on which you may exceed and get a bonus. We don't set out performance standards."[56] However, the amount of the salary offered for the coming year can include recognition of accomplishments of the past year. "We're not rigidly limited by dollars," says Coulton. "We don't want to lose anybody for dollars alone, so we do our best to maintain an environment where people don't want to leave. Salary is reviewed on an annual basis and changes based upon performance and market trends."[56] Decreases are rare.[66] Salaries are, Coulton says, "very competitive. Within specialties, salaries are based upon total contribution, not simply on a revenue formula. This allows each staff member to contribute across all areas and not focus solely on revenue production. We believe this results in the best patient care."[56]

Unlike most academic medical centers, the Clinic doesn't need a practice plan to coordinate the collection of professional fees and support the doctors' salaries. That's part of the responsibility of the group practice, which is, in effect, the Cleveland Clinic.[46] Any surpluses generated by the Cleveland Clinic Foundation are invested in improving the Clinic and not distributed to the doctors, as might be done in private practices.[9]

Robert Kay, as chief of staff, notifies each member of the practice by letter of his reappointment and compensation every year. The information is confidential, and few at the Clinic, including the chairmen of the departments and divisions, know how much their colleagues are paid.[9] Each year, a few members of the staff, but only a few, contest the amount of their compensation. After discussion with Clinic leaders, those who remain dissatisfied can appeal to the trustees. In the experience of former CEO Kiser, this has never happened.[9] With almost every doctor reappointed each year,[37] the turnover rate among the staff, excluding retirements, is very low, less than 4 percent.[56]*

Kay occupies a central role in the group practice. "Rob knows all the staff, unlike most chiefs of staff," says orthopedics chairman Iannotti.[66] Consequently, the staff will often complain to Kay rather than to their chairman.[66] "They know they are primarily Cleveland Clinic employees. I never felt that at Penn. There, I got paid based upon clinical revenue, but here, your salary is based upon nonclinical as well as clinical activities."[66] As examples of the work ethic of the staff, Iannotti remembers how construc-

---

*Consequently, stability is characteristic of the clinical staff, which also holds for the division and department directors, many of whom have held their positions for a long time.[30] "I'm a 'lifer'," says Muzaffar Ahmad, chairman of the division of medicine from 1991 to 2003. "Been here thirty-two years."[39] As nephrologist Donald Vidt, who has been a member of the staff since 1964, puts it, "Once you settle into the system, you don't leave."[25]

tively his colleagues responded when the Clinic needed physicians to practice at the other hospitals the Clinic owns and to see patients in the evening. "There were few objections." Rather, Iannotti has found, "they see
themselves as part of a team, here to serve the whole. No one says, 'They're
picking on me.' "[66]

Close attention to daily events characterizes Kay's job. "Rob called me to
discuss why one of my docs had cancelled patients today," remembers Iannotti. "We get reports every week with the number of times the phone rings
until it's answered, which of my docs was late for his scheduled operation
by ten minutes—that sort of thing."[66] The Clinic retains a company whose
"mystery shoppers" constantly review how the Clinic and its doctors are
delivering service.

Administration

Each division is a business unit, and the chairmen are responsible for the
operation of their inpatient beds and outpatient clinics. "We expect our
doctors in these positions to be managers," explains Muzaffar Ahmad. They
must supervise the nursing care in the outpatient department, where the
nurses report to the clinical department chairmen, not to the director of
nursing like the nurses on the inpatient services.[49] "Our division heads have
greater managerial freedom than what I've seen at most medical schools."[39]
Consequently, the Clinic tends to look for, in its future leaders, doctors
with administrative and financial experience, "not necessarily for the guy
who's done the most cases," according to Hahn.[68]

To improve the ability of chairmen and others with leadership responsibilities to deal with administrative issues, the Clinic supports their studying business and taking advanced degrees. "I thought it the biggest waste
of time when I did it, that I'd never use the stuff," says Hahn, who took a
two-year night and weekend M.B.A. at Case Western Reserve University
(CASE).[68] "It was tough, like doing calculus in college. I was terrible writing
marketing papers, so unlike the scientific papers I was used to writing." But
in time, Hahn came to appreciate the value of what he was learning despite
having to combine homework at night with surgery during the day. He
enjoyed "working with my classmates and being exposed to quality standards from other businesses. It helped me think in a very different way.
Now I realize how valuable it was."[68]

The Clinic delegates less administrative responsibility to divisions and departments than is often the case in academic medical centers. The board of governors retains all financial surpluses that the divisions may develop. Chairmen must apply each year for money to invest in equipment or for the recruitment of new members of the staff.[71] Furthermore, divisions may not assign bonuses. Compensation is a function of the governors. The Clinic believes that this method of operating allows the leaders to make changes quickly and, when necessary,[36] reallocate resources expeditiously.[69] "Fred's not in conflict with entrepreneurism," says cardiac surgeon Toby Cosgrove. "The dollars from the hospital and the doctors go into the same pot. And are plugged into the institution as a whole."[69]

Clinic members with long experience detect that the increasing complexity of Clinic operations has produced a less democratic style of leadership. "It's just not as workable now," says Marc Pohl, a thirty-year veteran at the Clinic,[29] and, presumably, not as effective. Loop remembers the vulnerability of the Clinic in 1989 when he became CEO and introduced a more centralized style of leadership. Nevertheless, Loop must develop a general consensus for changes he wishes to introduce since his ultimate bosses are his colleagues. To some extent, this requirement can slow change.[54] Along with his partners, he constantly studies what troubles and mistakes are roiling competing institutions and how the Clinic can avoid such difficulties.[36]

Transitions

During 2003, the incumbents of several senior positions changed, so many that one senior member of the administration said, "I've never seen anything like it," and heard many colleagues ask, "What in the world is going on?"[50] One thing that was going on, a retiring chairman said, "There was a movement from Fred [Loop] and the board of governors to change senior leadership for younger people."[78] Most of these changes occurred without rancor.

Muzaffar Ahmad, the chairman of the division of medicine since 1991, decided that "it was time. I had been chairman for thirteen years," he said.[76] Ahmad was in the third year of the five-year period between reviews of his chairmanship. "The decision simplified my life," he says with relief. He returned to his previous practice of pulmonary medicine. As with many academics and clinicians relieved of managerial responsibilities, Ahmad says, "The administrative stuff is gone. What a pleasure!"[76]

Ahmad estimates that he had to spend 75 percent of his time managing the division of medicine as chairman and found that the administrative demands significantly exceeded those he had experienced when chairing the pulmonary department previously.[76]* Consequently, those who lead the largest divisions such as medicine and surgery must be prepared to put aside much of the clinical and research work that they had done as department chairmen, the usual but not universal source of division chairmen.[76]

Like Ahmad, Joseph Hahn, who had been chairman of the division of surgery since 1987, feels "relief" in no longer having to administer his immense division. "It was time to change and okay with me," said Hahn.[78]† Now sixty-three, Hahn had become responsible for a $700 million annual budget and was constantly called on to resolve such administrative challenges as arranging how the surgeons at the Clinic, where the beds were continuously filled, could perform their 170 to 200 operations each day. "Day after day it was up to me to decide whether to cancel cases and which cases to cancel. Some days, we couldn't finish elective cases until after midnight. And then, there were the malpractice problems. It wears you out."[78]

Hahn now chairs Cleveland Clinic Foundation (CCF) Innovations, a newly established department, where he directs three small biotech companies. One deals with new cancer therapeutics, another with brain stimulators, and a third with a stent for treating abdominal aneurysms.[79] In directing this work, Hahn can apply what his M.B.A. taught him. He reports, for his direction of CCF Innovations, to the Clinic's chief financial officer, Michael O'Boyle. Hahn continues to operate on Mondays and sees outpatients on Thursdays. As a neurosurgeon he limits his operations to such

*Reminder: departments are subsidiary to divisions at the Clinic, not the reverse, as is the case at most medical schools.

†Hahn's successor as chairman of the division of surgery is Dr. Kenneth Ouriel, whom Loop had recruited six years previously as chairman of the department of vascular surgery from the University of Rochester, where he had concurrently been offered the same position. "I came to the Clinic because the program was substantially larger here—the Clinic has the largest fellowship program in vascular surgery in the country. Fred guaranteed to support my recruiting more surgeons and buying sophisticated equipment."[31] When asked whether he found working at the Clinic much different from the academic center he came from, Ouriel responded, "There's a fairly lengthy learning curve, but eventually you find that it's so much easier to work here. The M.D.s and the entity are one. We're all on the same team."[31]

elective procedures as those required on the spine and peripheral nerves. "I wouldn't want to get called to the OR in the middle of a touchy negotiation," he says.[78]

In some respects, the chairs of the divisions, though officially senior, have less authority for management than the leaders of the departments.[67,75] "The chief of the surgery division is not the director of specific patient management and care as in Europe or at academic medical centers," says Dr. Victor Fazio, chairman of the department of colorectal surgery in Hahn's (and now Kenneth Ouriel's) division.[67] In the Cleveland Clinic system, the division chiefs do not control the financial resources as do most department chairmen in academic medical centers. All the funds flow into one place, the office of the chief executive officer, and are distributed by the board of governors and the central administration.[80]

And not everyone wants to run a division. Fazio knows of several of the Clinic's specialists, in addition to himself, who declined becoming candidates for the position.[67] "Not for me," says cardiothoracic surgeon Toby Cosgrove, chairman of one of the Clinic's most successful departments.[80]

In the division of medicine, Dr. James Young, like Ouriel, was pleased when Loop appointed him to the responsibility of chairing the division. Young had directed the heart failure program since cardiology chief Eric Topol had recruited him from Baylor University in 1995. "I wanted to be at a place that had one of the largest programs in my field. Imagine seeing ten patients with amyloid [an usual form of heart disease] in one year!"[72]

Despite being the likely successor to his chief when Topol is promoted to his next job, Young accepted the medicine chairmanship. "I have the chance to build the division, to improve the quality of the house staff, and to influence the direction the new medical college will take. Frankly, it would have been hard to top what Eric has done in cardiology."[72]*

The Clinic can no longer require that doctors retire from administrative posts or cease practicing medicine at particular ages[81] as in the past. The Clinic had considered establishing terms of service in the chairmanships but decided that a better solution was reviewing each leader's work every five years, and, on the basis of the reviews, deciding whether to continue the appointment. This system allows the Clinic to retain in leadership positions for extended periods those whose work as chairmen continues to

*See the discussion later in this chapter.

be particularly valuable.[76] In the division of surgery, Hahn, as chairman, would regularly evaluate the records of colleagues to determine whether operative complications, infections, use of blood products, and readmissions to the hospital exceeded acceptable norms. On the basis of such data, he would decide whether to certify the surgeon to continue to operate.[78]

Although few members of the group practice fail to be reappointed each year, the axe can fall rather suddenly and unexpectedly on those holding administrative jobs at the Cleveland Clinic Foundation. Tom Seals, age sixty-three, the director of the department of protective services for the past nineteen years, is an example. On June 1, 2003, chief operating officer Frank Lordeman called Seals into his office and asked him to retire on December 31. Loop approved Seals's enforced retirement, and since, according to Seals, each of his annual reviews had been excellent and he had never been criticized about his work, he was surprised, distressed, and confused.[82] The Clinic had even recruited his replacement, a retired head of the Secret Service, without informing Seals. "What they did to me flies in the face of Fred's policy of 'world-class service,'" Seals said.[82]

The leadership had learned that a particularly attractive candidate for Seals's job had become available.[81] Not wanting to lose Seals without having a superior person to succeed him, management undertook the recruitment confidentially and determined in advance whether the new director would take the job—not the result that Seals would have wished, but understandable from management's point of view.

Another senior executive who was forced to leave during the eventful 2003 was Shawn Ulreich, chair of the division of nursing since 1998 and a Clinic nurse since 1984. It was chief of staff Robert Kay, to whom she, as well as the other division chairmen report, who gave her the news. Although her official reason for departing the Clinic is "for me, it was time to move on,"[50] several observers confirmed that she wasn't the person who initiated the change.

One of the issues that led to her leaving will be familiar to other nursing directors and hospital leaders. Ulreich, wedded to the concept of primary care nursing,[77] did not favor replacing registered nurses with personnel less fully trained, a change then occurring frequently in hospitals primarily to save money. She also felt it her duty to protect her staff from having to admit and care for more patients than they could adequately nurse, leaving some beds without patients in them. In the view of Loop's administrative council, she defended her positions too resolutely and without adequate flexibility, producing differences between Ulreich and the other executives sufficient to warrant her replacement.[83] The Clinic offered to create another suitable job for her, but, deciding that the continued presence of a former head of nursing would have been anomalous—"I can see my successor thinking, 'We don't need two wives living in the same house'"—Ulreich resigned from the institution where she had worked for nineteen years. "It's nice not having to get up to attend all those 6:30 and 7:00 a.m. meetings," she said.[50]*

Elimination of a department or activity can also produce redundancies. One employee who was caught in this web was Tom Risk, a twenty-year Clinic veteran whose job disappeared when one of his principal assignments to manage the facilities, engineering, and housekeeping at the regional practices was outsourced to an external commercial firm. In the process, Risk himself was also outsourced or "retired," the word the Clinic employed, in June 2004. In keeping with the Clinic's desire to minimize the agony of such events, Frank Lordeman told Risk that he would receive a year's salary after he left and would be guaranteed a job for at least a year with the company that took over the work.

Both Seals and Ulreich and about twenty other senior executives at the main campus, like all physician members of the group practice, work on one-year appointments, and their performances are reviewed annually.[77] The one-year contracts are not applied to executives working off campus at the outpatient sites and owned hospitals.

Finances

In March 2003, *The New York Times* took note of the Cleveland Clinic, but not as the Clinic would have wished. Confirming the story that Diane Solov had reported in *The Plain Dealer*[85] and the Associated Press had distributed three months earlier,[86] the *Times* gave further national coverage to the news that the value of the Clinic's endowment and pension fund had dropped significantly.[87] The falling value of the stock market had reduced the Clinic's endowment to about $500 million, almost a third of what the

---

*In April 2004, Ulreich became vice president for patient care services at Spectrum Health, a consortium of three hospitals in Grand Rapids, Michigan.[84]

fund had reached at its highest value. The loss led to criticism of the Clinic's investment policy, which had favored equities whose value had greatly increased during the 1990s but which fell steeply during the stock market break that followed.

In the 1990s, Al Lerner, the billionaire financier and generous Clinic supporter who then chaired its investment committee, and the committee members allocated up to 90 percent of the Clinic's investments to equities, although some trustees advised caution as the market soared.[14] This strategy increased the value of the funds to between $1.2 and $1.3 billion over six years.[88] Meanwhile, the Clinic withdrew $663 million from this burgeoning accumulation for the development of its health system; for the construction of the cancer center, eye institute, and research building; for improvements to other buildings on the main campus; and for the development of the Clinic's external network of practices and hospitals. None of this capital was used for operating expenses.[88]* Although the Clinic carries $1 billion in long-term debt, it could raise between $500 and $800 million more and remain within the limits the market requires.[88] The total assets of the Cleveland Clinic Foundation are about $3.5 billion.[89]

Gradually, the Clinic revised the distribution of the resources, so that by 2003, equities accounted for 65 percent of its long-term investments and 55 percent of its pension fund.[85] By the summer of 2003, half of the losses had been recovered, and the endowment had reached $800 million.[34] At about this time, the Clinic started Foundation Medical Partners, a venture capital subsidiary, in which some of the endowment is now invested. Mal Mixon describes it as "not a for-profit subsidiary. All the investments are in the medical field, and we hope to gain a greater return than we get on our stock portfolio."[12]

Another financial problem that the Clinic would have preferred to avoid was the settlement reached with the federal government in which the Clinic paid $4 million to reimburse Medicare for improper billing.[90] This assessment, which many academic medical centers and some individual hospitals have had to pay, resulted from the Physicians at Teaching Hospitals (PATH) audits conducted by the Office of the Inspector General into whether inadequate or inappropriate documentation of physician services

---

*Forty percent of the cost of the building program came from endowment, 40 percent from borrowing, and 20 percent from cash flow from operations.[34]

had led to overbilling of Medicare. Ironically, the integrated governance at the Clinic facilitated the work of the auditors.

In general, however, the Clinic's financial status is stable. "The Clinic has been a highly profitable clinical model," according to Kevin Roberts, the former Clinic treasurer.[47] Net patient revenue had risen from $2,113 million in 1999 to $2,838 million in 2002,* when the Clinic's net income was $33 million, operating income $98 million, and cash flow, as expressed in its earnings before interest, depreciation, and amortization (EBIDA), a very healthy $303 million. The cash balance was $993 million. Accounts receivable are well controlled.[91]

The balance sheet, however, is less strong and reflects the losses in its investments and pension fund. The Clinic had to absorb unrealized investment losses of $270 million in 2001 and $82 million in 2002. Its pension fund had liabilities of $368 million in 2002; in 2000, before the market broke, the fund had a positive balance of $111 million. The long-term debt is more than 50 percent of unrestricted equity, a figure slightly higher than the maximum considered best for such an institution.[91] In 2002, Moody's Investor Service downgraded the rating for Cleveland Clinic Foundation bonds to A1 from Aa3, thereby slightly increasing the Clinic's cost to borrow money.[92]† A year later, Standard & Poors downgraded bonds issued by the county for the Clinic due to "the effect of the weak investment markets on its balance sheet and financial profile," *The Plain Dealer* reported in quoting the S&P report.[94]

Clinic Care, Inc.

Clinic Care, Inc. is a not-for-profit management service organization, a wholly owned subsidiary of the Cleveland Clinic Foundation that is designed to administer and develop various activities not directly related to the practice of medicine.[95] The Foundation's real estate holdings, including the hotels, are based here.‡ Until 1999, the Clinic was its own hotelier. Now the Clinic contracts with Intercontinental Hotels Management Group to

---

*The Clinic's fiscal year ends on December 31.

†Moody's bond ratings for risk, lowest to highest: Aaa, Aa, A, Baa, Ba, B, Caa, Ca, C. Moody also adds numerical modifiers 1, 2, and 3 to each rating classification from Aa to Caa.[93]

‡The land and the buildings where the Clinic conducts its work, both on and off the main campus, are currently worth more than $2 billion.[95]

run the hotels but maintains financial control of the work in the offices of Clinic Care. Until the work was recently outsourced to a private concern, Clinic Care managed the facilities, engineering, and housekeeping activities at the regional medical practices.[95]

Clinic Care also provides services for Cleveland Clinic Medical Services Inc., doing business as Allogen Laboratories, which performs tissue matching for transplantations.[96] Formerly, the laboratory performed this work for University Hospitals as well until, as its director Dr. Daniel Cook remembers, "an administrator there, who wasn't particularly pleased that the Clinic was doing work for them, told us that they would do their own."[96] Financially, Allogen Laboratories breaks even.[96]

Marketing and Public Relations

One nonclinical activity that the Cleveland Clinic performs with consummate skill is marketing and public relations.[64] Even its competitors at University Hospitals acknowledge this.[64,97-99] "The Clinic's PR is tremendous. They're very enterprising in reaching out to the community," says Dr. Richard Aach in the medical school dean's office at CASE and the former chairman of medicine at Mt. Sinai hospital.[97] "It's the best [administrative] department at the Clinic," in the opinion of another member of the dean's office.[98]*

The Clinic's marketing department is large, about thirty employees, according to the director, James Blazar, whom Loop recruited from the Henry Ford Hospital in 1999. The annual budget ranges from $5 to $8 million, which Blazar says is relatively small compared with those of university hospitals of similar size.[44] Blazar and his associates are constantly asking each other: "Are we still the best hospital in the market? If we've dropped, why did we drop? Is the public's perception of us changing? To what extent are the health systems forcing the patients to go elsewhere, and what can we do about this?"[44]

The Clinic uses an advertising agency to help it develop its marketing material, such as promoting specific clinical programs with brochures, the

---

*One hears, when holding on a Clinic phone, the recorded voices of professional announcers touting the various services the Clinic offers, whereas at University Hospitals, music, usually Mozart, fills the time. As someone who has spent an appreciable number of minutes in this state, I must acknowledge preferring the music while recognizing the commercial value of the Clinic's technique.

Clinic's Web site, and graphic art. The department also promotes the Clinic's continuing medical education programs given at various sites throughout the country, but now consolidated to a great extent in the conference center in the new Intercontinental Hotel and Conference Center that the Clinic owns.[100]

To keep in contact with the almost 10,000 doctors who have completed at least one year of training there, the Clinic publishes a magazine three times a year. "It's also well read by the people who work here and the trustees," says Sandra Stranscak, the editor.[101] The Clinic maintains the alumni connection by holding receptions at many national professional meetings and a reunion every three to five years, formerly always in Cleveland, now sometimes in Florida. "We do this primarily for collegiality," says Robert Hermann, the director of the alumni association. "It's more to encourage patient referrals than for philanthropy."[75]

There is an alumni board of thirty-two directors, elected by specialties. The group meets twice per year, usually at the Clinic but soon at the Florida site. Although the Clinic offers to pay their expenses, many of the trustees contribute the money to the alumni fund. The first sizeable alumni fundraising drive helped to build and equip the Clinic's new Alumni Library, a handsome and comprehensive resource in the Lerner Education Building.[101]

Appearance and Service

There's no question that Cleveland Clinic is, and has been, managed in a highly centralized manner and that this feature of the place is widely recognized.[17,65,66,69,71] Although the group practice is the primary example of this, the control from the administrative offices reaches into functions that may surprise visitors from other large hospitals. The look of the Clinic is an easily observed example.

"Facility aesthetics and quality are synonymous," says Frank Lordeman, the chief operating officer. "Fred [Loop, the CEO] and I strongly believe this."[48] When Lordeman joined the Clinic in 1992 from a community hospital in Cleveland where he was the CEO, he found the place "worn" and concluded that his predecessors hadn't paid adequate attention to appearance. Using proceeds from cash flow, he and Loop have invested continuously in facilities. The Clinic, Lordeman says, "mustn't look like a patchwork of designers. The look of the place must be consistent."[48] Accordingly,

Lordeman and Loop closed the in-house design office and started to retain outside designers, whom they chose and instructed.

In the tall Crile building, named for the founder and his son, both of whom were Clinic surgeons, and in other buildings where outpatients are seen, the doctors use shared examining rooms near their offices.[37] This convenience to the staff reflects, as does so much at the Clinic, the effort to combine what works best for the doctors—for they started the place—with appropriate concern for the care and the comfort of the patients. The facilities for the immense and highly productive medical and surgical cardiac services, in the midst of the 1970s main hospital building, are all commingled, the doctors' offices, the patients' waiting area, the examining rooms, the clinical laboratories, and even the operating rooms. The cancer and eye services have their own buildings designed by the doctors working there for greatest efficiency and comfort.[37]

The centralized scheduling system contributes greatly to the efficiency with which patients are seen and the doctors' time most productively utilized. There are no individual secretaries making patient appointments for "their" doctors or a separate building for outpatients distant from the offices of the staff. The proximity of doctors in each specialty to each other contributes to the collegiality that many cite as characteristic of the Clinic.[7,37,75,102]

Pleased with Cesar Pelli's design of the Crile in the 1980s, the Clinic retained him to design each of the three new buildings constructed during Loop's reign. The Lerner Research Institute, Taussig Cancer Center, and Cole Eye Institute are striking on the outside and attractive and functionally successful inside. Even those at University Circle who have seen the buildings praise them.[103] Loop instructed the designers to renovate the atrium for patients and their families waiting for same-day procedures "like an airline executive club."[48] The chairs and couches are arranged into small units so that families can sit together with some degree of privacy. The Clinic's outpatient facilities in communities surrounding the main campus have been built or refurbished to a high standard. "They're gorgeous," Lordeman proudly states.[48]

For out-of-town patients, families, and visitors, the Clinic owns three hotels with facilities and accompanying prices ranging from modest to luxurious.[100] The latest one, the Intercontinental Hotel and Conference Center, has been built within the Clinic itself so that its guests can walk from their rooms to their doctors without going outside.[100] The hotel includes elegant, multiroom VIP suites.* The Clinic will hold its medical conferences, many of which were formerly conducted at other locations in Cleveland and in other cities, in the new hotel.[100,104]

The cost of the deluxe accommodations in the latest hotel has brought criticism from some members of the staff. "Do we need the marble floors when there are clinical departments without adequate space or money?" asks one critic of the latest addition. "We need central parking more than a hotel in the middle of the Clinic." Some of the trustees also criticized the capital investment in hotels, but understand that the Clinic could sell them if the capital spent on them needs to be recovered.[12]

Thanks to the building program, the Clinic now occupies a very large campus that requires an extensive security system. The Clinic's 162 officers, who are responsible to guard forty-five city blocks, including off-campus properties, have police power.[17] They can arrest people engaged in criminal activity although the detectives on the Clinic's force call in city police for the more serious crimes like homicide and drug offenses. The department of protective services also operates an inspectors' bureau, which investigates financial crimes, including check passing, fraud, and embezzlement. Operating and licensing of Clinic-owned vehicles occupies thirty more employees. The department's command center processes 17,000 calls per year.[17]

Unlike much else in Clinic protocol, the management of the patients' food is decentralized, no longer in a large kitchen in the basement with the staff cooking and distributing meals to the inpatient units. The Clinic now buys Stouffer's frozen food in those familiar boxes sold in supermarkets. At mealtime, the patient's choice is microwaved in a food distribution room for each patient unit and delivered fresh and hot on real, not plastic, plates to be eaten with metal knives, forks, and spoons. Patients can order any of the many Stouffer dishes the hospital stocks, thereby providing many more choices than when the hospital prepared its own food. The diets are liberal, the doctors and dieticians realizing there's little value in discomforting patients with low-cholesterol or low-calorie diets for the few days most spend in the hospital. The Clinic has computed that it costs less to feed the patients with packaged than with hospital-prepared food, and, according to internal surveys, the patients are more likely to praise than complain

---

*The hotel charges $2,000 per day for the presidential suite with its four bedrooms.[100]

about their meals. "Though we're obviously a hospital," explains Lorde-man, "we try to emulate the hospitality industry. Now, if we only had more single rooms . . ."[48]

As a final point in this litany of how well the Clinic runs, visitors cannot help but notice the excellent signage. Although one must walk several city blocks from one end of the complex to the other, it's hard to get lost. "We're detail fanatics," Lordeman admits,[48] and perhaps that helps to explain a lot.

Ombudsman

Patients' complaints of a nonfinancial nature flow to the ombudsman's office—the "office of clinical effectiveness," as a brochure given to every patient describes the unit—with eleven full-time employees who perform the work of what other hospitals may call patient "representatives" or "advocates." The office processes about 16,000 "inquiries and concerns" each year from the main campus and the regional medical practices.[105] "Our objective is to be as gracious as possible," says Virginia Rosselli, the director of the ombudsman's office since 1986. "We are not a punitive office."[105]

Although the ombudsman's office helps to provide what Fred Loop likes to call "world-class service" at the Cleveland Clinic, economics drive the need for this department. As Rosselli constantly reminds her staff, "Obtaining new customers costs five times as much as retaining existing ones," and a dissatisfied customer can deprive the Clinic of potential new patients by complaining to family and acquaintances. Surveys have shown that customers are more likely, Rosselli has written, "to take their business elsewhere because of perceived service problems than for price concerns or product or quality issues."[105]

Delayed visits to a Clinic doctor and rescheduling medical procedures and operations constitute some of the most frequent complaints brought to the ombudsman's office. In some cases the office will arrange that the patient and family, if from out of town, are lodged at the Clinic's expense during the waiting period. In addition to calming the aggrieved patient and family and helping them obtain what they need, Rosselli and her colleagues learn about problems, which she will then pass on to the department involved. The ombudsman's office keeps records of how many complaints are lodged against members of the staff each year. Most doctors receive none, and a few one or two. One, however, was deluged with ten. "Statistics have shown," Rosselli said, "that a physician counseled by his chairman has a significant reduction in complaints the following year at review."[105]

Hospital Records—Actual and Virtual

A common medical record for each patient, the ambition of many hospitals and practices, has long been the custom at the Clinic. Whether an outpatient or an inpatient, the patient's complete record, with documentation of all tests and services throughout the patient's entire medical history at the Clinic, is available to each doctor providing care. This service, so logical to the layman, defeats the ability of many other clinical enterprises in which the doctors' office notes are seldom consolidated with hospital records. Physicians, whether in solo practice, in a private group, or in a faculty practice plan at a medical school, usually work administratively separate from the hospital to which they admit their patients. So, for reasons that are often political, doctors and hospitals have their own systems for managing patients' records and assigning registration numbers.

At the Cleveland Clinic, the group practice runs the whole enterprise, allowing a common registration number and consolidated medical record for each patient. To provide the record for each visit or hospitalization, several employees, some in trucks, transport the charts to the sites on the extensive campus in Cleveland and to the external sites where patients are seen.

Among its other advantages, the group practice facilitates the Clinic's implementation of workable computer support for hospital records. Most of the record keeping for the 22 million outpatients who have or are now attending the Clinic's outpatient facilities in Cleveland—a similar program for inpatients comes next—is now computerized.[106] All clinical records and laboratory results regardless of their source can be read from the computer screen. The majority of the physicians type the information directly or through a template into the computer. The rest dictate their notes for transcription into the record. The Clinic is installing the computerized hospital record in each of its owned hospitals.[107]

One of the Clinic's latest computerized innovations is called "MyChart." This scheme allows patients with computers to view an abstracted version of their charts that includes such information as the patient's problem list, medicines, selected test results, and the date and time that tests and procedures are scheduled. Subscribers can also make or change appointments and request prescription renewals, all on-line.[108,109]

Physicians, and, less frequently, patients and potential patients anywhere in the world, can communicate through "e-Cleveland Clinic" and receive second opinions and other medical advice from Clinic specialists.[108,110] The Clinic charges for this service, which generated about $1 million in net revenue during its first year.[108]

The latest development, which Dr. Martin Harris, chief information officer for the Cleveland Clinic and its health system, describes with great enthusiasm, uses a "black box," which measures the flow of dialysis fluid into and out of the abdomens of children being treated for kidney failure. Its data are transmitted by telephone to the Clinic, where the doctors can monitor the data and instruct the families how to adjust treatment when necessary.[108]

"Picking up or hanging up the phone is the only old-line communication thing left," exclaims Harris.[106] "And," he adds, "it's so much easier here because this is one organization. My work happens more quickly here, and it's more satisfying."[106] Harris appreciates the advantages of advancing computer utilization more efficiently at the Clinic by comparing his employment in the same field previously at the University of Pennsylvania, where he went to medical school, trained in internal medicine, and earned an M.B.A degree in computer management from the university's Wharton School. "It's multiple entities versus our model. Here, patients are patients of the Cleveland Clinic Foundation, not of a particular division, department, or practice plan. People who have grown up elsewhere may not appreciate this."[106] Harris ascribes the relative ease of establishing information technology at the Clinic to the predominance of clinical practice at the Cleveland Clinic. The Clinic will more likely assign capital, which at an academic medical center might be allocated to research and education, to facilities and services that specifically improve clinical care.

Employees

Among the many things the Clinic does right, personnel management appears to be one. According to the executive director of the division of human resources Robert Ivancic, who, one must acknowledge, is motivated to make human relations look good, "Our turnover rate is about 50 percent better than the average. People take great pride in working here."[45] According to one of the doctors who had previously worked at a leading academic medical center, "The support staff have a better attitude than where I used to work. Their contributions are recognized, and they are treated well."[37] Ivancic praises the Clinic's "solid pay and benefit package, which is well above the competition,"[45] and which has helped thwart unions from organizing any Clinic workers. Like the doctors, employees are salaried and receive no bonuses.

The Clinic's workforce files only "a handful of discrimination charges each year," according to Ivancic. "We would expect many more in an organization our size. Before we give up on anyone, we give him or her every chance. But we have little patience for bad behavior."[45]* The Clinic has an internal grievance procedure for employees whom the Clinic is considering discharging and for other complaints.

The Clinic outsources few services,† and directly employs most of its workers because, explains Ivancic, "We want to make sure that the people who take care of our patients meet high standards and are very consumer oriented."[45]

Kaiser Permanente

In 1992, leaders of Kaiser Permanente Ohio approached the Cleveland Clinic about admitting its patients to the Clinic's hospital.[111]‡ Kaiser, at the time, owned an eighty-bed hospital that could no longer accommodate the plan's needs. Cleveland, however, was overbedded, and Kaiser knew that the state would not allow it to increase the bed capacity of its own hospital.

Kaiser had been sending patients to the Clinic for specialty care that its own doctors and facilities could not provide. "This would give us the opportunity to consolidate in one place the hospital care for our patients," explains Dr. Ronald Copeland, executive medical director of the Ohio Permanente Medical Group. "We already had contracts with the Clinic for

---

*The Clinic has 27,000 employees, 17,000 of whom work at the main campus.[45]

† Only parking and retail, but not patient food. For environmental services, the Clinic hires professional managers although the staff is employed by an outside company.

‡ The Kaiser component is the nation's largest nonprofit, prepaid health care delivery system. The Permanente corporation, separate from Kaiser, is a medical group practice, the salaried members of which provide care only for Kaiser patients. The name *Permanente* was taken from a river in northern California.[111]

specialty care, and then, there was its fine reputation."[111] The Clinic would benefit from the arrangement by filling its unused beds.

Affiliating with Kaiser Permanente, however, would include some provisions that conflicted with long-standing Clinic policies. Most important was Kaiser's insistence that its patients be cared for by the members of its group practice, not by the members of the Clinic's group practice. Kaiser could continue to refer tertiary care to Clinic doctors as it had been doing previously. Kaiser also needed a superior emergency department, a service that the Clinic had not emphasized previously, and an obstetrics service, a department the Clinic had closed in 1966 to provide space for its growing cardiac surgical service.[112]

The Cleveland Clinic Foundation had been established and run by doctors to provide the facilities the doctors in the group practice needed to practice their profession. The Clinic had never welcomed physicians who were not in its group practice to work there, so allowing Kaiser to take care of their patients there was, in Ron Copeland's words, "precedent setting for the docs there. While some saw it as an invasion, the senior leadership of the Cleveland Clinic and the majority of their physicians and staff embraced the new arrangement as mutually beneficial."[111] To accomplish the goals of both parties, a group of beds was allocated throughout the hospital to Kaiser, where the one hundred doctors on its staff would care for their patients. The Clinic would provide all the nonphysician aspects of inpatient care, including nursing. Kaiser would continue to care for its outpatients at its own clinics throughout the region.

Kaiser's need for an emergency department brought to the Clinic's leadership the necessity of resolving an issue that had, from time to time, earned the Clinic unwanted publicity.[25] The founders had built its small emergency department with a few examining rooms and beds to provide care for the group practice's private patients. The Clinic had not been started for the principal reason that most voluntary hospitals start—to provide care for those who can't pay for it themselves.

Although originally built in a posh area of the community, the Clinic had, for several decades, found itself among a minority population, many of whom were poor, if not destitute. They were not particularly welcome at the Clinic[25] and received most of their care at nearby community hospitals or at Metro, the county's general hospital on the West Side of town. Two ways of discouraging the attendance of such patients was to have neither an emergency department nor public clinics. To take care of its own patients who needed emergency care, the Clinic maintained a room of five beds, which the staff used as a preadmission area. Though the Clinic turned away none of the few non-Clinic patients who came to the department, no sign identified it to the community.[25,113]

Adverse publicity challenged this policy since public money, particularly Medicare, provided funding for the care of anybody who qualified, regardless of the source of the referral. To many, the Cleveland Clinic looked like an elitist organization unconcerned with the medical needs of the local population.[114] Despite the changes to be described, in 2000, the main Clinic campus derived only 1.7 percent of its patient revenues from charity care.[115] Its principal competitor, University Hospitals of Cleveland, only a mile away, was "always there for the public," Copeland said.[111]*

How could the Clinic continue its exclusive admission policies and avoid what many considered an important responsibility to its community, particularly now that two community hospitals that had served the poor were closing?[29] Kaiser provided the impetus that helped resolve the problem. If Kaiser were to have its emergency department on Clinic properties, the Clinic had to provide a similar service. Accordingly, the Clinic and Kaiser built adjacent emergency departments, which opened in 1994. Kaiser doctors staffed their area, and the Clinic hired emergency physicians for its department.[113,117] The Clinic provides the nonphysician staff and services for both departments. Finally, contrary to its earlier policy, the Clinic put up signs identifying its emergency department and, in effect, told the community, "we're open."[113]†

Wanting to offer a comprehensive hospital service, Kaiser insisted that an obstetrics service be reestablished at the Clinic.[112] Compared with the issue of the emergency department, this was fairly straightforward. Space was found for this purpose, and the service reopened in the spring of 1995. Gradually, obstetrics grew and developed at the Clinic, although it wasn't until 2000 that the Clinic developed a neonatal intensive care unit and

---

*Chief communications officer Angela Calman explains that, since the Clinic does not have a trauma center, "our numbers tend to be lower."[116]

†By 2006, Kaiser will close its emergency department at the downtown campus and move this service to a Kaiser facility in the suburbs, where it will build a new emergency department, and to the Clinic's community hospitals. Since the health plan is admitting fewer of its patients to the hospital at the main campus, "It doesn't make sense for us to also have an emergency service there," explained Copeland.[117a]

hired its own neonatologists to staff it.[112] Previously, newborns requiring such care had to be transferred to another hospital, so long as it wasn't to the Clinic's principal competitor, Rainbow Babies and Children's Hospital at University Hospitals of Cleveland.[112] The Clinic had retained its gynecology service when it discontinued obstetrics in 1966.*

Although the Kaiser relationship has, in general, benefited both the Clinic and Kaiser during the decade it has been operating, some problems have emerged. With the closure of several Cleveland hospitals in recent years, the overbedded city became an underbedded city. Competition for admissions at the Clinic now developed between and among the members of the two groups. On a typical day, seventy-five to one hundred Kaiser patients fill beds at the main campus, with fifty to seventy-five more at the Clinic's community hospitals.[111]

To relieve the pressure, Kaiser encouraged its doctors to admit some of their patients to one of the Clinic's community hospitals in surrounding areas. To some extent, this helps the work of Kaiser doctors since they may be able to take care of inpatients nearer the clinics where they see their outpatients.[111] The main campus is far from some of the Kaiser sites, and surgeons must cool their heels between cases, not having a nearby office where they can do paperwork or see an outpatient. Copeland, a general surgeon, finds that, in general, the operating rooms on the main campus operate less efficiently than at some of the Clinic's community hospitals and, as he remembers, than at the small hospital Kaiser previously owned.[111]

Another irritant has been the Clinic's removing interns and residents from some of the Kaiser services. The residency review committees (RRCs), which certify graduate education, have limited the number of house officers being trained in some specialties and the number of hours they may

---

*In 2005, the Clinic decided, once again, to close its obstetrics department at the main campus and relocate its birthing services to its community hospitals.[117b] The census on the main campus's obstetrics service was dropping, and Kaiser was admitting more of its patients, including its obstetrics cases, to community hospitals.[117a] Obstetrics and gynecology chief Michael Falcone was quoted as saying, "Space is at a premium at the main hospital campus, but Hillcrest, Fairview and Huron hospitals can easily absorb the additional patients."[117b]

This development troubled Michael Levine, the chairman of pediatrics, who feared that the census and size of his neonatal intensive care unit might decrease. He grew concerned that the Clinic's interest in his specialty on the main campus was waning.[117c] The administration, however, told him not to worry, that the Clinic would continue to support and develop the pediatrics program which Levine had come from the Johns Hopkins Hospital to direct. Premature infants delivered at the community hospitals and children needing specialized care would be referred to Levine's division at the main campus.[117d]

be on duty. Accordingly, the Clinic has had to modify their schedules, resulting in fewer hours that the house officers may work. Many Kaiser doctors miss the opportunity of continuing to work with competent interns and residents on the patients they admit to the Clinic.[111]

Emergency Department

With the opening of the emergency department, the Cleveland Clinic's patients began to look somewhat more like those who attend voluntary hospitals in the inner city. "About half of our patients now come from areas of the city with contiguous ZIP codes," according to Charles Emerman, the director of the Clinic's emergency department, "and half are African American. About 10 percent are uninsured, and 10 percent have Medicaid."[117] In the days of the unmarked five-bed receiving area, most had been referred by physicians and had insurance other than Medicaid, and few were black. By 2004, the number of patients coming to the Clinic's department exceeded 60,000 per year, while the Kaiser area received about 26,000.[117]

With the Clinic's beds often fully occupied, patients being evaluated for admission must wait in the emergency department. Partly to deal with this problem, the Clinic and Kaiser departments share the use of a large observation unit where preliminary diagnosis and treatment can be carried out. Many of these patients can be discharged without admission after studies reveal their illnesses can be managed safely outside the hospital. About 19 percent are admitted, "which is typical of general hospitals," Emerman says.[117]

Patients with possible heart attacks and other acute illnesses are often admitted directly to the hospital, "bypassing our unit," Emerman says. "Surgeons, however, like to evaluate their patients down here before deciding what to do."[117] As is becoming more common in emergency departments, the Clinic's unit has radiology, ultrasound, and scanning equipment to facilitate making rapid diagnoses of patients coming to the emergency department.

Emerman directs the emergency departments at both the Clinic and at MetroHealth, the county's general hospital. He supervises sixteen staff physicians, all but one board-certified in emergency medicine; one-third work at both hospitals. The Clinic and Metro also train thirty-five residents in a three-year program.[117]

Contracting for Managed Care Contracts

The Cleveland Clinic, like other medical centers, responded to the on-slaught of managed care by developing, in 1994, the Cleveland Health Network, a regional contracting vehicle to obtain business from insurance plans. By 2004, the network included twenty-nine hospitals and about 5,500 doctors in the Cleveland area in northeastern Ohio, south to Akron, west to Sandusky, and into Erie in northwestern Pennsylvania. Each entity signed a document that binds it to contract together with those payers who accept the type of rates the network offers.[118] The network has rights to negotiate the managed care contracts for members of the network, including a health plan for the Clinic's 27,000 employees. A board of trustees with one representative from each of its constituent members governs the network. The senior administrator is Dr. Alan London, executive director for managed care for the Cleveland Clinic Foundation.

By the summer of 2004, London and his staff of thirty were responsible for developing and administering 500 contracts from 108 payers, which generated $1.8 billion of revenue for all providers in the Cleveland Clinic Health System and accounted for 60 percent of the system's revenue.[119] London's operation, of course, cannot influence the rates paid by Medicare and Medicaid, which insure one-third of the Clinic's patients.

Risk contracting, "thriving in 1997," according to London, "is now dead."[118] Dr. David Bronson, chairman of the division of regional medical practice, remembers that "we all took a bath" trying to develop the in-frastructure for capitation with its gatekeepers and other administrative overhead. Most patients no longer require authorization for referrals.[120]

The office of the Cleveland Health Network also directs group purchasing for all the member institutions, an activity that London describes as "flourishing."[118] The system has also developed a group malpractice purchasing plan that offers malpractice insurance coverage to community physicians who practice at system hospitals.[119]

Regional Practices

Over the years, many patients have come to the Clinic on their own, at-tracted by its reputation or encouraged to do so by relatives or friends whose medical problems had been successfully treated there. Others are referred by their doctors, often to specific physicians and surgeons with local or national reputations for the care of patients with particular diseases. Not infrequently, patients ask their doctors to send them to the Clinic even before the doctor might suggest a referral. "In the Midwest," says Dr. William Michener, a member of the Clinic staff since 1961, "there's a tradition for patients in smaller towns to go to one of the big medical centers."[8] Furthermore, tradition in some families brings patients to the Clinic for ailments both complicated and routine. "My grandmother always came to the Clinic," Michener has heard more than one of his patients tell him.[8]

By 1994, concerned that purchases of practices and hospitals by for-profit and other entities would erode such referrals, the Clinic decided to compete directly in what was becoming a national trend.[120,121] Rather than buying practices, the Clinic invited suitable physicians working in Cleveland and surrounding suburbs—many, though not a majority, had trained at the Clinic—to become full members of the group practice. They have continued to work in their neighborhoods and admit to the community hospitals with which they are familiar, but have relocated to larger facilities that carry the Cleveland Clinic brand name. "We just paid for their capital equipment, not goodwill, all at a modest cost," Bronson explains.[120] The Clinic thereby avoided the capital expense—usually exceeding $100,000 per doctor for goodwill—to bring the doctors on board.

By the spring of 2005, the Cleveland Clinic Regional Practice (physicians not practicing at the main facility) included 324 practitioners, 207 providing primary care and 117 specialists.[121a*] The addition of these doctors to the group practice reduced the numerical dominance of specialists on the Clinic's rolls, a fundamental change from the type of practice that had characterized the Cleveland Clinic since its founding.[121] Before the regional practices program started, only 3 percent of the staff were primary care physicians. By 2005, 16 percent offered this type of care in the Cleveland area.

At the Clinic's main campus, the staff now includes 60 general internists—21 of whom are hospitalists—and 8 general pediatricians—also including hospitalists. Recently, the complement of outpatient general pediatricians has been reduced and refocused to hospital care; there were 37

---

*In 1994, consultants, using experience in California as a model, had advised that the Clinic would need 450 physicians in the regional practices to "survive" managed care.[120]

general internists—including hospital coverage—and 4 general pediatricians in 1992.[120] The Clinic has also appointed family practitioners—52 by 2005, and all in the regional practice sites—to the group practice. Formerly, none of these primary care physicians were members.[71]

The specialists in the regional practice facilities offer sophisticated services that they can perform in nearby community hospitals, some of which are owned by the Clinic, or in the suburban family health centers with imaging, radiation therapy, and ambulatory surgery centers. A significant amount of the more routine urological, orthopedic, and cardiac surgical procedures, for example, is carried out by these community-based specialists, each of whom is a full member of the group practice.[58]

The Clinic estimates that it "loses" $30,000 to $50,000 per year on each primary care physician. Unlike in most private practices, most of the auxiliary revenue from such procedures as blood tests and x-rays, for which a private doctor would perform and bill in his or her office, is credited to other departments or to the Clinic's main hospital, where the tests are performed and interpreted. The Clinic runs a courier service that picks up the specimens three or four times a day from each site. The results are then electronically transmitted back to the ordering doctor. A few of these tests are performed at the regional sites when the data are needed quickly, for example, in determining whether the dose of chemotherapy for cancer should be given on that day.

Other tests such as electrocardiograms, stress tests, and echocardiograms are performed at the peripheral sites and interpreted and billed for at the center. The Clinic is now expanding its capacity for such radiological procedures as computed tomography (CT)—seven sites—and magnetic resonance imaging (MRI)—six sites. At some of the locations, treatment with radiotherapy is now available. Patients from smaller sites may visit larger sites in the suburbs that have such equipment and facilities without having to travel to the main hospital downtown.

The Clinic computes that most of the primary care physicians who care for adults generate net income of about $30,000 in laboratory tests and $40,000 in radiology each year and about $4 to $5 million per year in gross billings for specialty services, hospitalizations, and testing. The pediatricians tend to use these tests less frequently, and they are "genuine loss leaders," Bronson explains. "We consider women and children as the gateway point for care."[58] Women, Bronson says, make most decisions about where to obtain medical care, and, if they are satisfied, will advise other members of their extended families to receive their care at the Clinic.

Of 2.4 million outpatient visits, half of those the Clinic accommodates annually now occur in the regional medical practices. Whereas most of the patients seen by the specialists at the Clinic's main campus were formerly referred by doctors not on the Clinic staff, currently 20 to 25 percent of all patients admitted to the Clinic hospital come from members of the group practice not working at the main campus. These referrals contribute significantly to the Clinic's financial success. During 2004, services to patients in the regional practices generated $267 million of net revenue at the main campus and $321 million of net revenue in the region, not including the community hospitals. Although some patients might have come to the Clinic anyway without the regional practices, Bronson believes that much of this business is new, "as demonstrated by an overall tripling of Clinic outpatient volume over ten years."[58]

To accommodate the requirements for contemporary outpatient practice, the Clinic constructed or renovated fourteen buildings in Cleveland and the surrounding suburbs along key highways.[120] Loop decreed that the sites be "A-1,"[118] and, accordingly, each has been appointed almost luxuriously. The sites run with the efficiency and courtesy that characterize the main clinic and hospital so that patients will know, Bronson says, "that they are attending a Cleveland Clinic operation."[120]

One of the A-1 sites is located in Beachwood, an affluent East Side suburb of Cleveland. The Cleveland Clinic acquired it when the Mt. Sinai Hospital, which had built it to provide outpatient care to residents of the community, went bankrupt.[73] The Clinic spent significant capital to upgrade the facility, now described by Michael Rabovsky, its medical director, as "gorgeous."[73] In addition to those providing primary care to adults and children, doctors in most specialties, all full-time members of the Clinic's group practice, also work there. Most of the specialists are also based at Beachwood, but some come from the Clinic's downtown campus. In addition to the doctors' offices, Beachwood provides radiology, clinical testing, a pharmacy, endoscopy laboratories, in vitro fertilization (IVF),[122] and a surgi-center of seven operating rooms where operations such as cholecystectomy by laparoscopy and lumpectomy with lymph node dissection for suspected breast cancer, among other diagnostic and therapeutic procedures, are performed.[73]

As an expression of Loop's "world-class service" concept, attendants at

Beachwood greet the patients and escort them to their doctors' offices, and the Clinic provides valet parking. The internal architecture now reflects the Clinic style, where patients waiting to be seen sit in attractively appointed but relatively large areas that serve one or more specialties of many doctors rather than in small rooms for the individual doctors in private practice when Sinai ran the place. Patients requiring hospitalization are cared for at the nearby Clinic-owned Hillcrest Hospital, about seven minutes away, or at the main campus of the Clinic, about fifteen minutes away.[73]

The Clinic Beachwood IVF program began with the arrival of several doctors with CASE appointments who decided to join the competition. A group of obstetrician-gynecologists, formerly full-time members of the clinical faculty at University Hospitals of Cleveland, now forms one of the larger specialty groups at Beachwood. In 2000, wanting to join the Clinic's group practice rather than continuing in the relatively unstructured system at University, Dr. James Goldfarb and seven of his colleagues left en masse and took their practices to Beachwood, where they use the nearby Hillcrest Hospital for most of their deliveries and surgical procedures.[122,123] "We are an ob/gyn practice that offers all primary care ob/gyn services and also offers tertiary services in perinatology, perinatal ultrasound, and infertility/IVF in a pleasant suburban environment," as Goldfarb describes his practice.[124]

Goldfarb, who had been acting chairman of the department at CASE, was offered the job on a permanent basis. Prepared for administrative responsibilities with an M.B.A., Goldfarb discovered that "being chair wasn't that much fun, that administration was more form than function. It means one less line in my obituary, but I'm having a better time."[122] Goldfarb describes the compensation between the two jobs as "a wash."[122]

The group delivers about 700 babies per year. Goldfarb, who concentrates on in vitro fertilization, describes most of their patients as "suburban with normal or high-risk pregnancies and some with cancer."[122] Unlike at University Hospitals, where as many as 30 percent of patients on the obstetrics service are insured by Medicaid, none of the group's patients are, a pattern that is typical of Clinic patients throughout the system, where Medicaid makes up only 6 percent of total volume.[122]

Dr. Wulf Utian, who had chaired the department at CASE before Goldfarb became the acting chairman, also left University Hospital for the Clinic. Utian had led the department of reproductive biology at the medical school and the department of obstetrics and gynecology at University Hospitals from 1989 to 1999. "Enough was enough," Utian said about his twenty years as an academic administrator, first at Mt. Sinai Hospital and then at the university.[125] Rather than becoming a professor without administrative duties at CASE and University Hospitals, Utian left. "I was tired of the dogmatic hierarchy there and that the dollars and power were in the hospital rather than the medical school."[125] When many of his colleagues moved to the Clinic, Utian joined them. Unlike most of the doctors there, he sees patients on a part-time basis and pursues his research interest in menopause independently.

An anomaly of the Clinic's structure assigns most of the doctors in obstetrics to the division of surgery, "the only place in the United States," says Tommaso Falcone, the chairman at the Clinic, "where ob/gyn is still part of surgery and not an independent service."[126]

A group of six ophthalmologists, who had previously practiced at Mt. Sinai Hospital, also joined the Clinic. "We saw how the winds were blowing, that private practice was not going to survive in Cleveland because of the loss of patients due to insurance issues," says David Sholiton, the leader of what he says was then Cleveland's largest group of ophthalmologists in private practice.[127] Needing referrals to fill his operating rooms and other specialized units, Hilel Lewis, the chief of ophthalmology at the Clinic and director of the Cole Eye Institute, was planning to establish primary ophthalmology practices in the suburbs. "I told him that this wouldn't be well received in the community," said Sholiton, "and besides that would take years."[127] The Clinic and the group decided that combining their resources would benefit both, and, accordingly, in 1999, Sholiton and his colleagues joined the group practice while continuing to see their patients in the suburbs where they had been previously working. Sholiton had become friendly with Lewis, whom he respects as an accomplished researcher and retinal surgeon yet someone who appreciates primary clinical practice. "I thought it would be neat to be part of the Cole," said Sholiton, who then adds, "we'd be free of all that paperwork and governmental stuff."[127]

Before finalizing such deals, the Clinic carefully evaluates the worth of the practice from the tax returns of the partners and the practice, analyzes the billings and receivables of the group for the previous two years, and appraises the value of their capital assets, in the case of the ophthalmologists, the expensive equipment that they use. In Sholiton's arrangement, the Clinic then paid the practice for its assets and replaced the computer with the centralized Clinic system. "The one hit we took was no payment for goodwill," Sholiton remembers.[127]

The members of the group are pleased with their decision, but their situation is not exactly as it was when they were on their own. "When in private practice, my time was my time. I could close the office when I wanted. Now I must officially request a vacation, though it's seldom rejected." The Clinic provides support to attend professional meetings in the United States and for purchasing prescriptions for the doctors' use, but not for such expenses as leasing cars or attending meetings overseas when the doctor is not presenting a paper. Before joining the Clinic, the members of the group could charge such expenses to the practice before taxes had been deducted. "So we lost a bit of money on that one," says Sholiton. "But their medical and retirement benefits are very generous."[127]

Michael Rocco, a former cardiologist at University, also moved to the Clinic and to Beachwood. Rocco, who had received his medical and subspecialty training at the highly competitive Brigham and Women's Hospital in Boston, had become disillusioned with the leadership at University Hospitals of Cleveland.* Wanting to stay in an academic environment but not leave the city, Rocco joined the group practice at the Clinic and moved his office to the Beachwood site. He spends about half of his time at the main campus, where he performs cardiac catheterization, sees patients on the preventive cardiology service, and attends on inpatients.[128] Rocco decided to reestablish his office at one of the regional sites rather than at the main Clinic campus because many of his patients lived near Beachwood on the East Side of the city. "Distance and location matter," he says. "It's a major inconvenience for some to go downtown."[128] Rocco has seen more and more of the clinical services formerly only available at the main campus now established at Beachwood and other Clinic peripheral sites.[128]

Owned Hospitals

The Cleveland Clinic Health System also owns hospitals.† The immediate impetus for this strategy, at both the Clinic and University Hospitals of Cleveland, was the threat presented by for-profit hospital-owning corpora-

*See chapter 4.
†See appendix 2.

tions.[129] "Your market is an aberration, Tommy Frist, the CEO of Columbia-HCA, told Cleveland hospital leaders in the early 1990s," Richard Pogue, a University Hospitals trustee, remembers. "We're coming in here and taking one-third of the market share in five years."[130] Often paying too much for the hospitals they bought, failing, after a very controversial effort, to buy Blue Cross/Blue Shield of Ohio,[131] and suffering from severe internal financial and operational problems, Columbia-HCA, by the end of the decade, had sold the hospitals it bought[132] and withdrawn from the market.[130,132–134]

Despite their failure to dominate the Cleveland market, the for-profits drove community hospitals in the region to seek protection with the larger nonprofit health systems.[133] Their executives and trustees feared that by not being part of a system, they would have difficulty obtaining managed care contracts and couldn't generate adequate capital for future development.[135] When the battle ended, the Cleveland Clinic Foundation and University Hospitals Health System survived as the dominant hospital-owning corporations in Cleveland and surrounding counties.[132,133]

Beginning in 1997, the Cleveland Clinic Foundation associated itself with a group of hospitals in the suburban areas surrounding Cleveland, all within Cuyahoga County in which the Clinic is located.[118]* Many of these not-for-profit hospitals were looking for relationships with a large, successful entity like the Cleveland Clinic as the financial turmoil of the mid-1990s roiled community hospitals, CEOs, and their boards.[71] The Clinic actively pursued such arrangements, a process in which senior members of the board of trustees participated. "There was a lot of competitive courting," remembers board chairman Mal Mixon. "Al [Lerner, then president of the Clinic board] and I helped influence some of the community hospital trustees to go with us."[12] Because of the competitive nature of these deliberations, Loop, Lordeman, and a small group of administrators handled the negotiations on a confidential basis and did not involve the board of governors in the details of the purchases.[38]

Most of the unions are structured as full-asset mergers in which each community hospital becomes a constituent part of Cleveland Clinic Foun-

---

*This represented an important change from the Clinic's earlier policy of not buying hospitals. The same shift in tactics occurred at the University of Pennsylvania Health System when Dr. William Kelley, the CEO, having pledged earlier not to buy hospitals, felt himself forced to do so when other medical centers threatened to control the market by buying hospitals from which Kelley's teaching hospital had been receiving referrals.[136]

dation, "doing business," as the legal niceties prescribe, as the Cleveland Clinic Health System.[33] The Clinic became the sole member of the boards of the community hospitals, and at least three members of each board come from the Clinic. In conjunction with the community hospital boards, the Clinic has the power to approve the budget and large capital expenditures and to discharge the CEOs. However, the Clinic assiduously avoids micromanaging the community hospitals. As chief operating officer Frank Lordeman emphasizes, "We're a group practice, not a hospital."[33]

Unlike the arrangements of the Clinic's chief local competitor, University Hospitals of Cleveland, which owns 50 percent of some of theirs,[134] the Cleveland Clinic Health System totally owns each of its community hospitals.[118] Most of the hospitals were already associated with the Clinic through the network, and some came on board after leaving their connections with University Hospitals.[33]

Unlike University Hospitals of Cleveland, which changed the names of the hospitals it acquired,[12] the Clinic retained the preacquisition names[12] in most cases[3] so as not to interfere with the association of patients and their community hospitals. The titles of the hospitals include a subsidiary identification of their association with the Cleveland Clinic Health System.[137]

The Clinic spent little capital to acquire the hospitals, although it did absorb their debts and pledged to support capital needs.[33] In each of the acquisitions—ten by the spring of 2005—the Clinic avoided taking over clinical services, and most of the doctors admitting to these hospitals have not joined the Clinic's group practice but continue to work in their established practices.[120] Some of the physicians, however, participate in the Cleveland Clinic Health System Physician Organization, which provides access to managed care contracts administered by the network and other services.

It appears that the addition of the health system's owned hospitals and regional practices has provided Alan London and his staff with significantly greater leverage when negotiating with the insurance carriers than when the network was first established without the health system to support it. "The size and scope of services offered by our network has become invaluable to the insurers," according to London.[118] The merger lets London tell the insurers that the owned hospitals cannot do business with them if their rates fail to cover the costs of treatment. Trustee Mal Mixon adds, "Thanks to the system, we can now negotiate more favorable rates with the carriers."[12] As 2004 ended, all but one of the community hospitals in the Cleveland Clinic Health System were profitable.[12] "This was due to our charitable commitments to the community," according to Frank Lordeman, chief operating officer of the Cleveland Clinic Foundation.[137a]

Meridia Health System

By the mid-1990s, the largest group of hospitals not yet part of one of the dominant systems was the Meridia Health System, itself a merger of four community hospitals on Cleveland's East Side. Blue Cross/Blue Shield, which had acquired the Meridia group, had tried to combine with Columbia-HCA and convert to for-profit status. The state's attorney general prevented this change, leaving Meridia without affiliation in a market becoming dominated by merging entities. When Meridia's board decided to affiliate with a nonprofit health system,[138] only the Cleveland Clinic Foundation and University Hospitals of Cleveland remained as the principal competitors.[139]

Charles Miner, the president and CEO of Meridia until he retired in 2003, remembers well the intensity of the competition between Fred Loop and senior trustee Al Lerner, negotiating for the Clinic, and Farah Walters, University Hospitals' CEO, and trustee Richard Pogue, leading the effort for University Hospitals.[140] By the narrowest of margins—11–10, according to one source with one trustee changing his vote on the last day—the Meridia trustees decided to merge with the Clinic,[141] a decision that angered Walters, who claimed that the Blue Cross members of the Meridia board swung the choice to the Clinic.[142]

To take advantage of its new relationship, the four Meridia hospitals added "Cleveland Clinic Health System" to signs and stationery while retaining their well-established hospital names in larger type above that of the Clinic. Public identification with the name of the Meridia Health System, which remains as an administrative unit within the Cleveland Clinic Foundation, disappeared.[137,140,143] The Clinic legally controls Meridia and its hospitals as their sole member, with the executive committee of the board of trustees of the Foundation also functioning as the executive committee of Meridia. The same trustees simply change hats and meet sequentially. The board of Meridia, the descendant of the group that directed the hospitals before the merger, meets once a year.[140]

Meridia delegates to its constituent hospitals "as much as possible," according to Miner.[140] Centralized through the Meridia office, however, are finance, registration, billing, and information technology. The clinical laboratories and pharmacy have also been unified as much as is practical. The downtown Clinic has not assumed direction of these functions because of intrinsic differences between how community hospitals, with most of their doctors in private practice, operate compared with a referral hospital, whose doctors are employed as part of a comprehensive group practice.[140] Data processing, which the Clinic has assumed, is, Miner says, "more in the nature of standardization than centralization."[140]

Meridia's Hillcrest Hospital, the largest and most successful in the chain, arranged that members of Toby Cosgrove's group at the main Clinic campus operate at the community hospital, thereby offering clinical experience and competence in cardiac surgery in which the Clinic is dominant locally and nationally.[140,144*] The cardiac surgeons in private practice at Hillcrest became full-time members of the Cleveland Clinic Foundation's group practice.[140] Among the reasons for the willingness of these surgeons, and a few other doctors, to exchange private for group practice were:[140]

1. financial relief from soaring malpractice premiums
2. the prestige of being a member of the Clinic
3. the Clinic's desire to have one group of doctors providing the care for patients on the very important cardiac surgical service

Apart from the financial considerations, the merger, senior doctors and administrators insist, must take the "high ground" and improve medical operations, thereby enhancing care of the patients. Informal groups meet regularly to review the results of diagnosis and treatment and such practical issues as reducing the amount of time each patient remains in the hospital ("length of stay") without endangering or lessening the excellence of care.[140]

The effect of the Meridia-Clinic merger on the local market has been substantial. Currently, the Meridia hospitals lead in each of the communities they serve with the group, as a whole, providing 30 percent of the care and the remaining hospitals dividing up what is left.[140]

---

*Meridia also employs radiation oncologists and some of the anesthesiologists from the Clinic's full-time group practice.[140]

Florida

In the early 1980s, with Cleveland in deep recession and losing population, the Clinic's leaders, prompted by a request by some doctors in Florida, began to investigate the wisdom of developing a satellite of the Cleveland Clinic there.[23,145] "This was a heady time for us," remembers William Kiser, then the CEO. "We followed the corporate model, like the local law firms that were establishing satellite offices elsewhere."[9]

The Mayo Clinic had created a branch in Jacksonville in the northeast corner of the state, and the Cleveland leaders saw the advantages of doing the same farther south. They hoped to attract Clinic patients who had migrated to Florida either permanently or for the season and others from Latin America, where the reputation of the Clinic flourished thanks to the presence in many countries of doctors who had trained in Cleveland. The Clinic also liked the demographics of one of the fastest-growing regions of the country and believed their unique group practice organization could offer quality of care not then available.[41] Kiser and his colleagues selected Fort Lauderdale on the east coast where, research seemed to show, the Clinic's name was better recognized than elsewhere in the state.[145]

Cleveland Clinic Florida started operations on February 29, 1988; several years of trouble followed. Obtaining privileges for the medical staff at local hospitals proved particularly difficult, as local physicians resisted the presence of the Clinic, seen as a potent competitor.* After much difficulty and significant financial losses, the Clinic moved its entire operation inland from Fort Lauderdale to Weston, and built its own 150-bed hospital and four-storey outpatient facility there. By 2003, the medical staff numbered 120 physicians and the facility had grown to include a twenty-four-hour emergency department and facilities for open heart surgery and kidney transplantation. For the first time in its history, the Clinic brought in a partner, the Tenent Health Care Corporation, to operate the hospital, of which it owns 51 percent and the Cleveland Clinic Foundation 49 percent. The Tenent responsibility includes, among others, nursing and the operating rooms, two of the departments that the Clinic directly supervises in Cleveland.

---

*For greater detail about the trials of the Florida venture, see chapter 20 in the 3rd edition of John Clough's book, *To Act as a Unit*.[145]

The doctors, of course, are fully employed, fully salaried members of the group practice of the Cleveland Clinic Foundation, just as are their colleagues in Cleveland.[41] However, there are differences. The attrition rate among the physicians in Florida, for some years, has been more than 20 percent, whereas the turnover, excluding retirements, among the doctors in the group practice in Cleveland is 4 percent.[56] "Doctors have different motivations in Florida compared with Cleveland," said Loop. "Some are restless and tend to pass through. We need time for the staff there to mature."[146]

Not content with this operation, the Clinic opened, in 2001, an outpatient building and seventy-bed hospital, described in the Clinic's advertising as "a full service, 170,000-square-foot hospital built with state-of-the-art technology and the feel of a luxury hotel," in Naples on the west coast of Florida directly across the state from the Weston facilities. Further research had revealed that the Clinic was better known there than on the east coast of the state, leading former Cleveland Clinic Florida CEO Melinda Estes to conclude that "we should have gone to the west coast and route I 75" from the beginning.[41] The leaders were further surprised to discover that most of the patients at Cleveland Clinic Florida had never previously been to a Clinic facility and were not, for the most part, transplants from Cleveland. "One of the lessons we learned," says Estes.[41] The Florida clinics continue to lose money, but the new hospitals in Naples and Ft. Lauderdale are, in Loop's words, "highly profitable."[2]

The leadership is committed to making the venture pay for itself although, from time to time, when continuing losses there seemed particularly onerous, the board of governors considered closing the Florida operation.[69] "It was partly pride that kept it open," trustee William MacDonald admits.[11] As for the staff, several members think the Florida project ill-advised from the start but don't expect the administration to abandon it. "Bad ideas die hard," said one critic of the venture. The memory of the Florida venture, coupled with the Clinic's plans to spend large amounts of capital and increase debt to build its expensive cardiac center on the main campus, has discouraged talk about opening another satellite.

International

Although only 3 percent of Clinic patients come from countries other than the United States, the Clinic has, for years, invested heavily in recruiting international patients. The process began in 1965, when the king and other members of the Saudi Arabian royal family came to the Clinic for cardiac surgery. Financial support by the king for treatment of other patients from his country followed, and the international center was founded, the first such organization and now the largest, according to Lisa Ramage, its executive director.[147] About 5,500 international patients[148] come to the Clinic in Cleveland each year and 3,000 to the Florida satellite, most of these from Latin America.

International patients come to the Clinic for treatment by leading physicians and surgeons whose names are known in foreign medical circles, partly through graduates of the training programs now practicing in their home countries. The reputation of the Clinic is further enhanced through overseas visits by leading members of the medical group who will treat or consult on influential potential patients where they live. Courses given by Clinic experts in Cleveland and overseas; an exchange program, funded by the Clinic, which brings practicing physicians to Cleveland to learn the latest techniques; and a specific Web site for the international patients helps to increase the awareness of what the Clinic offers to doctors and potential patients from other countries.[147]

The international center has forty-five employees, most of whom speak at least two languages. One-third come from Latin America and one-third from the Middle East. The center, which has interpreters for Arabic, Greek, Italian, Japanese, Spanish, and Turkish, employs travel agents to ease the arrangements for the medical travelers by securing their lodging, scheduling outpatient visits and admissions, assisting with passport and visa issues, and securing translators. The international center, not the Clinic's central office, completes all financial arrangements, including estimates of cost and collecting for payment. "We need to have all their care coordinated because time is an issue for them," Ramage explains.[147]

The Clinic provides security for heads of state and other VIPs when they come for care.[17] This service often supplements the secret service and national security forces that such patients bring with them. Officers may stand by in the operating room.[17]

Whatever the effort and expense, the international business has great value for the Clinic. Since most of the international patients pay full charges—few have insurance—their care adds 10 percent to the Clinic's net income.[147]

The attacks of September 11, 2001, caused the international business to decrease[148] by 75 percent, but, by a year later, 25 percent of the loss had been regained, including most of the Latin American referrals. Ramage believes that many of the Middle East patients, concerned about the safety of the flight to Cleveland, now go to London for treatment.[147] In response to the problem, the Clinic is seeking patients from a closer neighbor, Canada, where patients must sometimes wait a long time for elective procedures. Aided by physicians, formerly from Canada and now practicing at the Clinic, the international office has encouraged patients to receive their treatment at the Clinic, only an hour away by air or five hours by car.[44,147] Among more recent international center innovations are a "Gold Card" program, a medical concierge service for out-of-state visitors, and special services for VIP patients.[147]

The Clinic is expanding its international services by contracting with the King Faisal Specialists Hospital and Research Center in Saudi Arabia to provide computerized second opinions through the Clinic's Web site, www.eClevelandClinic.org. Physicians at the Saudi hospital transmit electronic versions of patient records, radiology, and other technical data to Cleveland, where, within forty-eight hours, Clinic physicians provide their analysis of the diagnosis and treatment of the case. This service is also available to anyone with suitable computer facilities and costs $565 per second opinion.[110]

The Clinic has also formed a partnership with a group of Indian hospitals to provide consultations on a fee-for-service basis. The scheme should increase the reputation of the Clinic in this country with a population of one billion people and lead to referrals of patients with complicated illnesses to Cleveland.[149,150]

Despite its national and international reputation, however, most of the Clinic's patients live relatively nearby. Seventy percent come from the city and the counties surrounding Cleveland and 20 percent from the rest of Ohio. About 7 percent are referred from elsewhere in the United States.[120] A few of the best-known specialists attract many of their patients from greater distances. For example, Victor Fazio, chairman of the department of colorectal surgery with an enviable reputation in the surgical treatment of several diseases in his field, attracts 5 percent of his patients from overseas. Of his American patients with inflammatory bowel disease (ulcerative colitis, Crohn's disease), 70 percent come from states other than Ohio.[67]

Development and Philanthropy

For the first seventy years of its existence, the Cleveland Clinic engaged in little fundraising.[69,151] "The Clinic was a bastion of medical excellence but also of independence," explains Bruce Loessin,* the current director of institutional advancement since 2001.† "There was a concern about too much dependence on outsiders."[151] Cash flow and, beginning in the 1980s, borrowing financed its growth. Eventually, the Clinic entered the development business, and, not surprisingly, has become very successful at it.

The first full-time director of the development office was William Grimberg who, at the time Loop recruited him in 1994, was working for Cleveland Tomorrow, "a group of more than thirty chief executive officers from the largest corporations in Northeast Ohio," according to its Web site, "who are committed to improving the long-term economic vitality of the region."[152]

Loop charged Grimberg to create the Clinic's first capital campaign, designed to raise $225 million in five years to build what became the Lerner Research Institute, the Cole Eye Institute, and the Taussig Cancer Center. "Under the leadership of Cleveland industrialist and Clinic trustee Joe Callahan, we did it in four," says Grimberg, "and raised $256 million, $200 of which came in cash."[153] Trustees, members of the group practice, and close supporters of the Clinic contributed 30 percent. The rest was raised through a public campaign. "We solicited every doc," says Grimberg, "and they all gave," several contributing more than $100,000.[153]

With the completion of the campaign, Grimberg left the Clinic to create a private equity firm. Loessin, who succeeded him, had been the chief executive with the development office at CASE for twelve years, so he knew Cleveland well. Loop charged him to "make our development program as good as the medicine we practice."[151]

Loessin needed to extend the volunteers beyond the trustees, who with the doctors, supported most of the previous campaign. He created "leadership boards," groups of Clinic enthusiasts initially in such areas of particular strength or need as cancer, urology, digestive diseases, the Lerner

---

*Pronounced "Lo-SEEN."

†"Institutional advancement" is the currently fashionable synonym for what was formerly called "development" and, before that, "fundraising."

Research Institute, pediatrics, and, of course, heart disease. The boards, each with about twenty to thirty members, all, according to Loessin, "very important people and potential or current donors," meet in Cleveland twice per year at the new Intercontinental Hotel within the medical complex. The doctors describe their latest treatments, often bring patients to the demonstrations, and, in Loessin's words, "spread the message."[151] The sessions have been so successful that the cardiac programs, and others to follow, are now being exported to cities such as New York, Chicago, and Palm Beach. Tony Bennett appeared at one, singing his theme song, "I Left My *Heart* in San Francisco."[151] Always using the Clinic's most valuable strength, its doctors, development at the Cleveland Clinic is most emphatically "physician-centered." To support the new medical college, Loessin's operation raised, during 2003, $1.5 million, and in many cases more, to endow each of nine chairs.

Loessin is proud that his operation is relatively small, "lean and mean," as he describes it, which keeps the overhead relatively low, about six cents for each dollar collected. "The average is much higher," he says.[151] At the end of 2003, Loessin employed sixty people, half of whom were professional development officers.* Compared with development work at University Circle, the Clinic's program is consolidated whereas the separate corporations of CASE and University Hospitals of Cleveland each conduct their own programs. Loessin describes the Clinic's constituencies as more national and international, whereas CASE depends to a greater extent on alumni support. "There is an overlap between University Hospitals and CASE."[151]

Cardiac Services

In 2004, the magazine *U.S. News & World Report* ranked the Cleveland Clinic's Heart Center as the number one hospital in the United States for heart and heart surgery for the tenth consecutive year.[155] The directors and members of the heart services take pride in noting that the Clinic stands higher than such esteemed teaching hospitals as Mayo Clinic, Brigham and

---

*For comparison, Johns Hopkins Medicine, the entity that includes both the hospital and the medical school, employs about a hundred people in its fundraising work—not called "institutional advancement" there, says John Zeller, associate vice president for development.[154] The Hopkins program is recognized as one of the most successful at academic medical centers.

Women's Hospital, Duke University Medical Center, Massachusetts General Hospital, and Johns Hopkins Hospital, which trailed the Clinic in positions two through six.

The program is certainly large. In 2005, its cardiologists performed over 10,000 diagnostic and interventional cardiac catheterizations and the surgeons carried out 3,602 open heart operations. Collections for medical and surgical cardiology services provide half of the Clinic's income.[155a]

In their efforts to increase the size of their own cardiac programs, cardiologists, cardiac surgeons, and hospital administrators elsewhere ask what the Clinic is doing right. History, talent, and a "passionate dedication to medicine and caring for patients"[156]* provide much of the answer. As for talent, two pioneers in the contemporary treatment of heart disease worked at the Clinic just as the specialty was entering the modern era.

Dr. F. (Frank) Mason Sones (1919–85)[157] discovered that contrast material could be safely injected into the coronary arteries, the vessels supplying blood to the heart muscle. The pictures taken during the procedure show whether and where these arteries are blocked by the plaques of atherosclerosis. A graduate of the University of Maryland School of Medicine, Sones was a pediatric cardiologist, although the work that would make him famous was conducted mostly on adults. Working at the Clinic, he produced the first coronary arteriogram by accident on October 30, 1958.[158] In a patient with aortic valve disease, Sones's catheter slipped into the right coronary artery, where dye was then inadvertently injected, producing a picture of the interior of the artery. Although Sones feared that the injection might cause the patient to develop a fatal arrhythmia, the heart only briefly stopped beating, and the patient appeared to suffer no ill effect. Sones had by chance discovered a method to definitively diagnose coronary artery disease and describe the vascular anatomy of patients with this disease.

Although Sones contributed many other important advances to the field, none were as famous as the first demonstration of coronary arteriography. "Collectively, all of the cardiological advances of the past century pale in comparison with his priceless achievement," according to Loop,

*In the words of Dr. Bernadine Healy, who directed the Clinic's research division from 1985 to 1991 (see chap. 6.) Healy, who trained at Harvard Medical School, Johns Hopkins, and the National Institutes of Health—to which she would return as director on leaving the Clinic—and was a former president of the American Heart Association, could analyze the Clinic's virtues as an outsider, perhaps influenced, to some degree, by being married to Fred Loop, the cardiothoracic surgeon who became the Clinic's CEO in 1989.

who knew him well.[158] "He was always doing something new," said Irving Franco, one of his trainees who subsequently joined the Clinic staff. "His mind was always in the future."[159]

Sones flourished at the Cleveland Clinic, a relatively small enterprise in the 1950s when he made his important discovery. He was exceedingly hardworking, "often at the Clinic at midnight," remembers Franco.[159] Though subsequently offered many opportunities to work elsewhere, he stayed at the Clinic during his entire career after he had finished his training. He liked the absence, through most of his career at the Clinic, of a rigid administrative structure and the independence it gave him. "He hated committees," remembers Dr. William Proudfit, "particularly if they interfered with his work."[160]* Sones chaired his own department, called "Cardiovascular Disease and Cardiac Laboratories."[161]

Sones was not the easiest man to work with, those who remember him say. He was a workaholic—"his hobby was his work," according to Dr. Earl Shirey, a close colleague of Sones in the cardiac catheterization laboratory.[162] Sones was outspoken and might be critical and abrasive when crossed.[159,160,162] He could be rude to the nurses and didn't have much respect for the surgeons; Sones had a troubled relationship with Dr. Donald Effler, the chairman of cardiac surgery.[7] "Language could be a problem sometimes," recalls Shirey.[162] According to Dr. Douglas Moodie, a pediatric cardiologist like Sones, "he fired people on the spot."[59]† At one point his troubled relationship with many hospital workers led the chief of staff to order him not to make rounds and to leave that work to his colleagues.[7]

Sones smoked in the cath lab—he would die of bronchogenic carcinoma[158]—and used a set of sterile forceps to pick up his cigarette during catheterization procedures.[160,162] "At a meeting, his cough would always tell us if he was present," remembers Shirey. "When he tried to get off cigarettes, no one could live with him."[162]

Sones's brilliance and constant commitment to the welfare of his patients assured him a high reputation at the Clinic and in the profession despite the peculiarities of his personality.[162] Both Shirey and Franco insist

---

*Proudfit, who joined the Clinic in 1940, was chairman of the clinical cardiology department from 1965 to 1974.

†"Mason would never have lasted at the Mayo Clinic, which is more homogeneous," said Moodie, who had trained at the Mayo Clinic but spent most of his career at the Cleveland Clinic, where he directed pediatrics from 1987 to 2002.[59]

that Sones was always honest with his patients.[159,162] "He told us," said Franco, " 'never lie to your patients.' Tell them the truth, and they'll be your friends. Just say, 'I made a mistake.' "[159]

René Favaloro (1923–2000) contributed the second fundamental original discovery at the Clinic for the treatment of patients with coronary heart disease. Favaloro was a thirty-eight-year-old general surgeon from Argentina taking advanced training in cardiothoracic surgery at the Clinic[160] where, in 1968, he reported the first series of successful coronary artery bypass graft (CABG) operations, which he had first performed the year before. In Favaloro's operation, the surgeon removes a vein from the patient's leg and connects it from the aorta to the coronary artery beyond the region of obstruction. Through the graft, blood can now reach an area of the heart formerly deprived of blood flow because of the atherosclerotic obstacle. When successful, the procedure relieves angina pectoris, the sensation of pressure and pain in the chest produced by heart muscle receiving less blood than it needs. Although surgeons, some at the Cleveland Clinic, had previously invented methods to relieve angina, Favaloro's technique proved to be the most satisfactory and soon became widely adopted.

These two techniques, coronary arteriography and the coronary artery bypass graft operation, each developed at the Clinic, brought an increasing number of referrals to the cardiologists and cardiac surgeons, a flow that continued to grow in subsequent decades. Although Favaloro returned to Argentina in 1971, his colleagues at the Clinic refined his technique, thereby contributing to the prosperity and fame of the Clinic and its cardiac surgery department, which had been founded in 1949 by Dr. Donald Effler and subsequently led by Floyd Loop. Since 1990, Toby Cosgrove has chaired the department, which has continued to grow as have the number of cardiologists, some of whom perform the work Mason Sones had initiated in the catheterization laboratories.

Cosgrove looks like a top cardiac surgeon is supposed to look. He is a tall, handsome, well-muscled man, attired in the white trousers, white shirt with collar, and white shoes that have become the ritual working garb of surgeons at the Cleveland Clinic. This uniform is his scrub suit, and he will wear it in the operating room underneath a sterilized operating gown. Not for the leading cardiac surgical team in the United States the unpressed blue scrubs so familiar to television audiences. Unlike the space where Loop now works, Cosgrove's office—it was Loop's when he was the department chairman—is bathed in light, the furniture gray and sterilely modern, everything in place, including the films of angiographic studies that have been performed on his patients and will guide him when he operates on them.

Cosgrove, befitting a surgeon, has strong points of view. "Sones and Favaloro should have won the Nobel Prize and would have if they had been more politic," he believes. "Our non-mainstream thinking began with Crile [George W. Crile, one of the four founders]."[69] That the Clinic accepted lumpectomy for treating breast cancer long before many other institutions or doctors did,[75] Cosgrove suggests, indicates a willingness to embrace what's new and effective in medicine.[69] George ("Barney") Crile Jr., son of the founder, had been performing less extensive operations for the disease[163,164] beginning in 1955,[165] and was operating for ulcer using the, as yet, not widely accepted technique of vagotomy and pyloroplasty.[75] "We don't stand on tradition," says Cosgrove.[69]

The cardiac medical and surgical services at the Cleveland Clinic have grown because of more than just the contributions of Sones and Favaloro, important though they were. "How do we do it?" Cosgrove asks rhetorically. "Doctors do doctors' work."[69] Cosgrove personally operates on 700 patients annually,* which leaves little time for administering the department, much of which he delegates to his colleagues, most of whom operate almost as much as he does.[102] "The more you do, the better you get" helps to account, he insists, for the low morbidity and mortality of patients treated in his department. Data provided by the Clinic suggest that the incidence of complications and death from cardiothoracic surgical operations is among the lowest in the country.[69]

The system the Clinic has developed contributes mightily to its success. In the words of one of its surgeons, who was later recruited to a senior position at University Hospitals of Cleveland, "It's a very nurturing environment. Soon after I started there, I remember having a problem during an operation, tried everything I'd been taught. Toby came in, cleared away the tissues obstructing the heart, and everything was fine from then on."[61] This same surgeon described the place as "a very pleasant place to practice. It's like getting on a train in motion. You're constantly surrounded by a tremendous depth of expertise."[61]

---

*And, according to *The Plain Dealer*, was the highest-paid member of the Clinic in 2002. His salary that year was $1.8 million.[69]

Although frequently recruited for senior positions at leading medical schools and teaching hospitals, Cosgrove and his colleagues prefer to work at the Clinic. "Couldn't do it at other places," he believes. "Here, if you can grow it, you grow it."[69] Although the staff complains about the workload, the drive to work particularly hard seems endemic at the Clinic. "This place attracts people who like a large volume of diverse patients," says Loop. "I just wanted to work, hated the weekends when I wasn't working."[24]

To bring new techniques to the Clinic, Cosgrove encourages his colleagues to study at centers where the staff is innovating new techniques. Early in his career, he worked with a surgeon in Paris who was pioneering an operation to repair faulty mitral valves without replacing them with prostheses. Cosgrove brought the technique back to Cleveland, improved it, and now he and his colleagues at the Clinic operate on more patients with this condition than anywhere else in the country.[69] Cosgrove has reported the results of this operation and his other academic work as author or coauthor of more than 400 papers. His department now includes 13 cardiothoracic surgeons on the staff, 8 residents, 8 clinical fellows, and 10 "clinical associates," fully trained surgeons, often from foreign countries, who work at the Clinic to learn current techniques and perfect their skills.[166]

Dr. Patrick McCarthy, one of the Clinic's most respected—one of his medical colleagues calls him "the most courageous"[51]—of the cardiac surgeons, likes that "we're encouraged to push the envelope either with new things or volume. There's little trouble here getting bigger."[102] McCarthy was offered the position of chief of cardiac surgery at one of the famous Harvard teaching hospitals plus an endowed Harvard professorship. He turned down both honors. "For me, it was a simple decision, though my wife wasn't all that pleased. She liked the idea of living in Boston. Here, I have a terrific relationship with the cardiologists. We're a team taking care of patients."[102] At the other hospital, McCarthy saw less emphasis on collegial patient care, a characteristic of work at the Clinic[35] of greatest importance to him. "Of course, we all work hard here, but everyone wants to support you. Besides, I saw our place as having more potential."[102]

McCarthy's day, which starts at 7:00 a.m. and ends "whenever,"[102] is so busy that he runs two surgical teams. One, which provides surgical management for patients with congestive heart failure, has a chief resident and a surgical fellow. His "regular" team has a chief resident and a junior resident. Seven physician assistants support both teams. One of the reasons for his doing 500 cases each year has been McCarthy's growing reputation for performing operations to cure the cardiac arrhythmia, atrial fibrillation, the irregular heart rhythm that can significantly reduce the heart's function.[167] McCarthy's standing in the surgical community now brings 80 percent of his patients directly to him. Some have discovered him through the Internet.[102] Unlike many surgeons who leave the job to residents, McCarthy dictates his own operative notes, "so I can include clues to what I did and might expect."[102]

McCarthy, however, was not immovable. The offers to become a boss had continued and, finally, he accepted the chance to become chief of cardiothoracic surgery and co-director of the cardiovascular institute at the Northwestern University Medical School in Chicago starting in April 2004. "I wanted to grow out of being primarily a heart failure surgeon," he explains.[168] At the Clinic the large number of cardiothoracic surgeons had led to subspecialization within the field. For example, in addition to McCarthy's doing the heart failure work, Toby Cosgrove concentrated on valves and another surgeon on arrhythmias. One was expected to respect the boundaries thus established. "Also, my principal colleague on the medical side, Jim Young, had become chairman of the division of medicine and clearly wasn't going to be able to be as active clinically as he had been." That Northwestern offered to invest $50 million in the medical and surgical cardiac programs helped McCarthy decide to make the change.[168]

The Clinic can perform so many operations because the system works so well. Patients are prepared for surgery in induction rooms, adjacent to the operating rooms. Then they are wheeled into the OR and the operations proceed. There always, or almost always, seems to be an operating room available, and delays are seldom a problem.[61] After the operation, a secretary sends what former Clinic cardiac surgeon Robert Stewart describes as "a routine letter with the OP [report of the operation] note to the referring doctor."[61]

Many patients needing cardiac surgery, Stewart found, are sent to surgeons who are favorites of the referring doctors, "but many come from the outside or from our cardiologists to whomever is available."[61] So many patients come to the Clinic that Stewart was able to operate on 300 cases during his first year after fellowship.

A Clinic cardiologist evaluates most patients before the surgeons will operate on them and then cares for them from when they leave the post-operative recovery room until they are discharged from the hospital.[65] Roger Mills was one of the cardiologists specifically recruited to care for these patients because the surgeons were complaining that the medical preoperative and postoperative care was inadequate. Because of the large number of patients the surgeons are called on to treat, much of the care during the postoperative period has devolved on the internists. "One of our jobs is to keep the surgeons in the OR," says Susan Rehm, an infectious diseases specialist who participates in this work.[38]

Until cardiology at the Cleveland Clinic reached its current eminence and could attract highly competitive residents, most graduates of American programs did not choose to train there. Medical schools tend to advise their graduates to take their residencies and fellowships in teaching hospitals that are part of academic medical centers, not at stand-alone hospitals un-affiliated with medical schools like the Clinic. Many of the cardiac surgical fellows then came from overseas, in particular, like Favaloro, from South America. Now, "the number one surgeon in each South American country trained here," Cosgrove proudly says.[69] In returning to their home countries, these graduates of the Clinic's training program do not practice where they can compete with the Clinic, a problem at many academic medical centers that train their competition, former residents who set up their practices locally. Rather, Clinic trainees from overseas refer their most difficult cases to their former teachers in Cleveland.[69] Although Cosgrove recruits for his staff the best surgeons he can find from leading academic medical centers, each potential staff member must spend at least one year training in, and imbibing the traditions of, the Clinic before being appointed.*

Although the surgeons attract many of the patients who come to the Clinic for cardiac care, the medical cardiologists receive their share for diagnostic studies and nonsurgical treatment, many self-referred by the patients themselves rather than by doctors. Dr. Eric Topol, chairman of the depart-

---

*The cardiothoracic service requires a year of fellowship training regardless of where candidates for staff positions have previously worked. Even training at the august Johns Hopkins Hospital didn't excuse Dr. Mark Gillinov from spending a further fellowship year absorbing the Clinic traditions before being appointed to the staff, where he then began a successful career applying surgical techniques to the treatment of cardiac arrythmias.[169]

ment of cardiovascular medicine, leads a unit of seventy-two staff colleagues—thirty-three when he arrived in 1991—and seventy-two fellows.* Unlike most of the Clinic staff, Topol did not train there and, in coming to the Clinic, entered a new culture. "Here," he finds, "the best clinical people are the most admired. At Hopkins [where Topol trained in cardiology] and Michigan [where he was a member of the faculty before coming to Cleveland], researchers are the most respected."[172]

In coming to the Clinic, Topol departed from the traditional pathway for highly productive academic cardiologists, which often leads to directing a division at a renowned academic medical center. "It had the most extraordinary potential. The outstanding care, exceptional surgery, and the heritage deeply impressed me."[172] Topol saw the large volume of patients ideal for recruitment into clinical trials, the coordination of which he was becoming a leader in. He liked that all patients are patients of the Clinic, not private patients in the traditional sense, and approved the administrative structure of a single employer.[172]

In the fourteen years Topol has led the cardiology department, the research productivity has greatly increased, so that now, the academic accomplishments of this previously non-medical school-affiliated† hospital's cardiac program compare favorably with those of the most productive cardiology divisions at leading academic medical centers.[128] As of the spring of 2005, Topol's name appeared as one of the authors of more than 900 original publications in competitive journals and the editor or coauthor of thirty books, an astounding degree of productivity. Much of this work appeared after Topol, described by Dr. Gary Francis, one of his colleagues, as "the most organized, effective executive I've ever known," came to the Clinic. "Eric doesn't bother people or micromanage, but he's engaged."[51] Not only is Topol an extraordinarily productive clinical investigator, he's an excellent bedside teacher, "very passionate about everything he does." Cardiologist Joel Holland, who previously worked at Mt. Sinai and University Hospitals and trained at the University of Chicago, finds Topol "a wonder-

---

*The department appoints forty fellows—thirteen per year—for the standard three-year training program required for subspecialty certification. Most of these fellows have been residents in internal medicine at leading American teaching hospitals.[170] The department also appoints thirty-two senior fellows for advanced training in the clinical laboratories and programs.[171]

†See chapter 6 for the Clinic's new medical college.

ful chief, and everybody thinks so. He's very supportive of us, leads by example, and works very hard.[173] Francis adds an unexpected compliment: "He holds fabulous faculty meetings."[51]

In addition to the medical and surgical cardiac departments, twenty-two staff anesthesiologists[174] and four radiologists[175] work in the cardiac program.

How large should the cardiac program at the Cleveland Clinic become? "We have no concern about one unit's being too big," answers chief of staff Robert Kay. "I tell the doctors that their goals will never be limited by us."[71] Because inadequate space now inhibits further growth in the heart program, the Clinic is constructing a building specifically for treatment of patients with heart disease. This will take at least four years to be completed in part because the new cardiac center—in which inpatient and outpatient activities and administration will be combined—will be built where a parking garage, which will need to be taken down and rebuilt elsewhere, now stands. The decrease in the value of the endowment affected the Cleveland Clinic in several ways but has not delayed the inclusion of the features desired by the staff, the size of which—projected to include 970,000 square feet—will depend to a significant degree upon the amount of money raised from philanthropic sources, now a major responsibility of the Clinic's institutional development department.[151]*

The larger heart service, when the new building is available, will help to accommodate the continuously growing demand for cardiac services at the Clinic and will provide, in addition to more laboratories and operating rooms, additional offices and examining rooms for the staff. This will allow the Clinic to hire more doctors and relieve, to some extent, the complaint of current cardiologists that they are overworked.[65] In the meantime, to provide space for cardiac care in the current buildings, the Clinic is considering transferring from the central campus to one of its other facilities such nonintensive services like rehabilitation.[71]

The accomplishments of cardiology and cardiac surgery are not isolated events at the Clinic, an institution that continues to embrace creativity, innovation, and big ideas; rewards innovation; and values long-term strate-

---

*As of the spring of 2005, $250 million of the $300 million required had been raised or pledged.[151]

gic initiatives.[116] "Here," says neurology chairman Hans Lüders, "everything is possible. If you want to change the structure, you can do it. Because of the group practice model."[26]

Urology

In leading the department of urology, the largest and most profitable of the Clinic's surgical units—"much bigger than cardiac surgery"[53]—Andrew Novick readily admits that he is "stubborn and focused."[53] Born in Montreal and educated at McGill University and its teaching hospitals, Novick came to the Clinic in 1974 for his urology residency and then specialized in kidney transplantation. In 1985, he became chairman of his department which now includes fifty-eight staff members, forty-seven of whom are clinical urologists. The group is so large that it employs more than 70 percent of Cleveland's urologists.* $11 million from the National Institutes of Health (NIH) support seven research laboratories. An $8 million donation has recently funded the Glickman Urological Institute, which Novick directs and will move into its own building in a few years.[53]

Only the department of urology at the Johns Hopkins Hospital surpasses the Cleveland Clinic's unit as far as *U.S. News & World Report* is concerned.[176] The director of the Hopkins department, Patrick Walsh, says Novick's department is "the largest in the United States, compared with the 'one-man show' at CASE," and this from a doctor who received his undergraduate and M.D. degrees from Western Reserve and is a university trustee.[177] Novick praises the efficient character of the Clinic's "monolithic organization with no duality" of direction between hospital and medical school. "I can get things done much easier than my colleagues at other academic medical centers. Patient care being so paramount makes us different from them," Novick said.[53]

Breast Center

A good example of the ability of the Clinic to develop a program so long as it has able doctors is the breast center. The director, Dr. Joseph Crowe,

---

*Novick says that his urologists earn about as much as those working elsewhere in the Cleveland region. "It was much less when I started."[53]

was recruited in 1994 from University Hospitals, where he was an associate professor of surgery with tenure and director of the breast unit. The Clinic attracted him by offering to develop a coordinated center with convenient, accessible support from the medical oncology, radiology, and radiation therapy departments. Crowe was also guaranteed that he would have to perform only breast surgery, his area of special interest. Crowe had trained at University and spent nearly nine years on the faculty. He was looking for another opportunity when the Clinic approached him. He admitted, "the decision to move wasn't difficult."[178]

The center now cares for 15,000 patients per year, three to four times as many as the unit at the university. Crowe's group consists of six surgeons, six radiologists, and two internists, each specializing in treating diseases of the breast.[178]

"It's very different here," says Crowe in describing how the Clinic works compared with the system he was accustomed to at the university. "We're a multispecialty group practice so there's one unit versus separate practice plans at CASE. There, what was good for the hospital was not necessarily good for the practice plans and vice versa."[178]* Crowe also finds that the operating rooms run more efficiently at the Clinic than at University, and he has more secretarial, technical, and administrative assistance to make his work even more efficient. "Although it took seven to eight years to get the whole program in place, now we have the clinical and research assistance we need and highly competitive residents and fellows."[178]

Neurosciences

One of those perennially recurring turf battles among doctors has recently arisen between neurologists, neurosurgeons, head and neck surgeons, and vascular radiologists. The invention of angioplasty and intravascular stents allowed invasive cardiologists to perform some of the work previously the province of cardiothoracic surgeons with their coronary artery bypass graft operations. Now the nonoperative treatment of cerebral aneurysms has already reduced significantly the number of craniotomies in which neurosurgeons opened the skulls of patients to clip these abnormal

---

*See chapter 4 for an explanation of how practice plans operate.

vessels and prevent their rupturing and producing disabling strokes or death.[179]

Although the Cleveland Clinic is not immune to such difficulties, Dr. Marc Mayberg, chairman of the department of neurosurgery, claims that, in his experience at the Clinic, battles over turf are attenuated. "We know that we provide better care if we integrate," and consequently, the neurosurgeons and vascular radiologists collaborate when a patient with an aneurysm comes to the Clinic. Mayberg says that about half of aneurysms are now treated with the endovascular approach. Although he operates 50 percent less often for this lesion than in the past, the collaboration with radiology has nearly doubled the total number of aneurysms treated at the Cleveland Clinic, so that the number of operative procedures has stayed about the same.

"This is a cerebrovascular floor," Mayberg says with pride. Doctors from all the relevant disciplines work together even though their appointments may be in different departments. "We also have a spine floor with neurosurgeons, orthopedic surgeons, and rheumatologists all together."[52] Mayberg credits this cooperativeness to the absence of direct financial incentives. The staff doesn't receive bonuses and the salaries, in Mayberg's experience, "are kept within competitive limits." Furthermore, the income goes into one entity, the group practice, and departments and divisions do not keep surpluses they may generate.[52]

Many of the patients refer themselves to the department of neurology, the way many patients come to the Clinic. If the doctors send them, "it's often in response to pressure from the patients. So we advertise directly to the patients," says chairman Hans Lüders.[26] Many have epilepsy, Lüders's special interest. About 200 per year undergo neurosurgery in which the surgeon, guided by the neurologist's studies, excises the source of the seizures in the brain. Lüders says the Clinic's program for this work is the largest in the country.[26]

Like several other Clinic leaders, Marc Mayberg in neurosurgery has been offered tempting jobs at well-known academic medical centers. "There," he comments about the other academic opportunities, "innovating and integrating would have been difficult, the finances were complex, and space was restricted."[52] So he stayed at the Clinic, partly because "this is a very doctor-friendly place to work. I can operate on the same number of patients in two days that took me three or four days" at the academic medical center where he previously worked.[52] Mayberg ascribes such efficiency to significant investment in the infrastructure "to make the processes work well." The Clinic has enough operating rooms and faster turnover of patients, "so I have less scut work to do."[52]

Eye Institute

Dr. Hilel Lewis was an associate professor of ophthalmology at the Jules Stein Eye Institute of the University of California, Los Angeles, when, in 1992, the Cleveland Clinic invited him to become a candidate to lead its department. Lewis, who was born and educated in Mexico, had trained at several of America's leading centers for research and clinical care in eye diseases, including the Stein center and the Wilmer Institute at the Johns Hopkins Hospital. His research in the treatment of retinal, macular, and vitreous diseases was bringing him international renown with many invitations to write chapters, chair seminars, and give lectures. Ordinarily, someone with Lewis's academic trajectory would wait until an invitation came his way to direct a department of ophthalmology at a leading medical school or eye institute.

Lewis initially declined the offer to chair the Clinic's department of ophthalmology. "After numerous interactions," he explains, "Dr. Loop eventually asked me what I would need to build the best department in the country."[57] Lewis provided Loop with a detailed strategic plan to create and develop what Lewis described as "the preeminent ophthalmology department in the country."[57] Like many others, Lewis bought Loop's assurances and moved to Cleveland in 1993.

Lewis, who had been offered six other chairs by this time, felt that "the Clinic under Dr. Loop offered me the best possibility of building a department that could be the best in the world by providing patients with the best outcomes and service, conducting translational basic and clinical research, and training the future leaders in ophthalmology."[57] Lewis wanted, in particular, to "create a new model for research, goal-oriented and interactive between basic and clinical scientists," and felt strongly that clinically oriented basic science should be conducted in laboratories adjacent to clinician investigators. "Our strength was then and has remained clinical care.

We had to bring the investigators closer since the questions had to be asked by the clinicians," says Lewis.[57]

Loop agreed, despite his preference that all basic research leave the clinical departments for the Clinic's research institute. The division of ophthalmology—Lewis also insisted on divisional status for the former department—then proceeded to recruit basic scientists whose work related closely to clinical research. Other basic research associated with vision but without immediate clinical relevance remained in what would become the Lerner Research Institute.

Lewis spent the next six years planning his ideal program and then, in 1999, moved the division into a new, beautiful, and functional building designed, like three other major buildings on the Clinic campus, by the eminent architect Cesar Pelli. The building was named the Cole Eye Institute for the Cleveland family that had founded what became the Cole National Company, the largest manufacturer of optical glasses and frames, and had provided much of the funding for the project.

The division's national reputation has steadily improved, with the department ranked sixth, according to a survey of ophthalmology chairmen.[180] Understandingly proud of his department and its accomplishments, Lewis says, "The Cole Eye Institute is the most advanced eye institute and cares for more patients than any other eye institute in the country. It also now has one of the best translational research programs, with funding exceeding $10 million in 2003."[57] During the most recent year, the institute staff received $4.8 million in funding from the NIH.[181]

Lewis and his colleagues also run what has become an increasingly competitive residency program. The institute appoints 4 residents into its 3-year training program, choosing them from 400 applicants and interviewing 60.[57] The institute also trains 5 clinical fellows in the subspecialties of ophthalmology and 15 postdoctoral fellows in the basic science program.[182] Lewis's professional staff consists of 21 M.D.s, one doctor of osteopathy, and 6 optometrists. Three of the M.D.s plus 12 Ph.D.s perform basic research.[182]

In recent years, Lewis has turned down offers to direct many other eye institutes and a few deanships. He is likely to stay at the Clinic because "it has the best model to practice medicine, superb leadership, and a commitment to being the irrefutable leader in academic medicine."[57]

Orthopedics

Dr. Joseph Iannotti first visited the Clinic as a candidate to become chairman of the department of orthopedics in July 1999. He was then professor of orthopedics at the University of Pennsylvania and had entered that phase of his career when he was being considered for chairmanships. At the Clinic, he found a financially sound department unlike many of the other departments he had visited with "tough financial problems and disgruntled faculty. This place was running fine, and the people were happy."[66] Iannotti was impressed with the excellent facilities in the Lerner Research Institute, where well-funded scientists were working although, for the most part, in fields not related to orthopedics. The quality of the residents was high, similar to what he was used to at Penn. By November, he had accepted, and he started work in April 2000. By 2003, his department had grown from forty-two to fifty-two doctors. That year, *U.S. News & World Report* ranked the department fifth in the country, despite the Clinic's being the only hospital in the top five without a trauma center.[183]

Iannotti, whose clinical interests are the orthopedic problems of the shoulder and, in research, tendon tissue engineering, saw "a chance to build an academic department" within a very busy clinical enterprise.[66] He sees himself as one of the "new breed" of Clinic leaders, chairmen with academic interests in addition to clinical competence.[66] He learned, however, that because of the dominance of the group practice over the divisions and departments, his power as chairman would be less than was typical at academic medical centers.

By the time he had been at the Clinic for six months, Iannotti, who had developed a national reputation for his area of special clinical interest, was receiving enough referrals, mostly from other physicians and surgeons, to fill his schedule. He operates on about 280 patients annually, fewer than at Penn, but that was before he had the administrative responsibilities that accrue to a chairman. Iannotti finds that the operating rooms work at the Clinic with about the same efficiency that he was accustomed to in Philadelphia, the delays between cases being typical of hospitals with large volumes. He doesn't do all his cases at the downtown campus, however, performing his arthroscopic procedures at one of the satellite locations near where he lives.[66] Iannotti particularly appreciates the ease of obtaining consultations at the Clinic, which was not his previous experience. "It's painless to send patients to another doc," he says. "One hour later there's an e-mail with a report and a 'thanks for the patient.' "[66]

Pediatrics

Pediatrics in Cleveland has long been dominated by Rainbow Babies and Children's Hospital at University Hospitals of Cleveland. For much of its existence, pediatrics was "a stepchild to the Clinic's principal mission," according to its current chairman, Michael Levine. The Clinic paid relatively little attention to the specialty, which was started to provide care for the children of the Clinic's employees.[184] Its growth was further inhibited by the Clinic's closing its obstetrics department in 1966 to accommodate the growing cardiac surgery program.[185]

By 1987, the Clinic had opened its own Children's Hospital, and under the leadership of Douglas Moodie, chairman from 1987 to 2002, and, more recently, Michael Levine from 2003, the division has grown along with many of the other departments and divisions at the Clinic.* Important to this development was the reentry of the Clinic into obstetrics in 1995.[186] As a reflection of the standing of pediatrics among the Clinic's activities, the unit had only departmental status within the division of medicine until 1994. Gradually, the division has gathered under its jurisdiction such subspecialties as pediatric general and cardiac surgery, which had been lodged elsewhere previously.[184] Loop and Kay have supported Levine's effort to create a more comprehensive children's hospital by opening discussions to bring pediatric neurology, anesthesia, orthopedics, and radiology into the division. What has slowed this process is a political reality familiar to deans and leaders of clinical departments at most academic medical centers. "There're not many dollars involved," says Levine. "It's mostly ego."[60]

---

*Levine came to his current job through a career pathway traveled by few pediatrics chairmen. He was trained as an internist, not a pediatrician, and before coming to Cleveland was the chief of the pediatric endocrine division at Hopkins. He imagined his relocation as having some of the adventurous characteristics of William Osler's move from the established University of Pennsylvania to the brand-new Johns Hopkins Hospital in 1889. He saw the Clinic as an institution "in transition" and that he would have the opportunity to build the division. Levine's research interest is calcium metabolism.[184]

Radiology

One specialty where recruiting and retaining doctors within medical schools challenges directors is radiology. "Radiologists can easily make 25 percent or more income in private practice," laments Dr. Michael Modic, the neuroradiologist who is the chairman of the division at the Clinic. "Interventionalists can earn half a million and more."[187] Nevertheless, few staff radiologists flee the Clinic for the greater income of private practice. "Most of our docs have bought into the concept of the group practice. We have the best equipment, fascinating pathology, and superb colleagues. It's hard to feel sorry for someone who's getting paid $250,000 to $300,000 a year for work at such a great place."[187]

During the past decade, radiology at the Cleveland Clinic has expanded far beyond the downtown campus thanks to extraordinary advances in the computerization of its equipment. X-ray film is becoming a relic, replaced by digital techniques that allow doctors to read the images from computer screens. This means that radiological information can be transmitted to any facility equipped to download such data. Accordingly, the results from many of the radiological procedures performed at the owned hospitals and outpatient clinics are interpreted at the main campus by Clinic specialists, and the interpretations are then transmitted back to the place where the procedures were performed.

The availability of this technology has allowed the Clinic to offer sophisticated radiological services to hospitals and doctors' offices everywhere. The Clinic calls this service "e-Radiology," which is administered by CCF Holdings, the Clinic's for-profit subsidiary.[79,95] "We formed e-Radiology, Modic explains, "to provide a revenue stream to support the academic work within our division."[187]

E-Radiology leases such devices as MRI scanners and other expensive machines, whose images often require sophisticated interpretations, to radiologists and other specialists throughout the country.[187] Clinic radiologists at the main campus interpret the data, which have been electronically transmitted there from the doctors' offices.[187] The Clinic will also provide billing services for the facilities with which it is linked. The local site retains the fees generated for use of the equipment, while the Clinic receives the

payments for providing the professional services interpreting the procedures. E-Radiology generates annually about $15 million in gross revenue
and is profitable.[95]

Loop's Leaving

In December 2003, Fred Loop told his trustees that "2004 will be my last
year. They were amazed, but I'd held the job for fifteen years."[146] Mal
Mixon, the chairman of the Clinic's board, would lead the search, and Loop
would serve on the succession committee,[188] not unexpectedly since, as is
commonly believed at the Clinic, "the trustees love him."[35]

Loop's spontaneous decision to leave—his two predecessors did not initi-
ate the actions that led to their retirement[47]—was received as "the act of a
class operator." Much admired for maintaining a balance between dollars
and clinical care,[187] Loop will "go out on top," said Michael Modic. "It'll be
very difficult to follow him. The bar is already at such a high level." The
change will, this time, be conducted "without panic, not in a willy-nilly
fashion," added Modic, himself a suitable candidate but "not interested in
the job."[187]

The new CEO "will have to juggle a lot of balls and suffer the egos to
make it work, and he'll have to quit practicing," Modic believes.[187] Changes
of this magnitude often bring turmoil. "I hope our model of the group
practice will provide the basis for stability," said Martin Harris, the chief
information officer.

The New CEO

On June 1, 2004, the Cleveland Clinic Foundation announced that Toby
Cosgrove,[189] a cardiac surgeon like his predecessor, would succeed Fred
Loop as CEO on October 1, 2004.[190] The October date was chosen so that
the veteran Loop, rather than his successor, would be available to coordi-
nate the review by the Joint Commission on Accreditation of Healthcare
Organizations scheduled for September.[191]

The selection process began in March 2004, after the local press revealed Loop's intention to retire as CEO.[188] Five trustees and five members of the board of governors who were not themselves candidates con-

stituted the search committee.* Loop found its deliberations "fair and balanced."[146]

"The broad view was that the institution was doing very well and didn't want to make any radical changes," said David Bronson.[191] This general consensus dictated that the new CEO would almost certainly be someone currently at the Clinic, the tradition at the institution since its beginning. "We had all the people within the Clinic we needed," said Mal Mixon, the chairman of the trustees and of the selection committee. "We decided that each candidate had to be a physician and had to declare his interest and compete for the job."[192] The committee conducted the deliberations itself without employing a headhunter or a facilitator. One of the chairmen, not himself a candidate, suggested that "the stature of the CEO will be improved because he will be chosen by peer review rather than by appointment."[193]

The committee invited all members of the group practice who thought themselves suitable to become CEO to apply. Seven came forward. Among those discussed in these pages were Cosgrove; Robert Kay, chief of staff; Andrew Novick, chairman of urology; Jeffrey Ponsky, head of surgical endoscopy and director, graduate medical education; and Eric Topol, chairman of cardiology.[194] This news received rapid distribution in the community, the Clinic giving the names to Diane Solov who identified the seven being considered in a *Plain Dealer* article on March 17.[194] At the Clinic, however, says Bronson, "We didn't know how the names got into the newspaper. It was assumed that some of the candidates had spoken to the press, and, of course, it was known at [the Clinic] who had thrown his hat in the ring."[191]

To obtain advice from the leading members of the Clinic, the committee interviewed the division chairmen, each for one or more hours, followed by members of the senior executive team.[191] The committee invited every doctor in the group practice to participate and more than forty did, each spending about fifteen minutes telling the ten members what issues he or she saw the Clinic facing. In these sessions, the committee did not invite comments about individual candidates, but, David Bronson adds, "many were of-

*The trustees were Thomas Commes, Stephen Hardes, William MacDonald III, Patrick McCartan, and Mal Mixon. In addition to Loop, the physician members were David Bronson, chairman of the division of regional medical practice; Linda Graham, chairman of the department of vascular surgery; Walter Mauer, director of the office of quality management; and Michael Modic.[191] The doctors selected represented different departments and divisions so that one component, surgery, for example, would not dominate the proceedings.[146]

fered."[195] Dr. Edward Hundert, the new president of Case Western Reserve University and a strong advocate for the Clinic's new medical college, also met with the committee and advised that whoever was chosen should be committed to developing the school.[192]*

The committee interviewed each candidate at least twice. Bronson characterizes the first session as "a 'who am I' session," in effect amplifying on each candidate's curriculum vitae. During the second meeting, the candidates were asked to describe their visions for the Clinic.[191] Every candidate was offered the opportunity of meeting with each member of the committee, and many did.[191,192]

"We had set a date to make our decision," said Mixon. "Each member of the committee named his preference, the five doctors first with Loop last and then the trustees."[192] Loop did not want to give an opinion—"I didn't have much to say," Loop describes his participation on the committee[146]—but two of the trustee members stated that unless he did, they would remain silent. So Loop voted with the others. Everyone favored Cosgrove. The trustees were impressed that, as Mixon said, "Toby had great support among the doctors."[192] Within an hour after the committee had made its choice, the board of governors and the trustees met and voted to approve the nominee. Then Mixon told each candidate about the decision.[192]

Mixon was pleased that the process had run so smoothly and that the choice had not leaked until he and Loop could notify the candidates. Soon afterward, the board chairman and outgoing CEO met with Solov, who reported the news in *The Plain Dealer* the next day.[190,192] "It was the most important civic contribution I ever made," a contented Mal Mixon said.[192]

As for the selection of Cosgrove, Loop, who was very pleased with the choice, said, "Toby's different from me. He's more networked. He has numerous patents, is known for his bright ideas, and gets along very well with the people in the corporate world."[146] When challenged about another cardiac surgeon in the executive office, Loop replied, "I'm actually embarrassed about that. I have no special allegiance to a cardiac surgeon for this job."[146]

Others interviewed for this book said:

- "A superb doctor. He's played by the rules and hasn't messed around outside his department."[191]

*See chapter 6.

- "Has executive and professional presence."[191]
- "An outstanding manager. Collaboration with other M.D.s extraordinary. Has recruited unbelievably able colleagues."[196]
- "A compassionate person. Terrific choice."[197]
- "Talented. Has been here a long time. Will look at the big picture and delegate well, but he'll face a big culture shock going from surgery to administration."[193]

What will Cosgrove emphasize during his tenure? Chief operating officer Frank Lordeman thinks he will stress "continued growth. He'll increase capacity and margin. If we can decrease the length of stay significantly, we would pick up the equivalent of sixty additional beds." Lordeman also believes Cosgrove will work toward increasing the ambulatory activities particularly at the family health centers, which should allow inpatient work to be more emphasized at the main campus.[196]

As for Loop's next job, "he might like to be surgeon general in a future Republican administration," speculates colorectal surgery chairman Victor Fazio. Loop responds that "Washington is not for activists. Bureaucracies don't encourage imagination."[146] Fazio adds, "His orchids [Loop's great hobby] won't be enough, but he'll stay around as long as Toby needs him."[193]

The biggest question in the minds of many was whether the highly successful cardiology chairman Eric Topol, having missed the top job, would stay at the Clinic. "At sixty-three years of age Cosgrove is likely to be a relatively short-term CEO," one senior member of the group practice suggested, "making the situation perhaps a bit more palatable for Topol,"[198] who was fifty years old during the summer Cosgrove was chosen. "No comment," was Topol's reply when asked about his future plans.[199]

What Makes the Clinic the Clinic?

Current and former members of the staff and observers from elsewhere praise the fundamental purpose for which the Clinic exists and the basic reason for its success.

- "We're completely geared toward providing a product that patients want, whatever it takes."[173]
- "Patient care is a primary priority."[74]

- "Most people here are clinicians first, second, third, and last."[72]
- "We're all paid out of the same account."[7] "There's a single bottom line and no practice plan."[74]
- "We're an aggregation of a large number of incredibly good, talented, workaholic docs who believe strongly in the group practice model."[38]

"It's our spirit of inquiry," says retired general surgeon Robert Hermann, who joined the Clinic in 1962, in describing another leading characteristic of the Clinic. "We admire people with new ideas," said a longtime member of the staff.[7] Thinking about Mason Sones and other pioneers, Clinic veteran Earl Shirey says, "We're been fortunate in obtaining some key men who made important contributions."[162]

Clinic partisans, often those who have worked or trained there, love to compare their institution with University Hospitals of Cleveland and other academic medical centers.

- "We're much more friendly."[73]
- "At UH there are people running around demeaning colleagues whose primary focus is taking care of patients."[173]
- "Many of the people running things at other places don't and shouldn't take care of patients."[72]
- "Here, we don't suffer from a leadership gap."[128]

Why did ophthalmologist Elias Traboulsi, whom Hilel Lewis recruited in 1996, leave his position at the famous Wilmer Eye Institute of the Johns Hopkins Hospital? "I specialize in pediatric ophthalmology and genetics, and Hilel guaranteed that I would be able to make an impact in these two areas at the Cleveland Clinic. I didn't realize there was so much here until I visited."[37] It's an immense operation, with a thousand doctors at the downtown facility. One result of its size, which few at the Clinic dwell upon, however, is the loss of some of the "personal touches."[200]

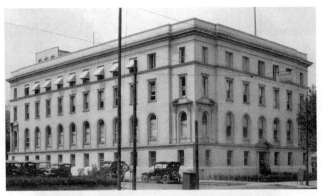

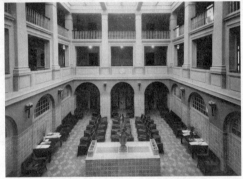

The Cleveland Clinic's first building (*top*), completed in 1921 for the ambulatory care of the patients of the founders and their colleagues. Interior view (*bottom*) of the waiting area, an atrium rising from the second floor and surrounded by the examining rooms. The Clinic's first hospital building opened three years later. *Courtesy of the Cleveland Clinic Foundation*

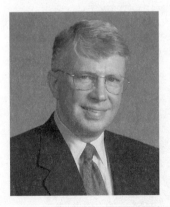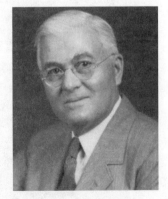

Dr. George Crile (*right*), the principal founder of the Clinic and its president until 1940. Crile's authority led to many calling his creation "The Crile Clinic." Dr. Floyd ("Fred") Loop (*left*), Crile's successor as the fourth physician chief executive of the Cleveland Clinic Foundation from 1989 to 2004. Both surgeons, Crile and Loop symbolized the dominance of this specialty at the Clinic. *Courtesy of the Cleveland Clinic Foundation*

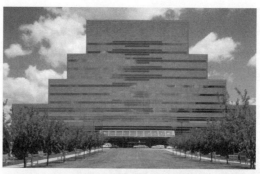

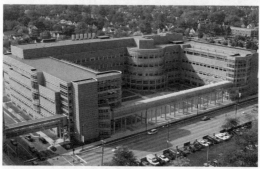

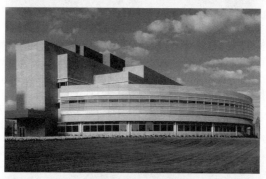

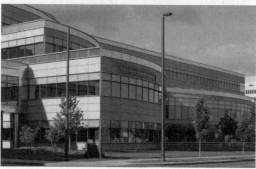

Four of the Clinic buildings designed by Cesar Pelli: (*from top to bottom*) Crile building for outpatients, Lerner Research Institute, Cole Eye Institute, and Taussig Cancer Center.
Courtesy of the Cleveland Clinic Foundation

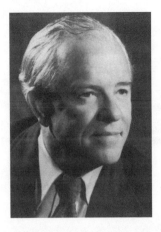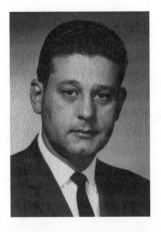

By developing coronary arteriography, Dr. Mason Sones (*left*) launched cardiology toward its current eminence at the Cleveland Clinic. While a fellow at the Clinic, Dr. René Favaloro (*right*) reported the first series of patients whose angina pectoris responded to the CABG (coronary artery bypass graft) operation. *Courtesy of the Cleveland Clinic Foundation*

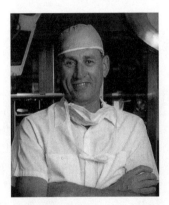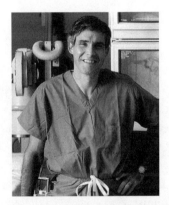

Looking like a cardiac surgeon should, Dr. Delos ("Toby") Cosgrove (*left*) succeeded Fred Loop as chairman of the department of thoracic and cardiovascular surgery and then in 2004 as CEO of the Cleveland Clinic Foundation. Dr. Eric Topol (*right*), the master of the controlled drug trial and chairman of the department of cardiovascular medicine from 1991, built one of the strongest clinical and academic cardiology programs in the country. As chief academic officer, Topol is responsible for the development of the Clinic's new medical college. *Courtesy of the Cleveland Clinic Foundation*

CHAPTER THREE

University Hospitals of Cleveland

Turmoil in University Circle

One mile east of the Cleveland Clinic, in an area of Cleveland called University Circle,[1] stands the Clinic's principal competitor for specialty care in the region, the University Hospitals of Cleveland, the primary teaching hospital of the Case Western Reserve University (CASE) School of Medicine. During the 1990s, a feud between the president of the university and the CEO of University Hospitals impeded the efforts of the deans and faculty in the school of medicine to develop their clinical practices and conduct research, caught as they were between the agendas of these two powerful leaders.

University Hospitals of Cleveland

On May 14, 1866, having decided to build a new hospital—it would be Cleveland's third—a group of Cleveland's wealthier citizens, predominantly Protestant, native-born, and Republican, elected a board of trustees to construct and operate Cleveland City Hospital, an entity that would eventually become part of University Hospitals of Cleveland.[2]* The city, which had been founded in 1796, was, by the end of the Civil War, an increasingly busy manufacturing center where industrial leaders such as John D. Rockefeller[4] would soon make fortunes.

Constructed on what was then called Wilson Street near Fourteenth Street and the Lake Erie waterfront, the new hospital was designed "for the reception, care and medical treatment of sick and disabled persons,"[2] which meant the poor and destitute since, at the time, most patients with money were treated in their homes or their doctors' offices. When Cleveland built a replacement for its publicly funded City Hospital, later called Cleveland Metropolitan Hospital, in 1887, the trustees renamed their institution Lakeside, by which it was to become widely known, and, in January 1898, opened a new plant modeled on the Johns Hopkins Hospital in Baltimore.

In 1914, the trustees of Lakeside Hospital and Western Reserve University began exploring the concept of constructing new hospital and medical school buildings adjacent to the university campus at University Circle east of the older parts of the city, where both the hospital and the medical school were then located. In 1926, a new board of trustees created a holding company called "University Hospitals of Cleveland, Incorporated" (UHC), which took over administrative control of the Maternity and of Babies' and Children's hospitals, recently built on the new site, and Lakeside, still downtown. As the hospital's historian Mark Gottlieb writes, "Although each institution maintained its own board and endowment funds, all were answerable to the University Hospitals corporation and its board of trustees, which included representatives from each of the hospitals."[5]

Finally, on February 1, 1931, the patients were transferred from the old facility to the new ten-storey hospital building in University Circle, where private patients would be cared for in the Hanna House and the other medical and surgical patients in the new Lakeside.† With the faculty of the

---

*See *The Lives of University Hospitals of Cleveland,* by Mark Gottlieb—on which much of this history is based—for a detailed description of the first 125 years of the hospital.[2]

I adopt the local convention of referring to University Hospitals of Cleveland as "the hospital" and not "the hospitals."[3]

†Many of the voluntary teaching hospitals of this period made special provision for those who could afford private rooms. Phillips House at the Massachusetts General Hospital in Boston[6] and Harkness Pavilion at the Columbia-Presbyterian Medical Center in New York City[7] were two other well-known examples of such facilities designed specifically to provide comfortable accommodations for the private patients of the hospital staff.

Western Reserve University School of Medicine occupying its new building on the campus since 1924, University Hospitals of Cleveland and the medical school now constituted a physically coordinated group of structures for education, research, and patient care, an arrangement that would later be called an academic medical center.

Case Western Reserve University School of Medicine

The medical school with which Lakeside would long be affiliated was founded in 1843 when a group of professors and the dean at a struggling medical college in Cleveland resigned from its faculty and asked Western Reserve College,* a small liberal arts institution, to establish a medical department in the city.† The college, founded in 1826 and located in Hudson, Ohio, about twenty miles southeast of Cleveland, responded so quickly that instruction began in the fall of 1843. Typical of the time, students were not required to attend the lectures. Each session of instruction cost $72. The students' first examinations were held at the end of a three-year apprenticeship, and those who passed were awarded their academic diplomas and licenses to practice medicine.

During most of the nineteenth century, Western Reserve College lent only its name and neither received funds from, nor contributed funds to, the medical department. All members of the faculty supported themselves with their practices, the only salaried employee being the janitor. At the end of each academic year, the teachers divided up the surpluses, if there were any left, after all expenses were paid.

Relations between the medical department and the college, according to the historian of the medical school and university, were "distant and sometimes hostile."[8] Each year, the trustees automatically approved the candidates proposed for graduation by the medical faculty. The president of the college, who furnished and signed the diplomas, did not preside over meet-

---

*Its name derives from the Western Reserve, sometimes called New Connecticut, 3.5 million acres in northeastern Ohio, which Congress allotted to the state in compensation for losses sustained by its citizens from actions of the British during the Revolution. The Reserve extended for 120 miles west from the Pennsylvania border and from Lake Erie south to the 41st parallel, which runs through current Akron. The space was larger than its parent state and about one-seventh the size of the current state of Ohio.[8]

†For further details, see *Case Western Reserve: A History of the University, 1826–1976* by C. H. Cramer, on which much of this history is based.[8]

ings of the medical faculty until 1891. Two years later, with the resignation of the dean, the appointment of deans passed to the president and board of trustees of the university.

In 1880, the trustees decided to move the college from Hudson to Cleveland and changed its name to Western Reserve University. The first building constructed on the Cleveland campus, Adelbert Hall, is still in use and now houses the president's office and the university's central administration. Its name recalls the former name of the men's college of Western Reserve University, upon which industrialist Amasa Stone had insisted when he funded much of the cost of moving the university to Cleveland. Adelbert was the name of Stone's son who had drowned while a student at Yale.[9]

For much of the university's first decades in Cleveland, women were educated at a separate College for Women in buildings eventually located across Euclid Avenue from the men's college. In time this unit became known as Flora Stone Mather College after Amasa Stone's daughter, who, with her husband, Samuel Mather, had been particularly generous supporters of the university.[10] Although the colleges would merge in 1971 into the Western Reserve College for both men and women,[11] the names persist on the campus. Adelbert Hall backs onto Adelbert Road. The Mather name appears on buildings on the former women's campus and on two hospital buildings, one of which was originally designed as a nurses' residence. The university chapel is named for Amasa Stone.

By the end of the nineteenth century, the medical department was occupying the third of three structures it would build downtown until moving, in 1924, into a new building, described as "the largest structure occupied by any medical school in the United States"[8] at the University Circle campus of the university. A four-year graded course was offered in 1895 and made compulsory four years later; by 1909 a bachelor's degree was required for admission. The Flexner report[12] praised the medical department—the name of which was changed to "school of medicine" in 1912—Abraham Flexner telling the university president that, except for Johns Hopkins, the Western Reserve school was the best in the country.

Although the school had, since its founding, been associated with several hospitals, in 1898, an official relationship was established with Lakeside Hospital—both were then still downtown—to become its principal teaching hospital. Consequently, as in more than 60 percent of American academic medical centers with privately owned medical schools today, different entities would direct the school and the main teaching hospital with which it was associated.[13]

As the twenty-first century began, the relationship between University Hospitals of Cleveland and Case Western Reserve University—the Case School of Applied Science had merged with Western Reserve in 1967, bringing about a change in the name of the university that continues to dismay some of the older faculty[14]—came under intense review and not for the first time.*

Education and Research

The association between the medical school and the hospital appears to have been comparatively stable in the 1950s, which allowed the school to revise its curriculum so comprehensively that the changes would bring national renown to the Western Reserve University School of Medicine and establish education as a primary emphasis of the school.

For much of the twentieth century, medical students spent most of the first two years of the medical course in lecture rooms and laboratories learning the scientific basis of the profession. Traditionally, they studied anatomy, biochemistry, and physiology in the first year; pathology, bacteriology, and pharmacology in the second. Correlation clinics, in which patients with diseases related to the science they were learning were presented, and introduction to clinical medicine—how to take a medical history and perform a physical examination—provided some relief from the heavy diet of medical science that filled each day.

This curriculum owed much to the effects of the Flexner report of 1910,[12] which emphasized the primacy that science should hold in the training of doctors. At the time, this advice gave a much-needed spur to the training of doctors, much of which was conducted in schools without university affiliations and the facilities to teach the new medical science then becoming discovered.

As medical scientists added to the amount of knowledge students should learn, educators came to realize that too much information was being crammed into the preclinical years and that, increasingly, more of it had

---

*For more effective "branding," the university administration adopted, in 2003, the name CASE to be used when referring informally to what is officially Case Western Reserve University. Accordingly, I will usually use CASE when referring to the university.

little relevance to what the physician needed to know to practice effectively. The teaching of the courses by departmental disciplines neglected to coordinate the information so as to emphasize the relevance of the information to the work of the practicing doctor.

Appreciating these problems earlier than the faculty at most medical schools, the leaders at Western Reserve decided to change the curriculum radically.[15-18] Strongly supported by Dr. Joseph Wearn, the dean and chairman of the department of medicine, and, to a great extent, developed by Dr. Thomas Hale Ham, a hematologist from Harvard, the new plan, instituted in 1952, introduced the concept of "organ systems–based teaching," in which the basic science departments collaborated in teaching the normal human structure and function of the different organ systems and, in the second phase, how these systems functioned in disease. For example, in the block on the heart and circulation, physiologists and biochemists together taught how the heart and blood vessels worked in the healthy individual. Later, the same teachers plus the pathologists and microbiologists taught how they malfunctioned in disease, with the pharmacologists describing how drugs would affect their function. In the standard curriculum, then in place in most other schools, the students would have learned about the physiology and biochemistry of the heart and circulation in separate courses.

In a particularly important departure, physicians from the clinical departments joined their colleagues in basic science to teach in the first two years, traditionally the purview of the scientists. These clinical instructors introduced earlier in the curriculum than was then typical concepts of diagnosis and management, thereby providing to the students, in the so-called preclinical years, more of the knowledge they needed to prepare for the work that had brought them to medical school. This practice, which Wearn's successors continued, was not spontaneously accepted by all the basic scientists then at the school or those appointed afterward.[19]

Supporting this concept of early introduction into clinical medicine, each student was assigned, on arrival, a pregnant woman whose medical progress he observed throughout the four years. This experience allowed the student to observe and participate in the care of the members of one family from the first day of the four-year course. Dissecting a cadaver, traditionally the course that rather traumatically introduced the medical student to his profession, was postponed until the second year. As Ham said,

"It was sounder to face their first great moment of crisis . . . in connection with a normal family . . . rather than a cadaver in a traditional anatomy laboratory."[20]

Other reforms included assigning a laboratory facility to each student to conduct the experiments for all his scientific courses rather than working in different laboratories for each discipline. The departments, as it were, came to the student rather than the reverse. The program also abolished grades and class ranking, introduced a preceptor system throughout the four years, and allowed greater time for elective experiences. Since the new curriculum required the participation of many members of the Western Reserve faculty in the planning and execution of the changes, the amount of time dedicated to teaching, particularly among the clinical faculty, greatly increased.

The M.D./Ph.D. program, which prepared students for careers as researchers in fields related to medicine, was another creative educational innovation at Western Reserve.[21] To receive both degrees, students spent at least three more years than were required for the M.D. degree alone.*

Western Reserve's pioneering innovations in medical education provided "a time of great collaborative feeling among the faculty," according to former dean Frederick Robbins (1916–2003).[22,23] Many of those involved in the teaching would regularly meet for dinner at the home of Dr. Wearn in Gates Mills, an upscale Cleveland suburb, to discuss the curriculum and other medical school topics. "Mrs. Wearn always served salmon," Robbins remembered.[23]

The programs attracted highly qualified students and advanced the national and international reputation of the school[23] as other schools applied many features of Western Reserve plans. Whereas one of the former department chairmen would describe Western Reserve's medical school in the 1920s and 1930s as a "local school without a national faculty," with the advent of the new curriculum, "Wearn's vision and recruitments created a famous school. As it improved, it overpowered the rest of the university."[14]

As the novelty of the curriculum passed and other schools began to

---

*One of the first students in the M.D./Ph.D. program was Ferid Murad, who won the Nobel Prize in Physiology or Medicine in 1998. Murad, currently chairman of the department of integrative biology, pharmacology, and physiology at the University of Texas at Houston, recently became a CASE trustee. To help pay for his medical education, Murad moonlighted "from 7:00 p.m. to 7:00 a.m." with the obstetricians at the Cleveland Clinic.[21]

surpass Western Reserve in research productivity and prestige, the national reputation of the school waned.[24,25] By the 1970s, many of the most competitive applicants, who might have chosen to attend Western Reserve during its heyday, now preferred other schools.[25] By the beginning of the twenty-first century, the unique attractiveness of the Western Reserve curriculum was spent[17,26,27]—fifty years had elapsed since the program was developed, and some applicants were choosing to attend Ohio State, a less renowned school, with a lower tuition.[26,27]*

"The school was seduced by the success of the education program," concluded one member of the senior faculty, "and thought it could carry the day."[28] The devotion of the institution to education decreased emphasis on research at Western Reserve[29,30] just as the NIH was beginning its extraordinarily generous support for medical research at the Institutes' laboratories in Bethesda, Maryland, and in the country's medical schools and research institutes. From 1970, the first year that comparative data are available, to 1993, the school never ranked higher than twentieth among all medical schools in the amount of research funded by the NIH.[31] During many of these years it only stood in the high twenties, and in 1975 and 1976 was thirty-third.[31] "Research followed the educational thing, time-wise," comments Daniel Anker, the associate dean for faculty affairs.[32] Some of the research programs, however, had national stature. Four of the basic science chairmen appointed by Wearn became members of the National Academy of Sciences.[28]†

During the 1980s, when Dr. Richard Behrman, chairman of the department of pediatrics and director of the department of pediatrics at Rainbow Babies and Children's Hospital, was dean, the administration of research in the medical school was centered in the dean's office. "The research administration was totally controlled by me," says Behrman. "We paid the hospital for use of space there for research. I received the bulk of the overhead

*A significant number of competitive students choose one of the state schools over CASE if offered positions at both because of lower tuition at the state schools. Currently, about one-third of the applicants admitted to both CASE and Ohio State matriculate at Ohio State, and about 20 percent of those admitted to both CASE and the University of Cincinnati's medical school attend Cincinnati, also a state school. Accordingly, only about half of those accepted by the private Case and one of those two state schools choose to attend CASE. Overall, about two-thirds of the students accepted by CASE eventually attend other medical schools.

†In 2004, school of medicine faculty members Lynn Landmesser, chair of the department of neurosciences, and emeritus professor Oscar Ratnoff were members of the academy. Frederick Robbins, also a member, died in 2002.

[that the university didn't retain], so I could support the clinical and basic science departments."[19] It was during Behrman's deanship that the school's new research building was planned.

Behrman found the basic science departments "in the doldrums, most not in the first rank compared, for example, with Columbia," the medical school in New York where Behrman had previously been chairman of pediatrics.[19] Aided by a grant from the Cleveland Foundation,[33] the dean recruited several new department chairs. "Behrman was fantastic," remembers Fritz Rottman, chairman of the department of molecular biology and microbiology and one of the scientists who were aided by the Foundation's support that Behrman obtained. "He would regularly meet with us and encourage us. The basic sciences thrived."[34] Rottman[34] and John Nilson,[35] former chair of the department of pharmacology, were not alone[36,37] in considering the Behrman decade "the golden years of basic science"[35] at CASE.

Conflict between the Medical Faculty and the University President

In 1987, the CASE trustees elected the university's new president Agnar Pytte (B.A., Princeton; Ph.D., Harvard), a physicist who had been chairman of the department of physics and astronomy and then provost at Dartmouth College. An academic administrator with "a very strong personality,"[38] Pytte enjoyed the support of many of the university trustees, including Dr. Patrick Walsh, who called Pytte "a fantastic person with the highest values, sound ideas about the medical school, and very impressive interpreting issues."*

According to longtime CASE trustee and former board chairman Allen Ford, "he [Pytte] was very interested in the academic side of the university, a very strong and involved president and leader."[40] "His priority was undergraduate education," said Scott Cowen, former dean of CASE's management school and now president of Tulane University.[41] "Ag [Pytte's universally employed nickname] left the professional schools to their own devices."[41] Pytte emphasized those entities at CASE with less prestige in a university oriented toward engineering and science.[41-45]

---

*Walsh, the renowned chief of urology at the Johns Hopkins University School of Medicine, is an alumnus of what was then Western Reserve University, where he had received his A.B. degree in 1960 and his M.D. four years later.[39]

The board had charged Pytte to develop an integrated academic, physical, and financial master plan. "He did a masterful job with this," said Ford. "Ag ran a tight financial ship, no deficits on his watch."[40] He raised funds very effectively,[43,46] and, according to Ford, "exceeded our expectations. Several new buildings we badly needed went up while he was president."[40]

Pytte greatly improved the university's alumni relations. "Ag put us in touch with our alumni and created twenty-nine alumni clubs where we had very few before him," remembers Elaine Hadden, a member of the CASE board for more than twenty-five years. "He was always available to faculty, students, and trustees. Ag was a very sincere man. He spoke from the heart."[47]

Pytte didn't, however, always keep his trustees informed about his plans. As one board member said, "Ag kept his own counsel. You never knew why he did what he did."[48] A quiet, not particularly gregarious man, Pytte could exhibit "a volatile temper,"[41] or, as one of the members of his staff put it, "Ag was not as long-suffering as might have been useful, but he usually kept his temper in check."[42]

Some of the strongest criticisms of the president came from the medical campus.[14,19,23,26,28,34,37,38,41,42,44,46–67] In the words of one of his critics in the medical school, "Ag didn't appreciate the stature of the school." Pytte had, "like many university presidents," an observer of the school said, " a love-hate relationship with the medical school," which spent 40 percent of the university's budget.[63] As a physicist, the president was more enthusiastic about supporting the sciences in the college than in the medical school.[38] Many at the medical school saw him "taxing the rich [the medical school] to feed the poor [the liberal arts departments]."[44]

The medical school with its practice plans and other systems were seen as "mysteries to him." One medical school chairman, stating an opinion shared by other chairmen and some trustees, thought Pytte had "a deeply based, irrational dislike of physicians," some of whom were earning more money than he. One hospital trustee heard him refer to the clinical chairmen as "businessmen masquerading as academics" or as "businessmen wearing a halo." Pytte was said to be "very unhappy" that members of the faculty had relationships with community leaders and members of his board. A severe critic of the president at the medical school added, "Ag was the first president I know of who took on the school. He wanted to take the school down a peg [and engaged in] surreptitious and middle-of-the-night kind of attacks." A consultant saw the president as "engaging in areas he didn't understand." He was continuously accused of "extracting" money from the school to support other university activities.[56]* When reminded how the University Hospitals and the clinical departments had subsidized the medical school, he replied with anger, "That's your obligation."[69]

Not everyone at the medical school, however, criticized the president so severely. Pytte won praise for supporting a distinguished senior member of the medical faculty whom Farah Walters, the CEO of the hospital, had fired from his hospital position. "Ag's a man of principle, a staunch supporter of the faculty and academic freedom," said Dr. Brooks Jackson, then a member of the affected department and now a chairman at the Johns Hopkins University School of Medicine. "He's got the granite of New Hampshire [where he worked at Dartmouth College and now lives] in his veins. Someone with less backbone wouldn't have stood up to her."[70] Jackson felt that most of the faculty, particularly those below the rank of clinical chairmen, supported the university that Pytte led. The hospital, however, Jackson concluded, "did not seem to understand that when it comes to faculty, the university has the moral authority and allegiance of the faculty over the hospital because the university shares the core values of the academic faculty and much of the community whereas the hospital under Farah Walter's leadership did not. The hospital board never seemed to have understood this fact until considerable damage had been done."[70] Walters and Pytte, "both rigid personalities,"[41] were destined to oppose each other whenever conflicts between the hospital and the university arose.

When Behrman left the deanship in 1990 for a job in California, Pytte appointed to succeed him Dr. Neil Cherniak, a distinguished academic pulmonary physician, who had significantly improved the small division[56] he had inherited as its chief. Many members of the faculty concluded that Pytte's motive in appointing Cherniak was his desire to have an accommodating physician as dean who, while building the research reputation of the medical school, would not shake up the school or the university or oppose the president's policies.[14,19,23,28,30,37,38,50,51] Because he was an original thinker, "who took a scholarly approach to the issues he faced,"[71] Cher-

---

*This was not the first time that the university was accused of "extracting" money from the medical school. Greer Williams, the author of the definitive study of the Western Reserve curricular reforms of the 1950s, describes an episode in which an earlier university president tried to divert funds that a donor had intended for the medical school to other university needs. When the dean apprised the donor of the president's plans, the donor transferred the funds to the University Hospitals, where the president could not control them.[68]

niak's transfer out of research and into the dean's office was seen by some of his colleagues to be a mistake. One critic called him "Pytte's puppet"—a subtle but weak leader.

Whether or not this was the case for Cherniak, Pytte had appointed strong deans to direct other schools in the university,[42] and not all observers agreed that Cherniak's leadership was ineffectual.[72] One of the division chiefs saw Cherniak as someone who greatly helped the chairmen improve the academic productivity of their departments.[71] Gail Warden, the CEO of the Henry Ford Health System in Detroit with which Cherniak developed an academic relationship, found him "good at keeping things under control. He was strong and could go toe-to-toe with Pytte because of his academic credentials. He appointed some very good people in the dean's office."[66] Someone told Walters, "Neil's effective because he's a good horse trader."[73]

Pytte remembers that Cherniak was recommended by the search committee on which sat several of the school's leaders, and that he simply followed its advice, "as I did for most deanships."[74] Cherniak, however, was not the committee's or Pytte's first choice. That was Dr. Roger Meyer, chair of psychiatry and executive dean at the University of Connecticut. Pytte offered the job to Meyer, but, after prolonged discussion, the negotiations fell apart.[61] By this time, Meyer, who admits having "stars in my eyes" about becoming dean at CASE, was learning things about Pytte that troubled him. "You don't want to work for Pytte," a colleague at Dartmouth, where Pytte had been provost before coming to CASE, told Meyer.[61] The problems that this colleague had identified at Dartmouth resonated with the experience that Meyer was having in his efforts to negotiate with Pytte. When Meyer was offered the deanship, Pytte had proposed a salary that was less than Meyer was then making at the University of Connecticut and copied key trustees on the letter, making any further negotiations, in Meyer's words, "very difficult."[75]

Among those considered for the deanship was Dr. Bernadine Healy, then director of the Research Institute at the Cleveland Clinic, who left a very strong impression. She wasn't recommended, however, "because she had the wrong address," said Pytte, "but, if the committee had nominated her, I might have appointed her."[74]

For his part, Pytte didn't take the criticism without responding. He once told a senior member of the medical faculty, "You guys want to take over the university." This perception of a dominant university administration directing a subservient medical school led many of the clinical chiefs and faculty to ally themselves more closely with University Hospitals of Cleveland.[76]

The Cleveland Foundation Commission

Conflict between CASE, University Hospitals, and other large hospitals had so alarmed leading citizens in the city[77,78] that the Cleveland Foundation[79]* decided to establish a study commission on medical research and education in August 1991.[33,80] The intensity of the clash "just didn't make sense to them," said Robert Eckardt, vice president for programs and evaluation at the Foundation who staffed the commission.[33] The project aimed to help the university and the hospitals resolve their differences and eventually consolidate the research and educational programs at CASE's medical school and biomedical engineering programs, University Hospitals of Cleveland, Metro Health Medical Center (the county hospital familiarly known as "Metro"), and the Cleveland Clinic.[40,74,81] The Foundation hoped that the commission could help create a highly productive hub of medical research which would, in part, feed the commercial development in biomedicine.[33] As a stimulus to the institutions to work together, the Foundation decided to award no grants to any of the institutions until they could resolve their differences.[81]

Dr. William Anlyan, chancellor of the Duke University Medical Center who chaired the commission, saw "a lack of clear authority" at the CASE/University Hospitals academic medical center and said, "If you can clarify that issue, then you have an opportunity for greatness."[49] Part of the difficulty, he noted, was that neither the university nor the department chairmen in the medical school wanted a strong dean.† Anlyan remembers his group advising "clean things up at home and decrease competing directly with the Cleveland Clinic."[49]

Another member of the commission, Dr. William Kelley, then executive

*The Foundation, established in 1914, describes itself as "the nation's second largest community foundation . . . a pioneer in the field of philanthropy with assets totaling more than $1.5 billion from over 800 individual funds."[79]

†Not an uncommon phenomenon at medical schools, where many chairmen prefer working for a weak rather than a strong dean and can influence, as members of search committees, the choice in that direction.

vice president of the University of Pennsylvania and dean of its school of medicine, thought that the institutions were "on a disaster course because of terrible relationships. The head of the hospital was competing head-to-head with the university."[78]

The Cleveland Foundation commission recommended that the medical school form a "primary" relationship with one major hospital and favored University Hospitals of Cleveland as that hospital. Under their plan, Metro would become a "principal" affiliate.[82] This definition, seen as making Metro "less equal" than University, did not appeal to its CEO, who wanted the chairmen at Metro to have equivalent standing with those at UHC.[82]

As the commission was deliberating, a joint committee of trustees from the university and University Hospitals began meeting in November 1991 to try to resolve some of the most pressing problems at their institutions. Consultants told the committee that the Cleveland region lagged behind the nation in "per capita biomedical research" and then stood at "60 percent of the average for the thirty-seven largest metropolitan areas."[82] When asked how "the Cleveland area with its strong medical institutions" could achieve the status of a leading center for medical care and research, the consultants advised that the medical institutions, specifically University Hospitals and CASE, needed leadership, recruitment of top researchers, and seed money.[82]*

The committee studied the financial data, which alleviated "concerns . . . that funds generated by UHC [University Hospitals of Cleveland] might be used to underwrite undergraduate education of the University" but noted "the absence of detailed information from each of the clinical Departments regarding their financial results of operations."[82] The group observed "management inefficiencies of the current system" and described an episode in which an employee, "who clearly should have been terminated promptly," was not discharged for almost a year.[82]

More comprehensive solutions were shelved. The committee advised, and leading trustees from both institutions favored, consolidating University Hospitals and the school of medicine under a vice president for health affairs for the university. The time seemed propitious since the CEO of University Hospitals of Cleveland, Dr. James Block, was then leaving to be-

---

*By 2002, Cleveland ranked eighteenth among cities in the amount of federal research grants that institutions in the city received.[83]

come president of the Johns Hopkins Hospital and Health System in Baltimore. The university president, however, rejected the deal even though, in Kelley's words, "he would have come out on top."[78] Anlyan said, "He [Pytte] wouldn't listen to anything."[49]

Harry Bolwell, the activist former chairman of the hospital board, favored the creation of a chancellor—which critics called the "C word"[84]— who would rule over both the medical school and hospital within a joint venture of the two institutions. "I was willing to let Behrman [Richard Behrman, dean of the school of medicine at the time] run it, but the university president killed it."[85] Block, the hospital CEO during the commission's work, "stonewalled us at every turn," said one of the members of the commission.*

The No Confidence Controversy

A comprehensive administrative solution seemed possible for a brief period, concluded Dr. Samuel Thier, whom the university board had invited to advise about the troubles at CASE and University Hospitals in June 1993.[76]† Thier's consultation—or "mediation," as some called it[87]—was prompted by the controversy produced by a letter of no confidence in Pytte,[87] which the clinical chairmen had sent to the university's board of trustees. The letter was drafted by David Bickers, the chairman of dermatology and chief of the medical staff at University Hospitals, and Adel Mahmoud, the chairman of medicine, who "rallied the troops."[37] After reviewing the document,[88] twenty-five of the twenty-seven chairs in the school of medicine, all present in Cleveland at the time, signed the letter.‡ While Farah Walters, the CEO of University Hospitals of Cleveland, supported the effort, though playing no specific role,[45] the leaders of the group found it difficult "to engage Neil [Cherniak, the medical school dean] in these discussions."[88]

---

*Block, his predecessors, and his successors ruled the hospital from what Douglas Lenkoski, the retired former chairman of the department of psychiatry and chief of staff, calls "Mahogany Row," a suite of "beautifully paneled offices" on the first floor of the original Lakeside Hospital building.[57]

†Thier, then president of Brandeis University—"perhaps making me more acceptable to Ag [Pytte]"[76]—later became president and CEO of Partners Health Care, the corporation that owns the Massachusetts General and Brigham and Women's hospitals in Boston.[86]

‡CASE trustee John Lewis remembers that, at a hospital Christmas party, "one of the clinical chairs had a clipboard getting signatures for the motion in the kitchen."[48]

Several complaints had caused the chairs to take this action:[34,37,59,88]

1. *Pytte's announcement that the fees the university charged the medical school would rise.*[87] The chairmen argued that while they were required to pay a tax to their dean, none of the indirect costs collected on the grants awarded to the clinical faculty were allotted to relieve the departments' expenses. The clinical departments, they maintained, were supporting the university, which gave them little financial assistance.

2. *Pytte's negotiating an affiliation agreement with Metro without the knowledge or advice of the department chairmen at University Hospitals and against the advice of dean Neil Cherniak,* the *causus belli* as one of the chairmen described the president's action.[37] The accord appeared to create an academically independent campus at the county hospital, removed the provision that the department directors at Metro should report to the academic chairmen at the University, and provided that the chairs of newly formed departments might be based at Metro rather than at University Hospitals.[74,89] In an article describing the turmoil, *The Plain Dealer,* Cleveland's daily newspaper, stressed how titles constituted one of the factors leading to the chairmen's unhappiness. "Splitting up the chairmanships made them mad. . . . They're afraid of losing power," the newspaper quoted a former chairman as saying.[89] "Not the issue," responded Robert Ratcheson, the chairman of the department of neurosurgery.[88]

3. *Pytte's opposition to a new affiliation agreement between University Hospitals and the university* that a joint trustee committee had developed and that the chairs favored.

4. *Suspected revisions of faculty benefits.* Rumors floated that such benefits as remission of tuition for the children of CASE medical faculty attending CASE might be revoked and that faculty holding Ph.D. degrees working in clinical departments might receive fewer benefits than Ph.D.s in basic science departments.

The letter so angered Pytte that he threatened to replace all the chairmen who had signed it.[88] "We were called to a meeting with Pytte, Cherniak, the university provost, and the chief financial officer," Ratcheson remembers. "The provost was upset that we had engaged counsel to help us and told us that this was not collegial. We replied that firing all of us was not col-legial."[88] Pytte called Mahmoud after the letter was delivered. "He said he was very disappointed in me," remembers Mahmoud. "I told him it was unfair to single me out, that the letter was the reflection of the collective position of the chairs. End of discussion."[59]

The chairmen's letter describing their grievances came to Karen Horn, chairman and CEO of Bank One and formerly president of the Federal Reserve Bank of Cleveland who was then chairman of the university trust-ees. At a meeting in her office at the bank, Horn encouraged them that they were "on the right track" and confirmed that the department chairmen would not be fired "as rumor suggested."[37] They had made it clear that, if Pytte fired one, all would resign. Horn then advised, "We will try behav-ior modification on the president."[28,37] Mahmoud replied, "Don't waste your time."[28]

Horn appointed a committee of the board to examine the chairmen's complaints.[88] Then at a tense three-hour meeting of the university board, the trustees considered the objections of the faculty. Rottman, who at-tended the meeting representing the chairs, explained their complaints and tried to frame it not so much as against Pytte but between the medi-cal school and the university. Despite the way Rottman tried to present the facts, however, the clinical chairmen's annoyance with the president was clear.[48]

For the heated discussion that followed in executive session, Pytte was asked to leave the room although "he was very reluctant to do so."[50] The trustees supporting Pytte rallied enough of their colleagues[50] so that the group backed Pytte but only by a narrow margin, according to several trust-ees.[54,63] Others said that Pytte received "generous support"[90] and welcomed him back into the boardroom with applause[40,42,91] from those who had supported him.[92] One of the trustees believed that, if there had been a secret ballot—the group had not voted on the question of relieving Pytte[40,42,47,92]— Pytte would have lost.[92] Horn, who by now wanted Pytte removed as presi-dent, explains, "I didn't have the time away from my 'day job' to discuss the issues thoroughly with each member of the board."[54]

Most of Pytte's support, according to trustee Richard ("Dick") Pogue, who believed as Horn did that he should go,[45] came from what Pogue described as "old-line Cleveland people, particularly the women who loved him. He had courted them very successfully."[63] Most, though not all, of the business members, Pogue observed, would have voted against him.[63] One who did support him was trustee Charles Bolton. "I thought the effort regrettable and that Ag wasn't being treated fairly."[93] Bolton saw most of the opposition coming from those trustees, like Pogue, who were also members of the University Hospitals board.* Others agreed. Longtime CASE trustee Elaine Hadden felt "Ag was sandbagged by the medical school because he hadn't been able to appoint a dean strong enough to control the chairs."[47] Pytte supporters suspected that not every member of the clinical departments, if given the choice, would have backed the chairmen in their effort to rid the university of Pytte.[42]

Pytte's position seemed impregnable to the medical school leaders, who would have preferred a less rigid, more supportive and helpful university president. "He seduced the trustees," one of the clinical chairmen believed, "and put his own people on the board." He was described as "a master controlling trustees, a real street fighter."[37]† As a result of the no confidence vote, Pytte saw the clinical chairmen "as his number one enemies," according to Farah Walters.[45]

This most recent contretemps effectively ended Karen Horn's influence on the board. Through trustees who supported him, Pytte prevented her reelection as chair and arranged that attorney John Lewis, whom Horn[54] and others considered "a Pytte person,"[54] succeed her. She remained on the board as an ordinary member but stopped going to the meetings. Soon afterward, Horn left Cleveland for New York to become head of international banking and a managing director at Bankers Trust.[54]

Horn had always been somewhat of an outsider to the traditional CASE trustees.[42] She came from out of town, had had no previous connection with the university, and probably suffered from the assumption by her less correct colleagues that she had been chosen to be chair because she was a woman. "She was trying to lead a board with a better understanding of the lo-

---

*Pogue comments, "Most of the opposition could not have come from the few trustees who were common to both boards . . . at the time there were only six common trustees, and two of them, Al Ford and John Morley, were the ex-chair and vice chair of the CWRU board."[94]

†This was not the first time that a medical faculty had voted no confidence in a university president. A few years before the CASE episode, the Advisory Board of the Medical Faculty, the senior faculty committee of the medical school at Johns Hopkins University, had passed a similar motion.[95] The irritation this time was a special assessment levied by the president on the medical school to help resolve a serious financial problem at the university. Unlike at CASE, the president did retire, the medical school's action having contributed to his decision.[13]

cal geography than she had and was caught between strong voices on both sides," observed Richard Baznik, a thirty-year veteran of the university staff.*

On becoming board chairman, John Lewis sent a letter to the medical school chairmen containing what came to be known as the "shut-up rule," instructing them not to talk directly to trustees again but to take their complaints to the dean. The doctors concluded that Pytte had "outmaneuvered everyone." "We saw ourselves as sophisticated managers," remembers Dr. Helmut Cascorbi, then chairman of the department of anesthesia and president of the council of clinical chairmen at the medical school. "Actually we were very naïve in presuming that the board would do something about Pytte."[96] The details never reached *The Plain Dealer* since the chairs had pledged to keep the conflict private.

"This was the point when the medical school went flat," remembers Rottman,[34] or, as another chairman said, "things deteriorated significantly."[88] Rottman came to believe that the school could have continued to grow if the president had "supported us or at least was neutral. At its best, this was a neat place to do science."[34] But now, one of the basic science chairs said, "the growth tapered off, and we became less functional as a collaborative group. We in basic science were just hanging on, funding ourselves."[34] The failure of the chairmen's attempt to change the presidency drove some leading faculty away.

In addition to prompting the chairmen's letter, the Metro agreement so increased the turmoil—some called it a "revolution"[84]—that William Reynolds, the chairman of the University Hospitals board, writing to Horn, on January 15, 1993, objected to the university's not "participating in the meetings of the Joint Coordinating Committee" and ignoring its recommendations. Pytte had infrequently attended the meetings.[92] "Our Affiliation Agreement contemplated that this committee would provide cooperative planning and guidance for our respective institutions."[97] The University Hospitals trustees then passed a resolution in which they stated their belief that in signing the new agreement with Metro, the university took actions "not done in good faith or in a spirit of fair dealing . . . and, therefore, constitute a material breach of the letter and spirit of the affiliation agreement" between the University Hospitals and CASE.[98] University Hospitals of Cleveland threatened to, but did not file, a lawsuit.[99]

---

*Baznik is currently writing a history of the university.[42]

To calm the hostilities, the university trustees then called in Thier, who recommended that the university resurrect the plan to create a strong vice president for health sciences whom Pytte would appoint to rule over the schools of medicine, nursing, and dentistry.[87] The plan didn't appeal to Joyce Fitzpatrick,[41] dean of the nursing school (1982–97), who objected to what she saw as the university's trying to make a change affecting her school without involving her and her colleagues.[38] One trustee felt that, like other nursing school deans, Fitzpatrick "had sought to bring the nursing profession out from under the dominance of the physicians."[91]

The hospital trustees, however, thought this a "grand idea,"[63] since Pytte would no longer exercise direct control of the medical school. Pytte tried to convince Roger Meyer, to whom Pytte had offered the CASE deanship in 1990, to take the new job.[75] "We've had a battle here," he told Meyer, "but I've come out on top, and I want you to be the vice president."[61] Meyer, however, wasn't available, having recently accepted appointment as vice president for medical affairs and executive dean at the George Washington University Medical Center in Washington, D.C.[61] Meanwhile, Pytte had named Jerry Shuck, the chair of surgery, as acting vice president, a solution that also failed. "Pytte never defined my authority," Shuck says. "Eventually, I quit, and the position died."[100]

Although Pytte and the university board had supported creation of the vice presidency,[101] neither followed through on Thier's plan.[40,76*] In trying to explain what didn't happen, Thier suggests that Pytte "had become a victim of his experiences at Dartmouth College." Thier saw the undergraduate experience as Dartmouth's principal concern[76]—a university with "an undergraduate culture," as a longtime staff member at CASE who was familiar with Dartmouth observed[42]—and the medical school, at the time that Pytte was provost, almost an "appendage." At CASE, "it was the jewel in the crown."[76†]

Consolidating authority for all the health-related activities of the university in a potentially powerful vice president or chancellor didn't appeal to Pytte or to influential members of his board.[38,41] Pytte feared that a vice

---

*Despite being paid "handsomely," as Thier describes his honorarium for the consultation, he was jokingly told by a colleague, who was visiting at CASE, "Never has someone so well thought of failed so completely!"[101]

†As for the university as a whole, one chairman of the trustees described CASE as "a small Midwestern university,"[48] and another as "a regional, second-rate university."[54] As was true of most CASE trustees, neither of these chairs had earned degrees from CASE.

president could become a second president—part of the scheme allowed the vice president to report directly to the trustees for certain matters—thus undercutting the authority of the president.[42] Richard Baznik, a longtime staff member at CASE who was close to Pytte, believes that the president was more interested in preserving the strength of his office than losing any personal power.[42]

Thier didn't think any of Pytte's actions were based on malice. "He just didn't understand, and he was wrong."[76] Dr. Kenneth Shine, then president of the Institute of Medicine and former dean of the medical school at the University of California, Los Angeles, found, from his participation on a CASE advisory committee, Pytte's "attitude toward the medical school, staff, and dean appalling to me."[102]

Many university trustees, however, remained pleased with Pytte's efforts to improve other aspects of the university's work and did not press him to follow the advice of the consultants for the medical school.[76,92] "Pytte did more good for the university than people realized at the time," said John Lewis, who was then chairman of the CASE board. "He gave 110 percent of his time trying to improve the student body and the faculty and raising money."[48]

University Hospitals under Harry Bolwell and James Block

Meanwhile, at University Hospitals of Cleveland, the dominant leader from 1978 was the chairman of its board of trustees, Harry Bolwell, the CEO of Midland-Ross, a large Cleveland manufacturer.[85,100,103–105] "We were drifting into nowhere when Harry came on board," said Dr. Scott Inkley, chief of staff from 1978 to 1982 and hospital president for the next four years.[69] Bolwell came in "like a missionary from business," says Jack Burry, a senior executive with the local Blue Cross/Blue Shield plans. "Harry considered the people running the hospital as if they hadn't yet come down from the trees."[106]

To improve the administration of his sprawling responsibility, Bolwell applied "the principles of the businessman to the hospital," as his successor James Block described the process.[104] Bolwell divided University Hospitals of Cleveland into six component parts—Lakeside (the adult general hospital), Rainbow Babies and Children's, MacDonald Women's, Hanna

Pavilion (for patients with psychiatric illnesses), the outpatient units, and the general administrative functions—and appointed directors of each. He replaced the former CEO with Inkley, but, as Bolwell says, "I ran it. I got into the management structure, costs—they had no idea about this when I started—but I stayed away from the professional side."[85] Under Bolwell, described as a "relentless" leader[107]—he was reported to have said to recalcitrant managers, "If you don't agree, leave your resignation on my desk"[104]—the finances improved from a loss of $15 million when he started to a surplus of $30 million when he left, nurses' salaries rose, and, he says, the care of patients in general improved significantly.[85] "As board chair, he was living on the wards," Block says, as the doctors at University Hospitals treated Bolwell's wife, a nurse, for cancer. "Harry concluded that hospitals weren't well run, that service was not that good."[104]

Block, close to the man who would choose him to be the next CEO, admired Bolwell very much. "He was totally honest, very smart, and capable. If Harry hadn't done what he did," Block says, "the Clinic would have eaten University Hospitals, which was then a very sleepy place; could have been in Texas as far as the city was concerned. The best thing they had was the quality of the medical school, and the focus at UH was education and research more than clinical care. The Clinic had no serious competition for specialty care."[104]

Although contributing much to the operation of University Hospitals, Bolwell did not promote good relations with the medical school and university. He regularly claimed, not that good-naturedly, that the hospital gave the medical school $45 million each year.[57] "If you need a medical school to be a great hospital," Bolwell was heard to say, "you won't be a great hospital." Bolwell was so partial to the hospital and censorious of CASE that he wouldn't read letters on university stationery. Surgery chair Jerry Shuck remembers the inconvenience of the 7:00 a.m. meetings Bolwell held with senior members of the professional and administrative staff on the top floor of his company's building rather than at the hospital.[100] "Managing Harry was a full-time job," remembers Scott Inkley. "He was short-tempered and irascible but smart and very supportive of good clinical care."[69] Even the school of nursing received "Bolwell-treatment." The dean of the nursing school had an appointment in the hospital as did the hospital directors of nursing in the school. "Harry initiated a move to separate the jobs," remembers Joyce Fitzpatrick. "He wanted more control over the nurses at the hospital and didn't want the same troubles he was having with the medical school."[38]*

"Harry saw those hospital CEOs who were doctors acting like quasi-university presidents, worrying about the quality of the faculty and student affairs rather than running a business," says Block. "All of a sudden, this thing had become a big business. Where was Harry going to find a doc to run a hospital as he wanted it to be run?"[104] Bolwell found his doctor/CEO in upstate New York, where James Block was president of the nine-hospital Rochester Area Hospitals Corporation. Block, however, had never run a hospital so Bolwell initially hired him as assistant to the president. "He told me I would become CEO after a nine-month pregnancy," Block remembers.[104] When Scott Inkley retired in 1986, Block became the president.[3,69,85] Within a year, William Reynolds, a Cleveland industrialist, succeeded Bolwell as chairman of the board.[3]

The hospital was now directed by a physician (B.A., Haverford College, 1962; M.D., New York University School of Medicine, 1966) who had worked in the office of the Surgeon General in the U.S. Public Health Service helping to develop health programs for community, migrant, and rural health centers. Block had trained in pediatrics and ambulatory medicine at the Strong Memorial Hospital, the University of Rochester's principal teaching affiliate. After practicing pediatrics and administering primary care programs in Rochester for eight years, he assumed, in 1979, the position from which Bolwell recruited him to Cleveland. He had had no previous association with University Hospitals of Cleveland or with CASE University School of Medicine.

Block began his tenure at University Hospitals during favorable financial times, when the hospital was generating surpluses as large as $50 million per year. "We made the place a thriving business," Block says. "We priced 5 percent below the Clinic, controlled costs, and made money hand over

---

*When the connection with University Hospitals of Cleveland foundered, the school of nursing turned to the Cleveland Clinic, among other hospitals, for training sites during one of the recurrent nursing shortages. Joyce Fitzpatrick, dean of the CASE school of nursing at the time, remembers building a smooth relationship with Loop's predecessor, William Kiser, for this purpose. Fitzpatrick, who regrets that Loop showed less enthusiasm for this linkage, believes that, when she was dean, nursing at University Hospitals of Cleveland was superior to that at the Clinic. "This was then the community's opinion," she says, "and it owed a lot to the presence of the nursing school on our campus."[38]

fist."[104] Block assigned part of the surplus to the faculty working in the hospital, but he gave it directly to the investigators rather than to the dean of the school of medicine to distribute. "Behrman [the dean] didn't like this. Harry wouldn't let me give it to Dick to decide what to do with it," says Block, who continued this practice after Bolwell retired.[104]

Block directed part of the surplus toward improving what were described as "dreary" facilities to which little attention had been given.[14] He hired a full-time architect and "took a substandard facility and made it more competitive, made it a modern and beautiful hospital," says Dr. David Bickers, chairman of the department of dermatology and one of Block's senior officers in the hospital.[14] An open space between the main hospital and the children's and women's units was converted into a large, strikingly attractive, and functional atrium linking together the different parts of the complex.[57] The women's and children's hospitals were rebuilt. The hospital, during Block's tenure, also added four floors to the new outpatient building named for Bolwell. "And I built a new entrance to Lakeside Hospital," Block says. "The earlier one was made of plywood."[104]

Further improvements to the plant completed during the Walters administration would include:[73,108]

- a new building for Rainbow Babies and Children's Hospital and a new pediatric surgery center in the old Rainbow building
- the Mather building and Lerner Tower into which many of the inpatient beds were transferred from the 1930s vintage Lakeside Hospital and Hanna House*
- conversion of Hannah House into offices and new clinical facilities
- renovations in the MacDonald Women's Hospital
- development of several facilities for the care of patients off the main campus

Seen by most of his colleagues as highly intelligent,[28] "Jim was a genius at blue-skying," according to Bickers, who was a member of Block's planning committee.[14] "He [Block] was always coming up with new ideas," dean Neil Cherniak remembers. "He'd lie on the couch in his office and talk about dreams like the hospital buying the medical school from the uni-

---

*To create space for the tower, a new garage, built during Bolwell's administration, had been demolished and a replacement built across Cornell Road.

versity or developing a medical center together with the medical school and Henry Ford. Jim had an almost aesthetic temperament, which I liked, while Farah [Walters, Block's chief operating officer and successor as CEO of University Hospitals of Cleveland] seemed more practical. He was certainly imaginative but perhaps at times a bit too imaginative."[52] Jerry Shuck thought Block "a visionary with great ideas, but he did love to delegate the details. However, he could pour oil on troubled waters."[100] Walters saw her mentor as "charismatic and not just a cheerleader. He has qualities that draw people in, and he becomes the center of attention."[109] It was Walters who was often called on to relieve employees which Block, who hated to fire people, didn't like to do. With respect to this turnover, Walters remembers hearing people say, when she first arrived at University Hospitals in 1986, "If you're a department director, don't buy, rent. If you're an administrator, don't unpack your suitcase."[109]

Block had his problems, some of which would plague him when he became CEO of the Johns Hopkins Hospital on leaving Cleveland in 1992.[13] "Jim could be incredibly manipulative, but you wouldn't feel the knife going in," said a professor who, otherwise, much admired Block and what he accomplished for the hospital.[14] Another said, "He was mercurial, could be easy or hard to deal with."[52] Block irritated his colleagues in Cleveland, as he would those in Baltimore, by frequently being late for, or even missing, scheduled meetings[14,57] and being unwilling "to share what was planned and what was going on."[57]

Block's relationships with some of the leaders at the university and medical school could be troubled. Richard Behrman, the dean during the first half of Block's tenure at the hospital, and Block repeatedly criticized each other at meetings.[84] As for the university president, "we started with monthly meetings," Pytte remembers, "but I terminated them because the discussion mostly had to do with misdeeds at the Cleveland Clinic. They just weren't useful."[74] Eventually, "they wouldn't even talk to each other," Neil Cherniak said.[52]

Despite these problems, however, the University Hospitals of Cleveland greatly benefited from James Block's seven years as its president and CEO. As his chief of staff David Bickers said, "He was the right man at the right time."[14] Block loved his time in Cleveland. "I should have paid UH to let me work there," he said. "It was so much fun, and they were so good to me. One thousand people came to my going away party at Severance Hall," the Cleveland Orchestra's concert hall.[104]

Affiliation Agreements

During the 1950s, the relationship between University Hospitals and the medical school was "very positive," Scott Inkley, a pulmonologist first appointed to the staff during that decade, remembers. "The president then [John Millis] was quite supportive."[69] The first evidence of potential trouble between the school and University Hospitals appeared with the appointment of Frederick Robbins as dean of the school of medicine in 1966.[69] Robbins, a distinguished pediatrician and virologist who had shared the Nobel Prize for Physiology or Medicine in 1954 for growing polio virus in culture, came from Cleveland's Metropolitan General Hospital, a major teaching hospital for the medical school of what was then called Western Reserve University.

Favoring his previous institution, Robbins was said to have created "a distance, which over the years has widened, between the medical school and University Hospitals"[84] and, according to a later dean, felt Metro "equal to University Hospitals in prestige."[52] Some faculty at University Hospitals sensed that Robbins brought with him from Metro an anti–University Hospitals bias, that "rich people on the East Side [where University Hospitals and CASE are located] were more important to University Hospitals than the poor people on the West Side," Metro's district.[69] In general, Metro felt itself "inadequately appreciated,"[52] despite being, at the time, the site of successful research programs in addition to its busy clinical services.[28] Though leading the school with a gentle style and by consensus,[28] Robbins acknowledged that "I was partial to City [Metro] and people felt it."[23]

The university president, when Robbins first became dean, was "very interested in medicine" and chaired the faculty meetings in the school, although his successor, with whom Robbins said that he also had a fine relationship, did not.[23] Robbins left the deanship in 1980—"I was dean for fourteen years. Too long. One gets a bit jaded"[23]—to become president of the Institute of Medicine of the National Academy of Sciences. His successor was Richard Behrman. Like Robbins a pediatrician, Behrman had received his medical degree from the University of Rochester, held a law degree from Harvard, and led the school with a more assertive style than had his predecessor.[28] Behrman,* described as "a talented administrator,"[30] "very independent, and a man who made decisions,"[56] remembers the relationship between the school and University Hospitals during his term as dean from 1980 to 1989 as "reasonable."[19] Behrman was able to work well with Harry Bolwell, the chairman of the hospital board and the dominant force in the hospital's management.[105] The dean sat with the management committees of both the university and the hospital boards, and both he and the hospital president had, in Behrman's words, "free access to the trustees on both boards, which restrained people from working against either institution."[19]

When Behrman's term began, the medical school and University Hospitals of Cleveland were operating under an affiliation agreement adopted in 1928. In an amendment of theoretical importance, the boards of the university and hospital agreed in 1976 that the chairman of any newly created clinical department and the head of the relevant clinical service at University Hospitals need not necessarily be the same person,[110] a concept that Robbins approved. In most schools with close ties to their principal teaching hospitals, the chairman of a clinical department in the medical school also directs the concurrent service in the hospital. Although the hospital certifies physicians to practice there, it is the chairman and his division chiefs, in most cases, who recruit and hire the clinicians. The clinical faculty in most schools look more to the dean of the school of medicine as their ultimate boss than to the CEO of the hospital. At only a few institutions— the teaching hospitals affiliated with the Harvard Medical School constituting the most famous examples†—does the CEO appoint the professional staff and control the direction of research and financing. This potentially controversial amendment was not implemented during the life of the agreement.

The titles of the leaders changed over the years, however, adding confusion and ill-will since, in academics, titles can matter a great deal. Since 1866, the leaders of the clinical services at what became Lakeside Hospital

---

*Behrman is now executive chair of the Federation of Pediatric Organizations.[19]

†The teaching hospitals affiliated with the Harvard Medical School, each of which is a separate not-for-profit corporate entity, operate quite independently of the school. The clinical departments in each hospital are led by their own chairmen, who consider themselves of equal administrative standing with the leaders of the departments in the other hospitals. Each hospital, not the school, pays its full-time doctors and collects the grant and clinical income they generate.[111]

and later University Hospitals of Cleveland had been called "directors."[112] When the Ohio statues were changed to permit boards of nonprofit corporations to call their members "directors" or "trustees," at their option,[94]* the designation "director" of the clinical service at University Hospitals was changed to "chairman." Farah Walters, the University Hospitals CEO at the time, preferred that they be called "chairmen" and not "chairs," regardless of the gender of the leader.[112] This decision meant that such individuals were "chairs"—the approved gender-correct designation in academic circles—of their departments in the medical school and "chairmen" of their services in the University Hospitals. This issue did not apply at Metro, where the service chiefs had long been called "chairmen" or "chairs."[112]

Whereas Frederick Robbins, when dean, favored selecting chairmen of clinical departments wherever the best qualified candidate was based—"not a popular decision at University Hospitals," he observed—he never appointed a chairman who would be based other than at University Hospitals. Behrman continued this policy[23] and expected the department heads at Metro to report to the chairmen at the medical school for academic matters.[52] Nevertheless, the conflict between Metro and University Hospitals for status within the medical school persisted as controversy continued over which chair, the incumbent at Metro or University Hospitals, was the more equal.

In 1980, Robbins and Louis Toepfer, the university president, decided to terminate the affiliation agreement with University Hospitals.[40,63,69] "Some of the basic issues of relationships between the university and its teaching hospitals remain and even grow in awkwardness," wrote Toepfer to the president of the hospital. "Thus it is time to review the amended agreement, and develop a better one."[113] The parties, however, never could create "a better one" and, once the agreement had been abrogated the next year, the university and hospital would operate without one for eleven years.[63,99] "It was civil war from then on," said Inkley.[69] The prolonged absence of an agreement appeared as "a huge black cloud," to trustee Dick Pogue.[63] Harry Bolwell did not help. "He walked away from an affiliation agreement," according to Dr. William Speck, the chairman of the department of pediatrics during Bolwell's time.[105] The conflict indirectly affected

---

*Despite the policy in Ohio, I continue to use in this text the widely employed word *trustees* for the members of the governing boards of not-for-profit corporations.

the basic science departments. "The acrimony at the top demoralized us as well as the clinical faculty," said Lynn Landmesser, chair of the department of neurosciences.[114]

Finally, a joint committee of trustees from CASE and University Hospitals of Cleveland agreed on a new affiliation agreement, which was inaugurated on May 12, 1992. Specific terms included the following:[115]

- There was formal declaration of the primacy of the affiliation with University Hospitals of Cleveland.
- Chairmen of current clinical departments would be based at University Hospitals. Heads of new departments might be based elsewhere.
- A Joint Coordinating Committee of trustees from CASE and University Hospitals of Cleveland would be created with, as nonvoting representatives, the dean of the school of medicine, the president of University Hospitals, and a clinical chairman.

Several other provisions that the Joint Trustee Committee on Affiliation recommended were not included in the affiliation agreement:[82]

- The name of the University Hospitals should be changed to "CASE Hospital."*
- Vice chairmen of the clinical departments should be appointed at Metro.
- The dean's tax—an assessment the dean charged each clinical department for other activities he deemed worthy of support—should be raised from 3 to 5 percent.†
- The departmental practice plans should be consolidated into a single plan.‡

---

*An image survey conducted by University Hospitals in 1990 indicated that "only 45.5% of consumers were aware that UHC is associated with a medical school" and that "only 34% identified CASE as the affiliate."[82]

†The dean's tax at CASE developed from the need for more research space, particularly for the clinical departments. Since the school of medicine would have to support the interest on the loans obtained for the building, the university trustees required that the clinical practices agree to pay a tax to the dean before approving construction of the new building.[116]

‡The 1992 affiliation agreement included an Appendix A titled "Joint Vision Statement." That statement, as summarized by Dick Pogue, "expressed the hopes of CWRU and UH at the time that:
• Greater Cleveland can develop an Academic Medical Center of preeminent stature;
• The heart of the center is the School of Medicine;
• From this academic medical core, the resource base for teaching, research and clinical practice can

The new affiliation agreement between CASE and University Hospitals lasted only eight years. On December 11, 1999, Henry Meyer, the chairman of the University Hospitals board, acting at the behest of Walters, advised his counterpart at the university that the hospital would terminate the affiliation in one year[118] as provided in the agreement, which allowed either party to withdraw twelve months after notifying the other of such intention. During this "cooling-off" period, designed to allow the university and hospital to try to resolve their differences, the parties could not agree, and, accordingly, one year later, the affiliation agreement of 1992 ended.[119]

A committee of trustees from the two institutions had been assigned to develop a new arrangement palatable to both parties. Hospital and university trustee Dick Pogue remembers "long negotiating sessions that went on endlessly." Organization, not dollars, seemed to separate them. "The issue was stature," Pogue recalls. "Who would be heads of departments and other organizational issues such as how much authority the hospital would cede to the dean."[63] One of the members remembers Pytte and Walters "as very antagonistic toward each other."[50] The committee tried to resolve the issue at the CEO level in a final meeting attended by Walters and the outgoing president—Pytte would retire on June 30. It was an unproductive session.[63]

Affiliation Agreements Continued:
The Short, Troubled Presidency of David Auston

The attempt to create a new affiliation agreement would ultimately contribute to the departure of Farah Walters from University Hospitals in 2002, but its most dramatic effect would be to limit to twenty-two months the presidency of Pytte's successor David Auston. An engineer with a distinguished research career in both industry and academics, a member of the National Academy of Sciences and the National Academy of Engineering, and a fellow of the American Academy of Arts and Sciences, Auston was provost of Rice University when he was recruited to CASE. He was seen as "a sane person,"[51] "a thoughtful man who appreciated the situation and had the right values."[26] "He got off to a great start," Pogue remembers, "but

---

be broadened and enhanced through collaboration with other medical institutions including the Cleveland Clinic;

• The leverage which is offered through this collaboration is enormous and the benefits are incalculable."[117]

then got sucked into the negotiations, which he found distasteful."[63] Those acquainted with both Pytte and Auston found the new president "more positively inclined to the medical school" than his predecessor.[65]

When he was hired, the executive committee told Auston not to be concerned about the affiliation agreement.[92] Auston hadn't run a medical school at Rice—a criticism that others, particularly those partial to Walters, would charge against the new president—and that the board would deal with the affiliation agreement.[120] When informed that a three-man trustee committee would soon resolve the issue,[40] Auston asked the committee not to complete their work on the affiliation agreement before he arrived.[48,92,121] When this controversy between the president and the trustee committee—which one observer described as a "time-bomb the trustees had placed on the president's desk"[120]—reached the medical faculty, some began to wonder who was really in charge of the university.[122] Meanwhile, Auston saw that the continuing conflict between the medical school with its weak deanship and the University Hospitals with its strong leadership was lowering the reputation of the medical school and causing difficulty retaining and recruiting faculty, a problem the trustees and doctors also discerned.[3,40,123,124]

Dr. David Korn, a senior officer at the Association of American Medical Colleges and the former dean of the school of medicine at Stanford University, remembers meeting Auston during a session of the medical school advisory committee when the president "took us to a long dinner in a private room at a restaurant."[125] Korn was told that Farah Walters felt the university had been disloyal to University Hospitals by sending its students to other hospitals, specifically Metro and the Veterans Administration Hospital, and depriving University Hospitals of patients. "I think the dinner was sobering to Auston, who dreamed naïvely that the Harvard system* was the answer. I told him that the Harvard system had matured over 150 years and had grown because the partners had worked it out together."[125] Korn, who had graduated from the Harvard Medical School and trained at its affiliate, the Massachusetts General Hospital, saw nothing positive coming "from trying to impose the Harvard system on the warring parties."[125]

The circumstances of Auston's appointment contributed to the problems that followed. During the selection process, attorney John Lewis, then

---

*See previous footnote.

chairman of the CASE trustees, phoned Auston to tell him that another candidate had been chosen.[48] Two weeks later, Lewis called again with the news that the leading candidate had rejected the offer, "for personal reasons," and would Auston be willing to be reconsidered?[48] He agreed and eventually accepted the job, but without fully realizing the intensity of the conflict between the hospital and the university.

Auston saw each party unaware of what each could add to the other and that the hospital's senior management and trustees were acting very independently. The conflict between Walters's administration and the Cleveland Clinic contributed to the disharmony between CASE and University Hospitals of Cleveland since, from the university's point of view, relationships with multiple institutions such as Metro and the Clinic supported its educational and research missions.[41] Some of the university's leading trustees, as well as Auston,[120] favored a closer relationship with the Cleveland Clinic, an anathema to Farah Walters and her supporters.[26]

The trustees had charged the president to talk with Fred Loop and see what could be arranged. He did so, and the first practical steps toward the founding of the medical college at the Clinic with an intimate connection with CASE occurred during Auston's truncated reign.* His efforts to develop a clinical affiliation with the Clinic, however, failed.[120] He probably wouldn't even have tried to accomplish this unattainable arrangement if he, like so many at the university, hadn't become so intensely angry with Farah Walters.[126] It was said that when Walters detected weakness in someone she exploited it.[41]

Dissatisfied with several policies of the board's executive committee[50] and the intense involvement of CASE trustees in the negotiations with University Hospitals,[94,120] Auston tried to have some additional trustees appointed to the board whose point of view coincided more closely with his own. An intense meeting of the nominating committee called for this purpose further harmed his already flawed relationship with John Lewis, who was participating very actively in the details of the university's operation.[62]†

Auston saw himself increasingly unable to exercise what he saw as the

---

*See chapter 6.

†In some respects, Lewis was trying to direct the university—thereby blurring the line between board and president—as did Harry Bolwell at University Hospitals when he was chairman of the hospital board from 1978 to 1986 and intimately involved in the day-to-day operations of the hospital.[120]

president's responsibility to resolve the affiliation agreement crisis and to frame important issues for the board's consideration.[120,121] Furthermore, Auston had come to feel that his executive committee[92] did not sufficiently appreciate the value of the grants and overhead generated by the medical faculty from the NIH.

Auston concluded that the proposed agreement, negotiated on behalf of the university by trustees Allen Ford, John Lewis, and Richard Watson, the chairman of the group, conceded too much to University Hospitals,[50,120,122] would erode the authority of the university president,[120] and, as he told a reporter at *The Plain Dealer*, "further diminish the stature and quality" of the medical school programs.[127] The president became as much concerned about the role of these trustees in the operation of the university as about the influence of Walters on the medical school.[120] He began to doubt whether the departure of Walters would, of itself, facilitate resolution of the affiliation agreement, among other issues.[120]

Auston was increasingly seen as "an unhappy man," overburdened and exhausted by the conflicts roiling his academic medical center[122] and unable to resolve them.[50] "I think the role of president is an absolutely, incredibly impossible role," the newspaper quoted Lewis as saying. "He [Auston] really became stressed out. He in fact told me so."[128]

On April 27, 2001, Auston resigned the presidency. The setting was a heated meeting with Lewis and Ford,[129] who were, as Auston and others[62] saw it, inappropriately interfering with his efforts to resolve the controversy. Lewis called an emergency meeting of the executive committee of the CASE board at his downtown law office to inform them of this unexpected development.[91] Several trustees then visited Auston at his home that night and tried unsuccessfully to convince him to change his mind and stay in the job or, at least, not to leave so precipitously a month before graduation.[48,91]

University trustee Malvin Bank, a lawyer, felt confident that if Auston had appealed to the whole board, he would have been supported.[50] Although other unresolved issues during his presidency contributed to his decision to leave,[48] Auston and Walters had, in Dick Pogue's view, "radically different views of the contributions of the hospital to the NIH research that CASE wanted to claim. Auston and others felt that these polar views were preventing a solution to the conflict over the affiliation agreement."[63] One observer suggested that if *she* had left before *he* had reached his decision to go, David Auston could still be working at University Circle.[126]* Those in the medical school dean's office felt Auston's departure "a real loss."[65]

Attempts to develop a long-term affiliation agreement continued during the interim presidency of James Wagner from May 1, 2001 to August 1, 2002.[128] Auston had appointed Wagner, the dean of the CASE engineering school, to be the university's provost in September 2000.

"I met each week that we could with Farah as soon as I became the acting president," Wagner remembers. "By August [2001], I was ready to negotiate."[130] Walters proposed two models. She called the one she preferred the "Harvard model" and the other the "Hopkins model."† Under the Harvard scheme, University Hospitals would shape its relationship with CASE similar to that between Harvard's teaching hospitals and its medical school. University Hospitals of Cleveland would independently appoint its clinical faculty and control the research conducted within the hospital and its new Research Institute. Under the Hopkins model, University Hospitals would be the dominant clinical affiliate with CASE. Some collaborative arrangement could continue between the university and Metro and the Veterans Administration Hospital, but no connection would be permitted with the Cleveland Clinic.[130]

Both schemes, Wagner concluded, "were competitive, not collaborative" and, he told Walters, "I'm trying to negotiate a partnership, and you're trying to negotiate a victory."[130] Henry Meyer, the chairman of the trustees at the hospital, sees such conclusions differently. "They're one-sided. It's unfair to see it solely as Farah personally winning. It's true she wanted to win for the hospital."[124]

At the Cleveland Clinic, the trustees postponed entering into an official relationship with CASE until its relationship with University Hospitals of Cleveland was resolved[130] and a new president of the university had been elected.[134]

---

*On leaving CASE, Auston become president of the Kavil Foundation and Institute in Oxnard, California.

†Walters was particularly familiar with these models as a member of a small group of leading eastern teaching hospitals whose CEOs and other officers met together annually. In addition to University Hospitals of Cleveland, the group includes the following hospitals: Johns Hopkins, New York–Presbyterian, Partners (Massachusetts General & Brigham and Women's), Strong Memorial (Rochester, New York), University of Pennsylvania, and Yale–New Haven.[131,132] Referring to the accusation by members of the faculty that she continuously fought developing relationships with the Clinic, Walters told the author, "If I was supporting the Harvard model, why would I be so antagonistic to the Clinic?"[133]

By the end of 2001, the talks had stalled[135] and, as 2002 began, trustees and officers from the university and University Hospitals abandoned their efforts to create a new, long-term affiliation agreement.[63,136] "It's pretty clear from everyone's perspective that the university is in transition," Meyer told *The Plain Dealer.* "They felt uncomfortable putting a ten-year agreement in place with a new president coming on board."[136]

The university and hospital, however, had to develop some form of agreement to prepare for the review by the Liaison Committee on Medical Education (LCME), the accrediting agency for the nation's medical schools, which was due to conduct its on-site survey beginning March 11, 2002.[137] Since Farah Walters held such strong views, the university officials worked out a solution with the hospital trustees rather than with the CEO and concentrated on a three-year deal.[122,130] Dick Pogue, who led the negotiations for the hospital, remembers how quickly it all happened. The group assigned to the problem could reach no agreement at a dinner on the Friday night preceding the meeting of the CASE board of trustees on the next day.[63] "Three said," according to Wagner, " 'let's walk,' and three said, 'let's do it.' "[130] "I proposed a two-year agreement, and they said 'no,' " remembers Pogue. "The dinner broke up without an agreement."[63]

The CASE president-elect, Dr. Edward Hundert, was consulted and asked to consider a one-year affiliation, "a band-aid," as university trustee Frank Linsalata described the arrangement. Hundert responded, "Let's go with one year," and that is what happened.[130,138] Hundert says, "I preferred a one-year agreement. Big issues can be solved better in one year than in three."[139] The short time would support his "trying to change the culture around these issues, rather than becoming a part of the old culture."[139] Hundert also felt confident that his discussions with the Cleveland Clinic, which had already started, could be concluded very quickly. The long-term agreement that needed to be negotiated with University Hospitals would be "a quite different, and more solvable problem, namely, creating the closest possible partnership with CASE's longstanding primary affiliate given the fact of a multiaffiliation model for the School of Medicine."[140]

At the CASE board meeting the next morning, Dick Pogue remembers, "Frank Linsalata and I worked out the final details of the one-year agreement in principle in a side room while the board was in session. Frank then walked into the board room and obtained the board's unanimous approval."[94] The University Hospitals board then adopted the one-year agreement.[130] Farah Walters had not participated in the negotiating sessions. The LCME accepted the arrangement but added, "you're on our watch list."[121] Development of a more permanent affiliation agreement would await the inauguration of Hundert as president of CASE and the departure of the former leaders of the school of medicine and University Hospitals.

CHAPTER FOUR

University Hospitals of Cleveland

The Farah Walters Years

Although University Hospitals' abrogation of the affiliation agreement in 1999 represented a nadir in the relationship between the hospital and university during the 1990s, for most of the decade, turmoil rather than calm best describes the state of affairs between the hospital and university. The leaders during much of this period were Agnar Pytte, president of the university; Neil Cherniak and Nathan Berger, deans of the medical school; and Farah Walters, CEO of the University Hospitals Health System (UHHS) and of the hospital at University Circle.

Walters, the protégée of James Block, succeeded him as hospital and health system CEO in 1992, when Block moved from Cleveland to Baltimore. Born in Tehran, Farah Moavensadeh Walters—she married Cleveland lawyer Stephen Walters in 1970—came to the United States at the age of nineteen to attend Ohio State University initially to study physics and then medical dietetics.[1,2] After further training at the Brigham and Women's Hospital in Boston, Walters became director of education in the nutrition department at Metro and moved to University Hospitals in December 1985 to direct the department of nutrition.[2]* By this time, she had taken a master of science degree in nutrition and an M.B.A., both from CASE.[2]

Although Block had met Walters previously, he says that he first discovered her skills through the food which, he says, was "excellent, as was the presentation of it. I went to dietary, and there was Farah."[4] Seeing executive potential in her, Block helped develop her career—"did a Pygmalion on her," as one observer of the scene commented[5]—eventually promoting her to chief operating officer and then recommending to his board that she succeed him. James Block and Farah Walters were different in many ways. Block was more politic but not as strong an administrator. "It was often hard to know just where he stood, which was never a problem with Farah," said a leading trustee. "Perhaps," he concluded, "that's why they made such a good team."[6]

Aided by an executive search firm, the trustees' committee to find a new CEO considered several contenders to succeed Block; the final list consisted of six candidates, including Walters.[2] "We saw some very good people," remembers William Reynolds, the chairman of the hospital board at the time. Several were chief operating officers at competitive university hospitals.[6] Reynolds also interviewed the chairmen of the clinical departments for their opinions and told Walters, ironically in view of later opinions of some of them, she "was their choice."[2]

Although the trustees recognized that Walters "could be quite difficult at times," Reynolds and his colleagues had learned that "she was a superb administrator and had a vision for the place."[6] The board had had the opportunity of observing Walters closely since she had been, in the words of one of the chairmen, "the effective leader" of the hospital for two years as James Block become increasingly involved in activities outside the hospital.[7] Accordingly, the trustees accepted the advice of the search committee and Block and appointed Farah Walters CEO of University Hospitals of Cleveland.[8] Walters would now become the first woman to lead University Hospitals, the first president of the hospital for a decade who was not a

*When the Walterses were planning to move to Cleveland for Farah's husband to enter a law practice there, her mentors at the Brigham advised trying to get a job at the Cleveland Clinic or Rainbow Babies and Children's Hospital, which they held superior to University Hospitals of Cleveland.[3]

doctor,[2] and the first woman in the United States chosen to head an independent academic medical center not governed by a state or university.[9]

Having favored Walters while he was CEO, Block would support her afterward because, as he says, "Cleveland was a very tough market, and Farah was a wartime general. I knew that under her, University Hospitals would not be pushed into the Great Lakes. UH was lucky to have someone like her in the war years of the 1990s."[4] Walters, however, knew that she was taking on a responsibility with more than its share of difficulties. "I was walking into a job that was troubled because the president so disparaged the medical school and hospital. To the university's leadership, I would become the villain because I supported the clinical chairmen."[10] She recognized that "ultimately the faculty takes the side of the university. The CEO has to play second, third, or fourth fiddle to the president and the dean."[2]

A Strong Leader for University Hospital

As one would expect of this highly capable and effective but strong-willed executive, Walters attracted critics as well as supporters.[1,4,5,8,11–63] Those admiring her describe Walters as visionary, uniquely persuasive, charming, a compelling speaker with a terrific memory, and "the single most impressive leader I've ever worked with." Many members of the faculty credit her for taking over the hospital at a difficult time and creating a health system where previously there had been only a group of teaching hospitals and a few external entities. "She had a vision about what a regional health plan should be," said Henry Meyer, chairman of the University Hospitals trustees since 1999. "Most of the acquisitions, the creation of QualChoice [the health plan owned by University Hospitals] and UPCP [University Primary Care Practices], she did."[45]

Many organizations recognized her contributions:[9]

- YWCA Lifetime Achievement Award
- Ohio Women's Hall of Fame
- First woman to be named Business Executive of the Year by the Sales and Marketing Executives of Cleveland
- First woman to receive the Business Statesman Award from the Harvard Business School Club of Northeast Ohio

- 1983 Distinguished Alumnus of the Year by the Weatherhead School of Management, Case Western Reserve University
- Named one of fifty individuals who were "changing the future of health care in America"[64]

"Farah is, without question, one of the most brilliant strategic thinkers with whom I have ever had the pleasure of working, and she had a vision for academics not held by most administrators," said Dr. Ellis Avner, chairman of pediatrics at the medical center's renowned Rainbow Babies and Children's Hospital from 1995 to 2003.* "She's also one of the most complicated people I have known, extraordinary on both good or bad days. Working with her was an exhilarating roller coaster ride."[14]† In a city that Avner saw as "an 'old boys' town in medicine, she made an extraordinary impact."[14]

One of the basic science chairmen, who strongly admired her, said that she had "three things against her. She was an Iranian, a woman, and not an M.D. And she was outspoken, a rare commodity in Cleveland."[52] Margot Copeland, a senior executive with KeyCorp, agrees. "With Farah, you knew where you stood. She's a woman of conviction . . . an effective leader in a difficult industry."[65]

Walters is convinced that being a woman, foreign-born, and not a doctor contributed to her troubles. "Cleveland did not have women in high positions," she said. "Cleveland and academic medical centers and hospitals are no place for an uppity woman. Could I have played the game better?—yes, but I couldn't afford to play favoritism. I thought the best thing to do was to tell people what was needed. I was wrong. The culture in academics includes much backstabbing, so I became the topic of many conversations by people who barely knew me. Whenever something went wrong, the issue was that I was a woman with a different cultural background."[66] Walters believes that "a woman in a powerful position becomes an enigma, with people asking, 'How did she get to this position?' Everything is subject to this. I don't want to whine about this, but it's a fact of life."[67]

"Despite knowing that she was unpopular because she had to implement tough decisions at Block's request," said Dick Pogue, chairman of the hospi-

---

*In 2004, Avner became director of the Children's Research Institute at the Children's Hospital and Health System in Milwaukee and associate dean for research at the Medical College of Wisconsin.

† Walters liberally supported Rainbow, one of the medical center's most visible components, with funds that other department chairmen would have preferred be directed to their activities.[47]

tal trustees from 1994 to 1999, during much of her regime. "We on the board respected her."[8] According to a physician member of her staff, "beneath the hard exterior was a softness for the underdog. Farah insisted on supporting the care of patients with AIDS."[23] Another of her associates asserted that "she always had the hospital at heart." "I love UH," Walters says, "because, throughout its history, it has been committed to what I most admire: caring for those unable to pay, taking care of the community, and teaching."[2]

University Hospitals Health System

University Hospitals began to respond to the growing menace of managed care during the latter part of James Block's tenure. He hired hospital administrator Terry White to develop relationships with community hospitals in the region to assure that patients would continue to be referred to University Hospitals. White, according to Farah Walters, selected hospitals to approach "on the basis of those where he knew people rather than according to a strategic plan. They signed one-and-a-half page documents," she continues, "which stated that they would contract together and share one board member. We found that wasn't going to work unless we had an ownership relationship with the hospitals."[68]

Beginning in 1992, the year Walters became acting CEO, she began the process of expanding her charge from the hospital in the University Circle to a comprehensive health system incorporating community hospitals and outpatient clinics throughout greater Cleveland. Although cash flow was still agreeable—the first installment of the Medicare cuts wouldn't hit the finances of hospitals until 1997—"doom and gloom is all we heard," she remembers. From a strategic planning process involving a consultant, trustees, and senior members of the hospital and clinical faculty, "we decided that we needed to serve one-third of the Cleveland market to be successful. That meant about 700,000 people, which was enough to feed the [specialists in the] clinical departments."[68]

To do this, Walters reasoned, University Hospitals needed close relationships with enough good primary care doctors. Studies suggested that, to reach the goal of 700,000 potential patients, the system needed one primary care physician for each 2,500 patients, including one per 1,000 insured by Medicare. At the time the hospital depended for many of admissions and referrals on private, insured patients from three practices: University Suburban Health Center, a group of private physicians working in an upscale suburb;* Mednet, a multispecialty group that Block had brought into the system when he was CEO; and the relatively few primary care physicians working full-time in the clinical departments.[68]

"The average patient doesn't automatically go to a teaching hospital," Walters explains. What happens involves several steps." The patient who needs specialty care usually first goes to a primary care doctor, then to a specialist, and "then maybe to a teaching hospital. Cleveland is very spread out, and we estimated that patients would be willing to drive fifteen to twenty minutes to get to us. So we decided to recruit outstanding primary care doctors and support them with primary care centers and a few community hospitals. What we most needed was getting access to patients—that was the scarce resource as far as we were concerned. Cleveland had too many beds. We didn't need more of them."[68]

Walters had to convince the heads of the clinical departments with primary care responsibilities—medicine, pediatrics, and family medicine in particular—that her hiring the doctors wouldn't impinge on their turfs. Since administering primary care in university hospitals almost always loses money,[69] Walters was able to persuade the chairs to let her develop the program and, accordingly, absorb the costs.[68]

The development of University Hospitals Health System constituted one of Farah Walters's most important contributions to University Hospitals of Cleveland.[60] "She caused UH to realize it was in a very competitive and challenging environment," Dick Pogue told a reporter for *Crain's Cleveland Business*. "She sensed earlier than many people in the industry that times were changing dramatically."[70]

University Hospitals Health System is the sole member of the boards of the eight hospitals that it wholly owns, giving the CEO and colleagues at University Hospitals ultimate control, to the extent they wish to exercise it, over their operations. These hospitals include the University Hospitals of Cleveland at University Circle, which consists of Lakeside, the general hospital; MacDonald Women's Hospital; Rainbow Babies and Children's Hos-

---

*See the discussion later in this chapter.

pital and Ireland Cancer Center; plus seven community hospitals, most within Cuyahoga County and two nearby counties.*

In addition, the system owns 50 percent of each of four "partnership hospitals," also located within the same area, and is "affiliated" in a non-ownership capacity with eight more hospitals. The system also owns 51 percent of a large comprehensive rehabilitation and assisted living center in northeastern Ohio.[71] After the sale of one of the hospitals that had consistently lost money, of the twelve hospitals owned wholly or in part by the system, eight were generating surpluses, two were breaking even, and one was losing money. In calendar year 2004, the system budgeted a surplus of $8 million from the wholly owned hospitals.

The University Hospitals system seems to direct its wholly owned hospitals more intimately than does the Cleveland Clinic. One president leads two or three of them and is charged to maintain a consistent approach in day-to-day operations.[71] Certain back-office functions such as purchasing have been consolidated. The local hospital boards continue to function with representatives from the system holding minority membership in numbers though controlling the hospitals corporately. The system negotiates for managed care contracting for the owned but not for the affiliated hospitals.[71]

Although many of the trustees of University Hospitals of Cleveland also served on the board of the system, and vice versa, Walters wanted each corporation identified as a separate entity and agreed with Dick Pogue's suggestion that the boards meet separately and in different locations.[3,72] The hospital board meets in the Bolwell building at the medical center and the system trustees at the Union Club in downtown Cleveland.[3]

Despite such efforts to give each an independent identity, the same person led both. As the system grew in the late 1990s, some questioned whether Walters should hold both positions. "Each became more than a full-time job," said Orry Jacobs, Walters's chief operating officer at University Hospitals from 1994 to 2002.[35] Seventeen people reported directly to her, "which was excessive for efficient governance," said one of the system executives. "It was too many, and despite this, she continued to be involved in all matters of the system. Her senior people met together infrequently."

The expansion of the health system had led to the incorporation of forty

*See appendix 2.

different boards of trustees into the health system. "She wanted to go to every board meeting and make every decision," according to one of the trustees. While he was chairman of the hospital board, Dick Pogue tried to convince Walters to relinquish the hospital job and concentrate on leading the health system. "She refused," he remembers. "I backed off. I told her I caved on this because I was not prepared to force her departure in light of the many positive things she was doing for the combined entity."[8] If Walters had remained in her job past her departure in 2002, she planned to appoint someone to the position of president of University Hospitals, she told the author.[73] She also favored having one chairman for the board of University Hospitals and another leading the board of University Hospitals Health System.[73] After Walters left, different people would be appointed to direct the hospital and the health system.

Finances

For most of the past ten years, the University Hospitals Health System has lost money on operations. However, when one includes investment income and other items, the "bottom bottom" lines have been positive, and it was on the basis of this figure that the trustees judged the financial success or failure of the health system's CEO. Operating losses in 2003 equaled $25 million, a substantial improvement over the finances of the past two years as the operating performances of the hospital and system steadily improved. None of the operating losses came from University Hospitals of Cleveland, which had a slight surplus that year. Losses in two of the owned hospitals accounted for most of the shortfall. As CASE health care economist J. B. Silvers summarizes the financial effects of developing the health system, "like the typical nonhospital acquisitions made by systems, most UHHS [University Hospitals Health System] expansions seem to have lost money."[56]

Concern about the financial performance of the health system led Moody's Investor Service to downgrade its bond ratings from A1 to A2 in 2001 and from A2 to Baa1 in 2003 and to assign it a "negative outlook" in both years.[74] Standard & Poors also downgraded University Hospitals' bond rating "due to declining patient utilization, medical staff turnover and faltering financial performance during the past two years," *The Plain Dealer* reported while quoting from the S&P report.[75]

Despite the effect of the ratings raising the cost of future borrowing—ordinarily a serious factor in determining an organization's financial strength[76] —the system's large balance of cash and investments of $700 million would please potential lenders should the system decide to borrow further.[77] Long-term debt, about $450 million in 2003,[75] slightly exceeded unrestricted equity, suggesting that the system was, however, somewhat overleveraged.

From 1992 to 2003, annual revenue for the health system increased from $400 million to $1.5 billion. Expansion of the system, not the shrinking of University Hospitals of Cleveland, accounts for University Hospitals' providing only about half of the revenue to the health system by 2003.[45] Furthermore, almost half of the admissions to University Hospitals now come through one or more of the entities that are part of the University Hospitals Health System, such as its health plan, its doctor networks, or the owned and affiliated hospitals.[35] Thus, the health system that Farah Walters and her associates built contributes greatly to the success of, and possibly the survival of,[78] University Hospitals of Cleveland.[35]

QualChoice

Care of indigent patients and the inefficiencies associated with training students and house officers required that University Hospitals charge rates that exceeded those at the Clinic.[2]* Deciding that the payments offered by one of the Blue Cross/Blue Shield plans were inadequate, University Hospitals did not contract with the Blues for that plan.[35] The Cleveland Clinic accepted what people at university call a "sweetheart deal" and became a principal provider for the Blues, a condition that continues more than a decade later.† This decision deflected many insured patients from receiving treatment at University Hospitals unless they paid an out-of-network charge.

Furthermore, the Blues had excluded University Hospital from an im-

---

*These high costs even caused Walters to advise family medicine physicians to admit some of their patients to the nearby, less expensive Mt. Sinai Hospital.[2]

†Despite having established a comfortable relationship with the current Medical Mutual CEO, Walters could not obtain a contract for University Hospitals of Cleveland because the insurer's agreement with the Cleveland Clinic included an exclusivity provision that will continue for another decade and which the Clinic refused to revoke. Furthermore, according to the contract, a "severe financial penalty" would be charged to the insurer if it changed the arrangement.[3]

portant insurance product in the 1980s.[73] The CEO of the Blues at the time infuriated Block and his colleagues by suggesting that Cleveland needed only one tertiary care hospital—the Cleveland Clinic, in his opinion—and that Rainbow Babies and Children's Hospital should leave University Hospitals of Cleveland and join the Clinic.[2] These actions, along with Walters's assumption that Blue Cross executives had swung the sale of the Meridia Health System of hospitals to the Clinic,[79] contributed to the litigious relationship of University Hospitals to Blue Cross, while the Clinic and the insurer were enjoying a smoother ride.[26,56,70,79]*

To respond to this challenge, Block and Walters formed in 1991 "Qual-Choice,"[70] a third-party administrator and provider-owned health plan, originally established to provide health insurance to the employees of University Hospitals and CASE.[18,33,56,80] As QualChoice expanded, many of its members came to be insured by Medicaid, a carrier from which the Cleveland Clinic receives little support.[56] When Medicaid, which had paid hospitals relatively well, started transferring their patients into its HMO in the mid-1990s—"a disaster for us," says Walters[2]—University Hospitals converted QualChoice into an insurance company. "QualChoice protected our patient base and gave us data about what was going on," Walters explains.[2]

By 2005, QualChoice had grown to include 185,000 members, many not employees of the health system or the university, and offered a variety of insurance products.[80a] QualChoice and, consequently, University Hospitals continue to receive little business from Medical Mutual, the successor company for the Blue Cross/Blue Shield plans.[56]

QualChoice is structured as a wholly owned, for-profit subsidiary of the University Hospitals Health System. It has its own nine-member board of directors. The chairman of the QualChoice board is the CEO of the health system,[33] first Block, then Walters, and, thus, the president of QualChoice reports to the CEO of the system.

By 2002, QualChoice finally "made a slight profit," according to Thomas Sullivan, the former president, on revenue of about $400 million.[80] A principal purpose of the carrier, of course, is to keep patients coming to the system through referrals of insured members to the hospital and to the

---

*Not that University Hospital lost all these battles. According to *Crain's Cleveland Business,* the hospital settled two suits with Blue Cross for $15.9 million in April 1999.[70]

doctors who work there. When one considers the business thereby obtained, QualChoice has been a productive part of the health system even though, as a stand-alone venture, it has, until recently, consistently lost money.[18,56,81]

University Primary and Specialty Care Practices (UPCP) and Mednet

In 1994, both Farah Walters at University Hospitals and Fred Loop at the Cleveland Clinic started acquiring primary care practices. The reasons were similar. In order to appeal to the insurers offering managed care contracts, the hospitals required a network of primary care physicians whom the patients would first consult. These doctors would act as "gatekeepers" and only refer to specialists or for hospitalization those patients vitally needing such care, thereby reducing the costs of care by avoiding unless absolutely necessary the expenses of sophisticated testing and use of hospital beds. Affiliated with University Hospitals, these practitioners would presumably refer to the specialists at University Circle. Both organizations hired their doctors on a full-time basis, at the Clinic as members of the group practice and at University Circle as members of University Primary Care Practices (UPCP), a subsidiary of the health system. Each doctor at UPCP receives a clinical appointment on the medical faculty at CASE. Most of the sites where these doctors practiced came to be owned or rented by UPCP.

For many years, UPCP lost money, as the system guaranteed the doctors' salaries regardless of the size or efficiency of their practices, a problem sustained by several academic medical centers that had bought primary care practices in the heyday of capitated contracts and gatekeepers.[82] To reverse what were called "run-away costs," UPCP developed a system that the president and chief medical officer Dr. Michael Nochomovitz says "is based on local physician authority and responsibility."[83] Even though the system owns their practices, the doctors lead what Nochomovitz describes as a "physician staff health care delivery team" in the day-to-day operation of their work.[83]

The doctors, not UPCP, hire and supervise the people working in their offices, although for administrative purposes the employees work for UPCP's management services organization. UPCP charges the doctors rent for their offices—UPCP either owns or rents the buildings where the doctors work—plus overhead to support the central administration. By efficiently managing many of the expenses of their practices, the doctors can increase their income. Nochomovitz has phased out the salary guarantees offered the doctors when UPCP started.[83]

Because of its size and expertise, UPCP can provide efficient billing operations and make available malpractice insurance, supplies, and computer support at lower cost than a doctor would have to pay if working independently. UPCP also provides advice to help the doctors practice the most contemporary medicine and reduce complications, thereby providing better care for their patients and reducing the costs of malpractice insurance. UPCP contracts with the insurers and the managed care plans on behalf of the doctors and can obtain more favorable rates than a single doctor or smaller group could acquire. The members of UPCP also gain the prestige of association with University Hospitals of Cleveland and CASE. To the extent that they wish to do so, they can teach students and graduate trainees in their offices and participate in clinical research.[83]

As of the spring 2005, UPCP employed about 300 physicians, 25 percent of whom were now specialists.[83] Although UPCP will continue to add community physicians to its roster and expand its outpatient facilities, the acquisition of additional hospitals by the system has stopped. Rather than emphasizing referrals for hospitalization, UPCP is now stressing what Nochomovitz calls "total delivery of health care, which will let us offer favorable comprehensive programs to insurers. In the future, we will try to provide more patient satisfaction and more medical information to the public."[83]

The financial strategy for the doctors' practices and for UPCP as an accounting unit is to break even. Whether this is currently the case, Nochomovitz would not reveal, saying, "It's confidential information."[83]

One unit for which the system is no longer responsible is Mednet, a multispecialty group practice of ninety physicians, who provided care for a predominantly blue-collar population on the East Side of the city near the medical center.[84] James Block had acquired it in the late 1980s to provide capitated care,[35] as University Hospitals' first external multispecialty group practice.[35] Farah Walters retained it with the expectation that the doctors, not members of the medical school faculty, would refer their patients to University Hospitals of Cleveland.[84] The practice consistently lost money and, as the use of capitation diminished,[35] was finally jettisoned in 2002. Some of its members joined University Primary Care Practices and admit many of their patients to hospitals in the health system.[35]

University Suburban Health Center

Another group practice, closely connected to University Hospitals and of greater vintage than Farah Walters's creations, had been operating for decades in the nearby suburb of South Euclid, where a group of four doctors, each trained at University Hospitals of Cleveland, had organized an outpatient clinic. The founders built their facility on Green Road at the site of the former Rainbow Hospital, a rehabilitation facility for children, which, in the 1970s, had combined with the Babies and Children's Hospital at University Circle. Named University Suburban Health Center, familiarly "Green Road,"[64] it opened in 1973 with a staff of thirty physicians and surgeons, each with the academic credentials appropriate to attend and teach at University Hospitals of Cleveland. "One of our purposes was to keep university-trained doctors from leaving Cleveland to practice elsewhere," explains Dr. Hermann Menges, a cardiologist and one of the founders of the center,[85] but, according to Charles ("Chuck") Abbey, the executive director since 1984, "We always kept the freedom to run the place ourselves."[86]

Each doctor who wants to practice there must be approved by the center's board of trustees—each a doctor—and be vetted by the appropriate department chairman for a clinical title on the faculty of the CASE medical school and for admitting privileges at University Hospitals. Most of the care at the center is given by the volunteer faculty*—about 60 percent of those who see patients there—each of whom is paid through the center and not by the departments at the university or hospital. About 40 percent are full-time salaried members of the university departments, but most work principally at University Circle and spend a minority of their time at the health center.[86] Medical students and residents from CASE regularly train there. According to Menges, "the students always give us rave reviews for our hands-on teaching."[88]

---

*Called "part-time" in Cleveland even though the university or hospital may not pay them.[87] I use the more widely applied *volunteer* or *voluntary* for these doctors, who support themselves with their practices and donate time for teaching and supervision at the hospitals with which they are affiliated.

Unlike at some academic medical centers, where members of the full-time faculty assisted by house staff and students treat most of the inpatients, the doctors at University Suburban Health Center—at least many of them until fairly recently—personally care for the patients they admit to University Hospitals. "I live near the hospital and can make rounds on my patients each morning at 7:30 or 8:00," says Menges. "Now it seems that more and more of the doctors here refer their inpatients to the full-time staff."[89] There are financial as well as personal reasons for this change. The fees generated by most physicians for the daily care of patients in hospitals have steadily fallen, and, as Menges relates, many of the younger staff at the center live farther out in the country, making the commute to University Circle long.[89] With the doctors at the center often unable to interrupt their outpatient sessions to commute back and forth to the hospital to perform consultations, most of this work is now performed by members of the full-time faculty based at the medical school.[89]

The University Suburban Health Center is structured as a not-for-profit corporation and is governed by a board of eleven physicians, elected annually. Nine come from the dominant volunteer faculty group and two from the full-time staff. Thirty-seven not-for-profit professional corporations employ the volunteer faculty, the number in each group ranging from one to twenty-two doctors.[86] Each corporation pays its physicians and staff according to its own schedule. Efforts to combine the professional corporations into one group have failed,[86] as have similar attempts among the corporations of the full-time faculty at University Circle.

The corporations share the cost of the general overhead required to operate the center by paying rent—$33 per square foot in 2005—for the services common to all the groups.[86] The internal medicine group's assessment, for example, amounts to about 20 percent of its collections.[85] The chairman of the board of directors is salaried for the work he performs on center business. "Bud" Menges estimates that he spent as much as 40 percent of his time on administrative duties when he was chairman from 1985 to 1997.[85]

Having paid for the original construction of University Suburban Health Center, University Hospitals owned the place until 1984, when, thanks to a loan and investments from each member of the professional staff, the doctors bought the center and created University Suburban Real Estate, Ltd., a limited partnership that now owns it. Even while the hospital owned the center, the doctors who worked there operated it, as they do today. During the past three decades, the owners expanded the physical plant, added an ambulatory surgical center, and appointed additional generalists and specialists so that by the beginning of 2005 the original thirty had grown to 145. The leaders tried operating but later closed an emergency care center because it consistently lost money. They considered but rejected adding a radiology oncology unit because of the large capital investment that would have been required.

Because of its success, several private companies and the Cleveland Clinic have proposed buying the program. "Farah became concerned," Menges remembers, "and gave us $5 million [in exchange for the health system's acquiring 49 percent of the building[64]] for further expansion provided we would agree to change our affiliation only with the approval of University Hospitals."[85] Walters's concern was reasonable since referrals from the doctors at the center accounted, at one time, for as much as 40 percent of the private admissions to University Hospitals of Cleveland. "Farah told me," Menges remembers, "that if it weren't for us, University Hospitals of Cleveland would be only a hospital for indigents."[85] With the development of the University Hospitals Health System, the fraction of private patients admitted to University Hospitals from the center has dropped to a lower, but still important, 15 to 20 percent.[89a]

The center records 500,000 visits per year, including many wealthy citizens who live in the surrounding communities. "We must care for one-third of the CEOs in Cleveland," says Menges.[85] University Suburban Health Center became the model for the Green Spring project, a similar off-campus outpatient facility that James Block built at Hopkins after he left University Hospitals.[90]

Criticisms of Farah Walters

James Block, Walters's principal sponsor, understood that she had deficiencies. Block had appointed Terry White to establish relationships with community hospitals and to oversee the master facilities plan while Walters was chief operating officer of University Hospitals. "They could not get along," Block remembers.[4] White, described by a senior faculty member who had worked closely with him as "a consensus builder,"[47] later became a highly successful CEO at Metro.

Despite her many vitally important accomplishments on behalf of University Hospitals and University Hospitals Health System, Walters was not universally admired, particularly by many, though not all, members of the medical faculty. They variously faulted her as autocratic, capricious, controlling, demanding, opinionated, overbearing, unwilling to listen or to compromise, given to micromanaging, and always having to win.*

"Farah knew how to use power," one of the senior faculty acknowledged, and, in the process, "created great distrust." "She publicly discredited her people," said one chairman, and "terrified her board," according to another. Walters responds to this accusation by asking, "Why would my executive team have such a low turnover if I acted this way? Why did three of them who left want to come back?"[73]

Critics claimed that she controlled what information the board heard. One trustee said that "you felt that she gave you only half of the story." A leading university official believed that Walters had seen to the appointment of many of the trustees who were, consequently "very beholden to her. She kept them thoroughly convinced by keeping the place in the black, and that except for her, the place would fail."

Meeting with her could be productive and cooperative or, as one of the chairmen put it, "a one-way dialogue, a 'unilogue.'" Another senior faculty member who knew Walters's operating style well, commented that when meeting to discuss such issues as "finances and patient access, she totally monopolized the meetings and didn't allow time for general discussion. She wasn't receptive to contrary opinions, and most chairs remained mute when they disagreed with her. When we were meeting about strategic planning related to acquiring community hospitals and so on, Farah was terrific, and there were excellent discussions. Every decision made was by consensus."

Walters was criticized for "not understanding the value of the title *pro-*

---

*I spoke with Walters six times (once in Cleveland and five times on the telephone) and received from her a detailed "review and rebuttal" of information in the chapters on University Hospitals of Cleveland.[64] She told me that many of the descriptions of her were inaccurate, "defamatory," in some instances, or constituting what she called "Farah-bashing."[64] After she left, and the hospital and health system had new leaders, Walters said, "I was told that people were saying, 'it was all Farah's fault.' If you'd written this book while I was still there," she said to me, "you would have written a different book."[66]

Despite her reservations, Walters's review and our conversations provided much useful information to help me present a more balanced description of her term as president. Walters, however, continues to disagree with the validity of what many people told me and with my interpretation of some of the events.

fessor," and believing that "doctors were interchangeable." Walters adamantly denies that this is valid. "If this were true," she said, "I'd have been fired in a year. A university hospital CEO can't have this point of view and survive."[73] Walters criticized some academic doctors whom she saw caring more about research and manuscripts than patients and frequently traveling. "Actually," said chief of staff Robert Daroff, "Farah was deeply committed to research. She would say that if we don't support research, we're just a high-cost community hospital."[23]

Walters ascribes much of the opposition to her role as a "change agent. My bosses told me to do this. And I did it well but didn't make friends in the process."[66] She responds to the criticisms by asking, "Why would so many bosses—Jim Block, Bill Reynolds, Dick Pogue, and Henry Meyer*—have supported me and praised me when I stepped down?"[66]

"What saved her," according to J. B. Silvers, a professor of management at CASE who taught Walters when she was taking her M.B.A., "was that she was so smart and usually right. It was her style, not her substance, that caused her trouble."[56]

The two greatest sources of controversy between Walters and the faculty involved which organization, the clinical leadership or the CEO of the hospital and health system, should control the clinical research programs and which should appoint and discharge the professional leadership at University Hospitals.

The Overhead Conflict and Control of Research

By the 1990s, the medical school, having little discretionary income, increasingly came to depend upon University Hospitals for the funds needed to recruit members of the clinical faculty and provide them with laboratory and office facilities.[23,27,58,63,91] "The faculty," chief operating officer Orry Jacobs thought, "were looking on the University Hospitals funding as an entitlement."[91]

Consequently, Walters felt she could claim their support for clinical projects she deemed important for the University Hospitals. A senior university official agreed, saying, "Farah owned the clinical chiefs through financial

---

*Reynolds, Pogue, and Meyer were chairmen of the University Hospitals trustees when Walters was CEO.

support. Her total strategy was to have total control," which she exercised by assigning the money directly to the chiefs of service and the investigators rather than giving it to the dean for distribution, a practice she inherited from Harry Bolwell and James Block.

Meanwhile, little of the money from the indirect costs or overhead* collected by the university on the federal grants obtained by investigators working in the University Hospitals returned to the investigators, the school of medicine, its departments,[63] or, Walters ruefully noted, her hospital.[23,68] Hospital officials estimated that the university collected between $9 and $11 million per year in indirect costs on the funded research conducted by investigators at University Hospitals of Cleveland.[8] Faculty and administrators blamed the president for this practice as an expression of Pytte's antipathy for the medical center. The former president explained, "I did not change the overhead distribution system from what I inherited," and "I reject the idea that I didn't support the medical school."[92]

Walters and her associates knew that the surpluses from clinical revenue would soon be dropping and, when this happened, the hospital would have to start rejecting requests from the clinical chiefs, who were increasingly dependent on the hospital for developing their programs.[35] The University Hospitals executives looked at the overheads generated by clinical investigators working in University Hospitals, which the university, in their view, was hoarding and seemed to have no intention of sharing with the hospital.[35] According to one of her closest associates, money, in Walter's judgment, "was flowing from the medical school to feed the university,"[35] rather than being directed to the clinical departments and the hospital where the research supported by the grants that produced the overhead was being conducted.

Only by creating its own research enterprise, Walters reasoned, could University Hospitals of Cleveland recover the cost of at least some of its investment in the clinical departments.[23] Already, the hospital, rather than the medical school, administered grants obtained from commercial organizations such as pharmaceutical companies and collected any indirects asso-

---

*Some granting agencies pay "indirect costs" to compensate the organization where the research is being conducted—in this instance, CASE University—for the operations of the laboratories, including such charges as light, heat, and maintenance and for certain administrative costs related to the research. Indirect costs supplement the direct costs that the investigator has requested to conduct his research.

ciated with these grants,[63] an arrangement different from what was typical at many academic medical centers.

Accordingly, Farah Walters, supported by her trustees, established, in 1999, the Research Institute of University Hospitals of Cleveland, a wholly owned subsidiary of the hospital and health system.[35,36,63] Walters planned that the faculty working in the hospital would direct their research grants through the new research institute rather than the school of medicine, giving the hospital control of the indirect costs associated with the grants. Walters told her board that this maneuver could generate up to $10 million per year of "profit," thanks to her lower administrative costs. As a concession to the school, Walters agreed to share the overheads the research institute would generate.[10]

As its first director, the hospital appointed geneticist Huntington Willard, a member of the CASE University faculty since 1992. In this capacity, Willard reported to Walters, not to the dean.[63]* In establishing what was often referred to as "her"[38] research institute, she was attempting to duplicate the power of only a few well-known teaching hospitals, such as the Massachusetts General Hospital and the Brigham and Women's Hospital in the Harvard system, which run their own research and professional programs, independent of the medical school with which they are affiliated.[38] It was, in the opinion of one consultant, "Farah's declaration of independence."[38]†

Pytte, of course, strongly opposed Walters's plan, and found the whole project illogical from even the hospital's point of view.[28,92] "Farah believed you could make money on sponsored research." Pytte knew better. "This simply isn't true," he said.[92] Walters assumed that indirect costs, computed

---

*Willard left Cleveland early in 2003 to take what he called "the job of a lifetime" as director of the Institute for Genomic Sciences and Policy and vice chancellor for genomic sciences at Duke University.[63,93]

†The hospital's decision to build its own research building and, thereby threaten the financial security of the medical school by diverting the overhead funds to the hospital helped to convince Dr. Herbert Pardes, then dean of the Columbia University College of Physicians and Surgeons, to reject the invitation to succeed Agnar Pytte as president of CASE in 1999. (Pardes was the first candidate offered the position. It was a later nominee who had accepted and then rejected the presidency which led to David Auston's appointment.[43]) Pardes also reasoned that the hospital leadership's intense opposition to working with the Cleveland Clinic would probably prevent the university from affiliating with the Clinic, an arrangement that he believed could be very useful to the medical center. Pardes concluded that Pytte's successor faced "one tough job."[94]

as a fraction of the direct costs obtained by the investigator to support his research, would remain at the amount negotiated by the university. Knowing that she could operate the institute more economically, she could develop surplus funds to support more research or other hospital needs.

"This is insanity. It's a scenario out of hell," thought David Korn, who had heard about this plan while serving on a CASE institutional review committee.[38] Korn proceeded to tell the members of the committee how the NIH determines indirect costs. During negotiations between the NIH and the organization where the research will be performed, the institution requests indirect costs at a figure computed by its financial staff often supported by an analysis provided by an accounting firm. The NIH staff then conducts its own review of the data and, based on its determinations, awards indirect costs sufficient in the agency's judgment to cover the costs associated with the research but not large enough to permit the "profit" Walters anticipated receiving.[38] In addition, to fully cover the expenses of their research faculty, a recent RAND study has found, universities, and, presumably, teaching hospitals that administer their own research programs, must contribute, on average, about 25 cents from their own funds for every dollar the investigators receive from federal grants.[95]

"The University Hospitals trustees present sat there with their mouths open," Korn remembers. "The university president and provost were smiling. A deathly silence followed. Nobody challenged me. It was a very tense meeting."[38] It appeared to Korn that what he said was having little effect on the hospital trustees who were present.[38] "The situation had gotten lethal," Korn concluded. "The battles were tearing the place apart. Everyone was losing."[38] Clearly, observed one of her supporters among the clinical chairmen, Walters's research institute became viewed as "inflammatory or visionary, according to your point of view."[14] Undeterred, Walters and her board proceeded to construct their own research building with 309,000 square feet of space[62,96] across Cornell Drive from the hospital. It was completed in 2003.

While hospital executives regularly vented their annoyance that the full-time clinical faculty did not adequately appreciate how much University Hospitals was contributing to their work, the clinical faculty and its leaders found themselves torn between loyalty to the school of medicine and the hospital, an allegiance that Walters demanded in return for her support of their programs. In the view of one of the university trustees, she "held the medical school captive, preventing the university from controlling the school."[97]

Not every faculty member had to be convinced to accept Walters's point of view. Huntington Willard, the talented medical scientist whom she had chosen as the research institute's first director, so strongly championed Walters's approach[98] that some faculty saw him "adopting Farah's style and 'ramming through' such rules as flowing grants through the hospital and not the medical school."[57] The tensions on all sides became fierce.[98]

Recruiting Clinical Faculty

In addition to controlling the flow of research funds, Walters, many members of the faculty felt, challenged the primary right of the medical school to direct the appointment of faculty to the medical staff and to leadership positions at the hospital. To the annoyance of those clinical chairmen whose power to appoint faculty she was attempting to super-sede—"not her role," as former dean Frederick Robbins observed[51]—Walters recruited local clinicians with practices to fill the beds in the hospital. "It was my impression," said James Schulak, then the head of the abdominal transplant service and later Jerry Shuck's successor as chairman of surgery, "Farah Walters had the final say over who would be selected as department chairs."[53]*

The hospital and, therefore, Walters controlled how many of the en-dowed chairs for clinical faculty would be assigned. Money for these en-dowments had been raised through fund drives sponsored by the hospital that had been so successful that the number of such chairs increased from four to twenty while Farah Walters was CEO of University Hospitals.[9] Wal-ters and medical school dean Nathan Berger usually concurred on the as-signment of these chairs, often used to recruit new faculty or to convince faculty being recruited elsewhere to stay at home.[99] Nevertheless, because of what one senior faculty member called the "attitude problem" afflicting the center, chairmen and division chiefs had continuous difficulty recruit-

---

*In the text that follows, readers should understand that Walters denies that she exercised un-due control over the appointment of clinical faculty. She also refutes the charge that she fired many of the senior faculty, citing only the chairmen of pathology and surgery and the director of the cancer center.[64]

ing senior colleagues from other institutions. The absence of an affiliation agreement, current University Hospitals president Fred Rothstein remembers, also contributed to this problem.[100] Walters denies, however, that the hospital had particular difficulty recruiting doctors while she was CEO.[66]

Relieving Chairmen

Disaffected members of the staff also criticized the CEO when she relieved three of the service chiefs, Nathan Berger, director of the cancer center,[101] and Michael Lamm, chairman of the pathology service, and arranged the premature retirement, as he saw it, of Jerry Shuck, chairman of surgery.* The affiliation agreement allowed the hospital president to remove service chiefs.† Walters removed Shuck from the surgery chair by convincing her board to adopt a rule that chiefs must retire from chairing their services when sixty-five years old.[50] In each case, the displaced physicians continued in their university roles. Berger went to work in the dean's office, Lamm retained the chairmanship of the department of pathology and Shuck his title of professor of surgery.

Michael Lamm had become chairman of the CASE academic department of pathology and director of the pathology service at University Hospitals in 1981 when Harry Bolwell was chairman of the hospital board and eleven years before Walters became the CEO. Walters, and Block before her, wanted to trim the hospital pathology laboratories and have hospital administrators, rather than the pathologists, manage them and the offsite,

---

*Walters was thereby adopting a maneuver that George Crile had used in 1906[102] to force the eventual retirement of his chief, Dr. Dudley Allen. Later, the same rule would help prompt his founding of the Cleveland Clinic since Crile would have to resign the directorship of surgery at Lakeside when he reached the mandatory retirement age, which was sixty then, that he had had established for Allen.[103]

†Four chairmen left voluntarily during the Walters administration. David Bickers, the chairman of dermatology, was offered the chair at Columbia University, generally considered to represent a step upward academically, and Adel Mahmoud, the chairman of medicine, went into industry as president of Merck Vaccines and a member of the management committee at Merck & Co., Inc. "I didn't leave because Pytte pushed me out or because of him alone," says Mahmoud, who had had a problematic relationship with the university president. "I realized we couldn't advance because of the weak leadership everywhere, at the school and the university. Also, I'd been chair long enough [1987–98]."[44] William Speck left the chairmanship of pediatrics to become president and CEO of Presbyterian Hospital in New York City,[104] and Dr. Charles Schultz retired from the chair of psychiatry. "Given that I served as president and CEO for a full ten years," Walters writes, "the fact that only four chairmen/directors chose to leave UHC . . . shows . . . how distorted is the characterization . . . of a supposed 'culture of fear.' "[64]

private outpatient laboratory that the pathologists owned and had set up at the request of the former hospital administration. Walters, Lamm said, "insisted that the clinical laboratories accept markedly lower payments for the professional services the department supplied and, when I refused, fired me from my role in the hospital."[105]

Walters explains, "People were complaining that the department responded slowly with pathology reports, and Lamm wasn't interested in fixing things. He was putting all his money into research. He even threatened to shut down our ORs if we didn't do what he wanted."[10] Furthermore, she claimed that Lamm was "misusing funds," a charge that he denies.[39*] Dean Neil Cherniak, acting vice president Jerry Shuck, and the joint coordinating committee supported her action, Walters said.[67] Despite the decision she felt she had to make, Walters says, "I had much respect for Lamm as a researcher and scientist."[66]

Opposing Walters's action,[68] Pytte supported Lamm's remaining as chairman of the department in the medical school and agreed to pay the academic department part of the money that would be lost with the demise of Lamm's practice plan.[34] The clinical pathologists also performing research either transferred into the academic department or left for other positions.[34] In view of the weak, unfunded status of the medical school, the dean at the time was "not a key player" in this Pytte-Walters controversy,[34] which hospital trustee Dick Pogue characterized as "a classic example" of the strife between the president and the CEO.[8] "The dispute was ultimately resolved by the Joint Coordinating Committee, a group from both boards that had been established in the 1992 affiliation agreement for conflicts just like this one," Pogue said.[72] Farah Walters comments about this episode: "This was Ag Pytte wanting to settle scores with University Hospital and with Pogue who had tried to fire him."[66†]

As a result of Pytte's support, Lamm continued to direct at CASE one of the leading academic departments of pathology in the country, a department that stood number three in NIH grants in 1997. Attesting to the quality of the faculty he recruited and supported, three of his colleagues would become chairmen of the departments of pathology at such leading

---

*Walters wrote in her "review and rebuttal" for the author, "This situation riled people so much that one prominent doctor, reflecting the views of his patients and other physicians, asked, 'Why don't you give Dr. Lamm an eye patch to wear so everyone will know him for the pirate he is?' "[67]

†See the section titled "The No Confidence Controversy" in chapter 3.

academic medical centers as Johns Hopkins and the universities of Pennsylvania and Virginia.[39] Walters then recruited, with difficulty, Lamm says,[39] a clinical pathologist without superior academic credentials or a desire to perform research to run the hospital laboratories.[34,39] Lamm voluntarily retired from the departmental chairmanship in 2001, retaining his endowed professorship.[39] Finally, in the summer of 2003, with the university, medical school, and hospital under new leadership,* the school formed a search committee for a chair of pathology who would head a reunited department combining both the academic and clinical aspects of the specialty.[100,105,105a]†

As the pathology episode illustrates, Walters took a leading role in relieving those chiefs who were forced out of their positions, although, she says, she discharged no directors without the concurrence of the dean.[66]‡ These actions led one member of the senior clinical faculty to observe, "The morale here has become so bad." After Jerry Shuck was ousted as chairman of surgery, he said, "I wasn't enjoying the job anymore."[55] He wasn't alone. Victor Goldberg, the much respected chairman of orthopedics, resigned the chairmanship after leading the department for thirteen years.§ "Many things were changing," he explains. "Revenue was dropping, and expenses were rising. There wasn't time to focus on research, create a productive academic environment, and maintain my own clinical work. However, if things were more stable, I might not have stepped down."[107]**

The chairmen retreated from trying to displace Walters. Beaten in their attempt to rid the university of Pytte, they concluded that any effort to do the same at University Hospitals would fail. "She stepped right into our defeatist attitude," one of the chairmen said. "There was fear that she would

---

*See the discussion later in this chapter.

†The medical school and hospital recruited Dr. John Lowe from the University of Michigan to lead the combined department of pathology.

‡Walters had a precedent in firing chiefs of services. Scott Inkley, when hospital president, remembers taking the leading role in relieving one of the chairmen of his administrative position. The dean at the time, Richard Behrman, agreed with Inkley's action.[106] According to the affiliation agreement of 1992, Walters shared, in collaboration with the dean, the responsibility for appointing and discharging leaders at the hospital,[73] a common policy at many academic medical centers.

§Rumors traveled through the hospital that Walters had discharged him, but both Goldberg and Walters deny this.[2,107]

**Goldberg is not alone in suggesting that the terms of those holding such medical school positions as dean, department chairman, and section chief should be limited. "Ten years sounds about right, but they'll need some assurances of security afterward to get the best to move and take such jobs."[107]

find out and make us pay for it."[50] "There was nothing subtle about it," said Brooks Jackson. "We can make it very financially attractive for you if you join us," he said in describing how Walters convinced chairmen to support her initiatives. "It was big carrots, big sticks."[34]

Directing an institution with its own board of trustees and independent financial resources, Walters acted as she thought best, fiercely protecting her charge and fighting to keep the hospital administratively separate from the university. Although Walters denies this is true,[66] one of her critics claimed, "she wouldn't even mention CASE in her talks." In a brochure that Walters prepared at the completion of her ten years as CEO,[108] reference to CASE was seldom included. She wanted research conducted in the hospital credited to University Hospital[109] rather than to the university where, in most academic medical centers, it resides.[110] In a table of "NIH funding to Ohio Institutions," Walters listed University Hospitals of Cleveland in second place with $80 million just behind CASE's "$94 million." In the NIH ranking for 2001, faculty in the medical school generated $174 million.[111] She then published another table that puts University Hospitals of Cleveland in the same list with such renowned teaching hospitals as the Massachusetts General ($209 million in 2001[112]) and Brigham and Women's ($178 million in 2001[112]) and wrote:[113] "To put into a national perspective the potential strength of The Research Institute, we can think of it this way: The $80 million in NIH funding to UHC-based faculty in 2001 would have made UHC the eighth-largest hospital-based medical research center in America if UHC had received recognition for its research."

"By like token," University Hospitals board chairman Dick Pogue says, "Mrs. Walters and I often complained to the university trustees and the dean that CASE seldom mentioned University Hospitals in press releases or other publications where a UH-based faculty member was discussed. Both sides felt that better communications policies were in order."[114] Walters added that "CASE never gave appropriate recognition for research performed at University Hospital."[66]

The custom of members of the clinical departments, when giving talks at other institutions, to identify themselves primarily as members of the faculty of CASE diminished recognition of Walters's institution.[115] At one point, she proposed that University Hospitals buy the medical school, and failing this, threatened to stop teaching CASE students and affiliate with Ohio State's medical school,[24,57] a proposal that the clinical chairmen at CASE quite understandably particularly disliked.[24]

"We shot that down," said Dr. Richard Walsh, chairman of the department of medicine who had a particularly prickly relationship with the CEO, "because I championed the tight affiliation model [between CASE and University Hospitals of Cleveland]."[62] Walters had put Walsh on probation[73] and tried, according to Walsh, to separate the cardiology division from his department,[62] a charge that Walters denies.[66] Finally, to relieve the clinicians of some of their teaching obligations so that they could care for more patients in the hospital, she proposed that the school send students to the Cleveland Clinic, usually her nemesis, for instruction.

Choosing Deans and Vice Presidents

Walters's term as CEO corresponded with a time when the leadership of the medical school was subservient to the university president and not independently strong. Cherniak had been succeeded as dean by Dr. Nathan Berger,* a hematologist/oncologist with a distinguished investigative career in oncology,[54,116,117] "a brilliant manager of extramural support,"[40] very committed to the institution[118] and to students.[11,118] Reviewing his tenure as dean, Berger emphasized the following advances:[119]

- expanded the faculty, established four new departments, and appointed seventeen new department heads
- increased the number of endowed professorships from thirty to sixty-seven
- constructed a new 50,000-square-foot research tower
- increased funding from the NIH from $104 million in 1995 to $184 million in 2002
- revised the curriculum, established several new degree programs, doubled the size of the M.D./Ph.D. program, which trains physician-investigators, and created scholarships for high-caliber students and underrepresented minorities
- conducted a capital campaign which, by the summer of 2004, had achieved its goal of raising $300 million two years ahead of schedule[120]

*CASE had recruited Berger from Washington University in St. Louis in 1983 as chief of the hematology/oncology division. In 1985, he became director of the Ireland Cancer Center and, two years later, successfully applied to the NIH for designation as a Clinical Cancer Center. Under his leadership, the cancer center and the division developed highly successful programs in fundamental research.[17]

- received "the highest marks possible" in the 2002 accreditation process; among the strengths, the reviewers listed its "well-respected," "accessible," and "integrally involved" dean and other administrators, and committed faculty who show "a persuasive enthusiasm for curriculum improvement"

In choosing Berger, university president Pytte had selected the person whom Walters had removed from the directorship of the hospital's cancer center in 1993. She charged that he was concentrating too many resources on expanding research capacity and inadequately building the clinical component of the oncology service.[17,41,101,121,122] Berger, like directors of oncology in many academic medical centers, wanted to make his division a separate department,[73] a prospect guaranteed to aggravate other departments, particularly medicine, where oncology was then assigned. Berger became associate dean and, after guiding the medical school through a successful reaccreditation process,[54] became an obvious candidate to succeed Cherniak.

As dean, Berger, described as someone who "wanted to protect everyone like a father but didn't have the resources to do it," was "caught in an impossible situation between Pytte and Farah,"[118] making his job "excruciatingly difficult." Furthermore, comments Stanton Gerson, the chief of the division of hematology/oncology, "Nate was not weak, but he had a very strong CEO and chairmen to handle and a university president who was not particularly interested in cancer."[30]

Walters had supported Pytte's selection of Berger as dean, "so that she could control him," according to one observer. Understandably, Berger's appointment in 1996 assured a degree of animus between the new dean and the hospital CEO since Walters and her associates "wanted to call all the shots" in the clinical departments, "and the medical school would have to adjust to this."[54] This "we-they thing," thought Robert Shakno, assistant vice president in the medical school from 1997 to 2001,* "damaged both the hospital and the medical school."[54] "Actually," says Robert Daroff, who as hospital chief of staff had regular contact with all the principal players, "Farah liked Berger though she thought him a poor administrator."[87] Walters didn't believe that the deans' problems reflected conflict with her or weak leadership on their part.[73]

---

*Shakno, now president and CEO of Jewish Family Services Association of Cleveland, had been CEO of Mt. Sinai Hospital before coming to the medical school.[54]

Pytte appointed Berger after candidates from outside the university had rejected the job when offered to them. One was Dr. Harvey Colten,[41] who had received his medical degree from Western Reserve in 1963 when, thanks to the new curriculum, the school was "one of the most selective in the country."[123] Chairman of the department of pediatrics at the Washington University medical school in St. Louis during the dean's search, Colten withdrew, despite repeated entreaties from leading members of the university board, because "a critical relationship with Agnar Pytte could not be forged. He [Pytte] had no appreciation of the issues affecting the school."[123]* Walters agrees. "Because I supported the clinical chairs, Pytte fought me," she explains. "I truly believe that at University Hospital our commitment to the mission of the medical school is what saved it in spite of Ag Pytte."[73]

Pytte also offered the deanship, with the vice presidency attached, to Roger Meyer, now considering for the third time a senior position at CASE. "I met with Pytte," Meyer remembers. "Unlike my experience in 1990, Pytte initiated the discussion by promising no games about salaries."[124] When he was offered the deanship the first time, Pytte had proposed a salary that was less than Meyer was then making. This time Meyer wanted a five-year contract, and Pytte agreed.[125]

Then Meyer met Farah Walters. "She began the meeting," said Meyer, "by saying that I was used to running everything, and that I would want to do it here."[125] Meyer's previous job at George Washington University had included jurisdiction over the hospital, the medical school, the practice plan, and an HMO. But in Cleveland, "the present structure between the hospital and the school required joint accountability."[125] Meyer thought that a potentially successful structure for trustee leadership would rotate the committee chairs from the school and the hospital, annually or biannually, but only if the present chairs of the two boards remained to assure a smooth working arrangement. "This was doomed," Meyer said, "when Pytte removed Karen Horn, the chair of the university board of trustees, and prohibited [future][76] trustees at the university from serving on the University Hospitals board."[125]

Horn had invited Meyer to meet with the university trustees. Meyer advised them, "If you do what Pytte wants—complete separation of the university and the University Hospitals—that's not functional."[124] In the mid-

---

*Colten later became dean of the medical school at Northwestern University.[123]

dle of Meyer's presentation, Pytte left the meeting—not the first time he had done so. "Though he had a very gracious manner 90 percent of the time," Karen Horn said, "for the rest of the time, he didn't."[126] Later Meyer would be told, "he does this all the time whenever he's angry. His doctor says it's better for his health."[124] Horn confirms that Pytte would leave meetings "whenever he didn't like what was going on."[126] Story Landis, then chair of the department of neurosciences and of the committee searching for a vice president for health affairs,[127] attended the trustee meeting at Horn's invitation[126] and remembers, "It was very unpleasant."[128]*

Roger Meyer, seeing only trouble in the job as Pytte had structured it, left CASE for the last time, having rejected three opportunities to work there.[124] Thus, it is true, as Pytte says, that, as with Cherniak, the president had tried to appoint one of the candidates the search committee had recommended.[92]

University Hospitals of Cleveland versus Cleveland Clinic

Competition and strong feelings between the trustees, administrators, and doctors working at University Hospitals and at the Cleveland Clinic have persisted since George Crile founded the Clinic in 1921. "You can't imagine the animosity toward the Clinic," said a former senior faculty member at University Hospitals. "It was a very bitter thing." Former dean of the CASE medical school Frederick Robbins, who observed the conflict for more than fifty years since joining the Western Reserve faculty in 1952, concluded that it was "the competition for patients and dollars that prevented our full cooperation. I tried to get them together . . . but when it came to patients, everything broke down."[51]

Farah Walters saw Cleveland to be a very difficult market for an academic medical center like University Hospitals to compete in because "the Clinic's right down the street," an observation that was also a favorite of James Block. "Elsewhere," Walters said, "academic medical centers compete with academic medical centers."[129]

"UH had two types of patients," Walters says of the hospital's clientele

---

*Pytte's lack of support to create the vice presidential position after a two-year search discouraged Landis.[87] In 1995, she departed CASE for the NIH to become scientific director of the National Institute of Neurological Diseases and Stroke. In 2003, the NIH named her director of the institute.[87]

before the 1990s. "Medicaid and the uninsured came through the emergency ward and filled many of our beds and our huge public clinics. On the private side came patients from the Menges's group [University Suburban Health Center] with its old blue-blood families. An interesting mix of the poorest and the wealthiest, but not the middle class."[129]

Most of the Cleveland Clinic's patients, it seemed to Walters and to many at University Hospitals, were private and well insured. The Clinic had not had an effective emergency ward to which local uninsured patients might come until the arrangement with Kaiser Permanente required the Clinic to develop one in the 1990s.* Many Cleveland CEOs, Walters observed, "thought the Clinic was for-profit and UH not-for-profit."[129] As one of the University Hospitals chairmen, who has previously worked at the Clinic, said, "The places serve totally different classes. We care for all from the knife and gun club to the carriage trade."[130]

Over the years, the faculty and staff at University Hospitals developed a party line.[26,41] "They regard the Clinic as a commercial venture and second-rate academically" compared with the purity and academic superiority of the university, according to Robbins.[51] Some University Hospitals doctors still refer to the Clinic as "that group down the street."[131] They see the Clinic doctors as employees rather than independent professors.[84] Clinic doctors harbor an "inferiority complex," other University Hospitals doctors claim, because they're not primary members of a faculty despite believing that "we're better than anything."

CASE clinical faculty think the doctors at the Clinic are "under more pressure than us to see patients,"[84] and that the Clinic may be a less friendly place for a doctor to work at compared with the university.[12] "The Clinic doesn't partner, it takes over," says Dr. Michael Devereaux, a University Hospitals neurologist, in expressing what many of his colleagues believe. "If you deal with them, keep your hands in your back pockets," he warns.[26] Devereaux sees the Clinic "more Republican in medicine—they have a corporate approach—we're more Democratic."[26]

However, an important advantage of working at the Clinic, says Dale Adler, the chief of cardiology and a busy practitioner at University Hospitals, is "you don't have to worry about how the office runs and where the patients will come from. The docs there are more pressured to see all those

*See chapter 2.

patients referred to the Clinic,"[12] which leads to an oft-repeated characterization at University Circle of the difference between the two hospitals: "patients go to the Clinic, but they come to University Hospitals' doctors."[31]

University president Agnar Pytte was "always being told horror stories about the Clinic. Never seen such intense dislike, which I think was more on the UH side than at the Clinic."[92] His counterpart at University Hospitals was clearly one of those for whom the Clinic was the enemy, and Farah Walters's enmity was evident for all to see. "Mention the Clinic, and she went up in smoke," said one CASE faculty member. "Beating the Clinic became her life's passion," said University trustee John Lewis,[43] an obsession that many faculty members thought destructive.[58] Walters interpreted efforts by hospital executives or trustees to cooperate with the Clinic as evidence of disloyalty. CASE was making overtures to, and awarding titles to, doctors at the Cleveland Clinic, further irritating Walters and her colleagues at University Hospitals.[91]*

Despite the criticism, many at University Hospitals admired or have been forced to admire, how the Clinic operates. Harry Bolwell "envied their structure."[19] "They're much more effectively structured," acknowledges Richard Aach, an associate dean and former chairman of medicine at Mt. Sinai Hospital.[11] In the opinion of James Block, "the Clinic is a business, very much a business. Even by 1990, we still couldn't even spell 'market.' Cleveland Clinic was spelling it in the 1970s and 1980s."[4]

The recruiting process at universities frustrated Block as it does many a teaching hospital CEO. "If I wanted to bring in cardiac surgeons, it could take years. The culture of search committees slows down recruitment by twelve to thirty-six months." Exaggerating to make his point, Block envied how Fred Loop and his predecessors could "do what they wanted to do." But this ability to decide rapidly could lead to mistakes. Cleveland Clinic Florida, was, Block says, "like a tar-baby" and contributed to the end of the reign of Loop's predecessor as CEO.[4]

Scott Inkley, who preceded Block as president of University Hospitals of Cleveland and is a native of the city and career-long member of the medical faculty, said, "At the Clinic, they know what business they're in. We operate

---

*However, university trustee Richard Watson believed, "If Farah were president of CASE [rather than of the hospitals and health system], she would have affiliated with the Clinic."[132]

with three responsibilities—teaching, research, as well as patient care. It became increasingly difficult for a busy executive to see a doctor here since so many had their research to do. The Clinic does it much more realistically. So we keep the old families, but the executives go to the Clinic."[106] Meanwhile, the Clinic prospered under consolidated management, "a great advantage," says hospital trustee Dick Pogue, "but an anathema to many academics."[8]

Despite the often repeated critical comments about the Clinic emanating from University Circle, however, several members of the staff at the university find the characterizations of work at the Clinic unhelpful. "It's a rivalry, more than a competition," according to Dr. John Ferry, a former senior University Hospitals administrator, "and is felt more by the top managers. The docs know many of the docs at the other institution. We all live in same small group of towns, and our kids go to school together."[28] Walters found the faculty's feelings about the Clinic "absurd. If you favored the Clinic, you were an enemy. I took the Clinic seriously."[3]

When the Clinic decided to develop a pediatrics service despite the dominance of Rainbow in the community, Walters saw an opportunity of creating, as she puts, it, "a community asset," by some sort of mutually advantageous relationship. "Fred Loop and I met over salads in his office," she recalls. "I suggested that the Clinic not develop its children's hospital[9] and we would not compete directly in cardiac surgery." Loop responded that the Clinic was committed to pediatrics, and the discussion ended.[3]

In 1994–95 Walters made the unexpected suggestion, considering the intensely competitive spirit she and her colleagues felt toward the Clinic, that University Hospitals of Cleveland and the Cleveland Clinic Foundation merge. "I remember saying to Al Lerner [the businessman-philanthropist and a generous contributor to both institutions] that we could create a powerhouse if the Clinic's surgical leadership was linked to our prominence in medicine." Although Walters saw antitrust considerations and cultural differences as potential barriers to the deal, Lerner, Loop, and Walters suggested that the three have dinner together to discuss this and other possibilities. "I never heard anything further," she said.[3]

At the Clinic, senior members thought that "Walters hated us." Saying "the Clinic should have paid her salary,"[133] Loop seemed to revel in Walters's animosity toward his institution. "UHC is not our competition," one staff member said. "We compete against ourselves to be better and hold to our own standards." A close associate of Loop added, "Fred doesn't think much about UHC; Farah's always talking about the Clinic."[134] Another observer said, "Loop pretended that the Clinic doesn't compete with UH. This burned Farah, who saw conspiracies everywhere."* Nevertheless, many at the Clinic were bothered about an attitude they believed the doctors at University Hospitals and the medical school felt about their institution. As one of the Clinic staff physicians said, "They're always thinking of us as 'second tier.' There's a clinic over there, and they're just cranking them out."

As an expression of these strong feelings, the CEO of the Cleveland Clinic had never been invited to tour University Hospitals of Cleveland, Loop once told John Lewis, who, in addition to his board memberships at University Circle, was a member of the law firm that was outside counsel to the Clinic. "Of course," comments Dick Pogue, "Mrs. Walters was similarly conscious that her chairman's two suggestions to his counterpart at the Clinic that some trustees and management of the two institutions get together to 'break the ice' were ignored."[72] Lewis thought that Loop "didn't worry much about UH," whereas the people at University Hospitals, and particularly Walters, "worried about the Clinic all the time."[43]

Critics at University Hospitals and CASE faulted the wisdom of Walters's retaining such intense feelings about the Clinic. "She should be planning what University Hospitals should do and not be so reactive and always try to emulate what the Cleveland Clinic did." Walters agrees, "Our job was not reacting to what the Clinic was doing but doing what we should do. Our strategy should not be a 'me too' strategy."[67]

Meanwhile, over the objections of much of the clinical faculty,[133] Pytte worked consistently, though relatively unsuccessfully, to bring the medical school into closer union with the Clinic.[126] His predecessor had "blanched at the idea of linking with what he considered to be the nonacademic Cleveland Clinic."[133] The officers at University Hospitals, Edward Hundert, the new CASE president, would learn, "were always trying to prevent the university from relating to the Clinic."[135]

---

*Ironically, in view of this opinion, Walters considered taking a job at the Clinic in the mid-1980s. She rejected the opportunity, concluding that "there really wasn't a job there for me. They just wanted a token woman in a senior administrative position."[2] Despite her competition with Fred Loop's establishment, she acknowledges that, at least during the 1970s, "Cleveland had three things that were great: the Clinic, the orchestra, and the Browns."[2]

Individual relations between physicians and investigators at the Clinic, Metro,[136] and University Hospitals of Cleveland, however, had prospered for decades when mutually advantageous for those concerned. These productive associations continued during the period when Walters was competing so strongly with Loop and augured well for cooperation when the new medical college opened.[41,135] Nevertheless, problems persisted for which Walters bore some responsibility. "Farah seemed too willing to punt when needs were expressed by the medical staff, saying 'that's a university responsibility,'" according to psychiatrist Douglas Lenkoski. "It was often Farah's combative style, not the content, that drove the medical staff up the wall."[41]

This ill will preceded the Walters administration. When the university entered into an agreement with the Cleveland Clinic to develop a joint program in biomedical engineering, the hospital objected, and James Block, Walters's predecessor, asked the chairs to call trustees whom they knew to complain.[137] The chairs met with Allen Ford, who was then the chairman of the university board, and, as described by Robert Daroff, the chairman of neurology at the time, "complained to him. Then Pytte called a meeting of the chairs and read us the riot act."[138] Pytte told the chairs never to go over his head to the board again.* The problem, Pytte said, was not an issue for the hospital since it was the engineering school, not the medical school, which was developing the program. "Thus," Daroff concludes, "Block got the chairs . . . to fight it out with Ag."[138]

In a talk to Cleveland civic leaders, Pytte emphasized the university's connections to the Clinic, the VA hospital, and other institutions. A picture of Pytte and Loop shaking hands appeared on the cover of a local magazine. The hospital leaders saw Pytte's actions as efforts to minimize the affiliation of the university with the University Hospitals.[23,36] Pytte saw the university benefiting from better relationships with the Clinic[25,139] and concluded that Walters and certain of the clinical faculty were preventing such accommodations from developing because of fear of the Clinic's clinical power.[92] Nevertheless, some of the leaders continued to believe that the Clinic, CASE's medical school, and University Hospitals could unite, in some manner, into a single unified academic medical center, and the three entities held futile discussions during 2000 and 2001.[140-142]

---

*The chairs clearly did not remember this admonition, for they would petition the CASE board again, this time to remove Pytte as president (see chapter 3).

Practice Plans and Faculty Salaries

At most medical schools, practice plans coordinate many of the clinical financial activities of the full-time clinical faculty. These organizations bill and collect for their professional services and may pay the salaries of the practitioners, develop benefits, secure malpractice insurance, and contract for managed care for the doctors. Such corporations have been deemed necessary so that the clinical faculty could develop pension plans and other benefits based on their earnings from clinical income as distinguished from support obtained from grants or paid directly by the medical school. Most, but not all, are organized as 501(c)(3) not-for-profit corporations and, accordingly, are charitable and tax-exempt organizations.[15] Organizing such plans as partnerships would have precluded the inclusion of pension and profit-sharing plans.[15] The leaders are often the chairmen of the clinical departments. When a new chairman is appointed, direction of the practice plan usually transfers automatically to the new incumbent.[15]

Individual departments and divisions initially developed their own plans, often through the creation of corporations frequently dominated by one or more of the senior faculty. Beginning in the 1960s, university academic officers, usually deans, attempted to gain control of these plans by consolidating them under their jurisdiction. This process often involved intense political maneuvering. The chairmen[44] and chiefs resisted relinquishing their authority over this vital function while the deans strived to gain control for general administrative reasons and so that part of the income could be spent to develop other missions in the medical schools.*

During the 1980s, dean Richard Behrman set the salaries of the chairmen and approved what the rest of the faculty were paid.[116] He discussed data frequently with the head of the hospital, if, for no other reason, than "to prevent faculty from going around me."[116] Hospital director James Block was giving annuities to favorite department chairmen at Christmas. "I insisted that they had to reduce their salaries by the value of the annuities," Behrman remembers. Each of the chairmen "eventually gave in," and Block

---

*I have described this process at the University of Pennsylvania in a previously published study.[90]

stopped paying the annuities.[116] But when Behrman tried initially to establish a dean's tax,[137] the chairs, according to his successor, said they would "hold meetings to discuss the tax on the Wednesdays of the fifth week of the month."[21] The deans lacked the power to enforce the tax,[20,128] which some departments consistently refused to pay,[20] or to consolidate the departmental practice plans under the deans' aegis.[13]

This relatively weak authority of deans of the school of medicine,[84] particularly with respect to the practice plans,[119] followed from the university's not wanting to be involved in the practice of medicine.[13,16,68] If the practice plans became one of the deans' duties, then the school and ultimately the university could be held accountable for their success or failure, and the university's leadership did not want to assume that responsibility.[39] "The university had decided that financing the clinical departments was a bottomless pit and stayed out of it," Walters said. "Pytte figured that failure of the practice plans would not affect the university. The hospital would have to bail them out."[68] Consequently, as one of the clinicians said, "The dean has no stick since he gives the departments no money."[84]

Thus, in recent years deans at the CASE University School of Medicine have had the least power of the leaders of the three entities with which the clinical chairmen deal—the school, the hospital, and the practice plans. Deans, however, can claim, what one chairman called "the spiritual thing," even though the CEO of the University Hospitals of Cleveland exercises more authority on the clinical faculty. "She could hire, fire, and not pay me," said one of the clinical chairmen, "but when I travel, I am introduced as from CASE, not UH."[20]

This lack of coordination among the plans contributed to some peculiar developments. In the department of dermatology the chair, David Bickers, had formed in 1979 University Dermatologists, Inc., to bill and collect for the professional services of the full-time faculty.[18] Bickers had personally borrowed $30,000 to establish an outpatient practice for his faculty. Untypical for such organizations, University Dermatologists was organized as a for-profit corporation because Bickers wanted to be able to take the practice with him elsewhere "if politics intervened."[15] To further protect against potential future institutional encroachment, legal counsel advised that Bickers became the president and sole shareholder.[15,18] When Bickers left CASE in 1994 to become chairman of dermatology at the Columbia University College of Physicians and Surgeons in New York, he sold the shares for $1,000 to Dr. William Lynch, his colleague and close friend[15] who had been appointed acting chair at CASE,[18] and as Bickers testified, had virtually co-founded the practice with him.[143]

When Dr. Kevin Cooper arrived from the University of Michigan to succeed Bickers, Lynch, then the acting chair, would not turn over the practice plan to him as Cooper had been told that he would[144] and Bickers wished him to do.[18] Cooper and University Hospitals—Farah Walters supported her new chief of service in this action—sued the former acting chair to force him to sell his shares to the new chairman.[15] It was said that Walters had become very angry with Lynch and "wanted to teach the doctor a lesson. Don't fool with me!"[15] Kevin Cooper points out that this statement was reported by Malvin Bank, the attorney for Lynch's practice, and, therefore, "not a disinterested party without conflict of interest."[144]

The case eventually reached the Ohio Supreme Court, which ruled that University Hospitals of Cleveland had no claim on the shares of University Dermatologists, Inc. The relationship between Lynch, his associates, and the corporation with the University Hospitals and the medical school ended with the "eviction," as the trial court stated, of Lynch's group from the hospital.[106,143] His corporation continues to function as an independent entity, and the court determined that the former acting chair was not obliged to sell the shares if he chose not to do so.[15,143–145] Cooper proceeded to create for his department a new practice plan called University Hospitals Dermatology Associates.[144]

When Dr. Wulf Utian, chairman of the department of reproductive biology at CASE and of obstetrics and gynecology at University Hospitals, retired from these positions, James Goldfarb, the acting chairman, assumed leadership of the practice plan. Then when Goldfarb and several of his colleagues left to join the Cleveland Clinic, Goldfarb took the practice plan with him, and his successors at University Circle had to create a new one.[115,146]

In another aberration from what has become routine at most academic medical centers, University Hospitals of Cleveland created its own practice plan for pathology. When Farah Walters sacked Michael Lamm as chairman of pathology in University Hospitals and revoked the hospital's contract with his department,[34] the practice corporation that Lamm directed lost its sources of income since the hospital pathologists no longer reported to him. Accordingly, Walters had to establish her own plan to collect the professional fees generated by the clinical pathologists, whom she would directly employ.

Dr. Brooks Jackson, then director of clinical pathology at the hospital and vice chairman of the department of pathology, remembers the time well. "It was an incredible mess," he recalls. "After Michael was fired, I reported to a hospital vice president and therefore indirectly to Farah."[34] Uncomfortable with the changes, Jackson looked for other opportunities, and in 1996, moved to the Johns Hopkins Hospital as deputy director of clinical affairs for pathology. In 2002, he became chairman of the department of pathology there.[34*]

By the beginning of the twenty-first century, the process of consolidating the practice plans and developing a coherent system for paying the full-time clinical faculty had barely reached University Circle despite a single practice plan being one of the stated goals of the affiliation agreement of 1992. Each of the clinical departments and even some of the divisions, several within the department of surgery alone,[10] still operate their own plans, some as 501(c)(3) not-for-profit corporations, a few as for-profit corporations.[28] Some are financially successful, others in, what one trustee called, "desperate straits."[78] One frustrated surgeon, who, after being recruited to University Hospitals of Cleveland, stayed for only three years, describes the state of affairs as "a collection of practices with doctors who think they work at an academic medical center." The surgeon had not met his department chairman before his appointment.[147]

The practice plans directly pay the salaries of most of the clinicians rather than flowing money through the university, which charges 11 percent to handle the funds and issue the paychecks.[20] Each clinical department at University Hospitals has developed its own formula for compensation.[148] The chairmen, in effect, decide how much to pay themselves and their colleagues and also determine what benefits, which differ from practice to practice, to provide through their practice plans.[149] All are virtually autonomous of oversight by the school of medicine and its dean. Dr. Martin

---

*Jackson is very happy to be at Hopkins rather than at the University Hospitals of Cleveland. "It's such a pleasure to be here," he says. "The place is run by physicians, which makes such a difference. One doesn't have to go hat-in-hand to hospital administration for permission to do something. It could take weeks to get the smallest things approved at University Hospitals."[34]

Resnick, chairman of the department of urology, admits that "the arrangement does permit chairs to abuse the system,"[148] or, more accurately, what one might call the "nonsystem."

Practice Plans: Some Degree of Coordination

Though prizing their independence and harboring suspicions about the activities of some of their colleagues, many of the chairmen recognized that their lack of coordination decreased the likelihood of their department's obtaining contracts from managed care companies. Insurance carriers wanting to develop relationships with physicians from University Hospital had to negotiate separately with each department, in addition to the hospital, a condition calculated to discourage them from signing contracts with the doctors. The hospital and the doctors saw themselves at a particular disadvantage in competing for managed care contracts with the Cleveland Clinic with its unified administrative structure.[148]

The presence of multiple plans also helped to prevent the Blue Cross/ Blue Shield insurer from dealing successfully with University Hospitals of Cleveland. "I was never able to make a package deal at UH," says Jack Burry, the former CEO of the insurer, "whereas at the Cleveland Clinic this was easy to do."[150] Burry and his associates found it very cumbersome to deal with each practice corporation as well as the hospital. The Clinic's unified administration, which could negotiate for the doctors as well as the hospital, removed this roadblock.[150]

"So we came together informally," explains Martin Resnick, "encouraged by the hospital but with little input from the medical school."[148] Recognizing how disorganized the practice plans were, Farah Walters saw, in the inability of the medical school to assume a leading role,[29] an opportunity for the hospital to direct the plans,[5,62,84] a project that she thought would be in the best interests of the departments as well as the hospital.[10]

The chairmen of the clinical departments proceeded to consolidate some of the practices' functions through the corporation the departments created in 1998 to contract as a group with the insurance carriers.[62,148,151] Resnick, as president of the group, and his colleagues later took on the function of negotiating for malpractice insurance on behalf of all the departments.[148]

With each department generating its own bills, patients often received many invoices from each of the doctors attending them and from the hospital. Recognition of this problem—an important difference from the single bill that the group practice at the Cleveland Clinic generates—led to the creation of University Hospital Faculty Services (UHFS), a management service organization (MSO) organized as a joint venture of the University Hospitals and University Physicians Faculty Association (UPFA), the independent practice association (IPA) representing the doctors. The hospital and the doctors each control 50 percent of UHFS.[10,28,151] A board of three chairmen of clinical departments from UPFA and three executives from the hospital direct the MSO. The chairmanship alternates between the two groups. The president of UHFS, Keith Coleman, reports to the board of trustees of the joint venture and specifically to its chairman, who is currently Dr. Resnick.[151]

Gradually, the hospital and all but two of the practices transferred their billing function to the MSO, with the hospital assuming much of the cost of computer support since it uses the computers for other functions as well. The MSO employs and administers the wages and benefits for about one hundred people. Most of the departments assigned their staff members, who were previously employed directly by each of the practice corporations, to the MSO, leaving the practice corporations employing only the doctors. Because some grants supporting faculty salaries flow through the university, affected members of clinical departments receive two paychecks, one from the university and the other from the practice corporation.[148]

The practice plans reimburse the MSO for the expenses of employing the staff and for the other services that UHFS performs, including its common expenses. The departments divide these costs so that the MSO generates neither a profit nor a loss.[151] The MSO, which also coordinates malpractice insurance and risk management for the doctors in the practice plans,[151] is developing a common scheduling system for patient appointments in all the departments. The separate practice plans, however, still buy health insurance for their members independently, thereby missing the opportunity to consolidate and negotiate lower premiums because of larger volume, and the doctors in their offices and the hospital continue to generate separate patient records.[84]

In deciding whether to consolidate further, the faculty have considered at least one, rather paradoxical, advantage to remaining separate. It may be that the lack of unity among the practice plans helped the clinicians and their institutions avoid being subjected to a Physicians at Teaching Hospitals (PATH) audit by the Office of the Inspector General. These reviews on whether the doctors working at teaching hospitals had correctly followed the regulations for billing patients with Medicare resulted in fines to many academic medical centers.* As of June 2005 the government had not yet surveyed the multiple independent plans at CASE and University Hospitals of Cleveland.[153a]

Financing the Medical School

That the administrations of the university and medical school had their differences at CASE would not surprise any who have worked in senior positions at academic medical centers. The principal issue is usually money. With CASE expecting each school to operate on its own income, the medical school received little support. For example, the university, which Neil Cherniak, the dean from 1990 to 1995, described as a "fiscally conservative place," obtained the bonds for construction of the new research building, but held the school responsible to pay the interest on the mortgage and the costs of amortization, totaling $5.7 million per year.[21]

The school in Cherniak's day depended primarily on income on its sizeable endowment. The state contributed $5 million in return for the school's admitting 60 percent of the class from Ohio residents.[21] Although more than one observer and faculty member has advised phasing out this provision to reduce the dependency of the school on Ohio applicants and improve the ability of the school to attract top students from throughout the country,[44,61,62,154] financial considerations have, until recently, dictated otherwise. "We have to work hard at recruiting students," said one of the basic science chairs. "It's Cleveland and low national visibility."[154]

The indirect payments developed on the research grants obtained by the faculty flowed through the school of medicine but little was left after the school paid the costs that the indirects were designed to cover. The university also levied an assessment on all the school's expenses, which the university insisted upon receiving—"a value-added tax," as Cherniak[21] and his colleagues[52] saw the payment, but one that Agnar Pytte says was in

---

*The first institution so reviewed, the University of Pennsylvania, agreed to pay $30 million to settle a charge of false billing of Medicare by some of Penn's full-time physicians.[152] The Cleveland Clinic paid $4 million,[153] its audit made relatively easy for the government by the Clinic's unified administration.

effect when he arrived as university president and claims that he did not change.[92] Cherniak remembers that the president raised the tax by about 2 percent.[155] Consequently, the school had little discretionary income for Cherniak to recruit faculty that he thought the school desperately needed. "I felt that the school had lost its research luster despite Behrman's recruiting some good basic science chairs," said Cherniak. "I was in a major financial bind when I became dean, so I concentrated on trying to increase research funding and raising money from donors."[21]

The clinical chairmen refused to support the school further since their funding from the school had not increased. Deans had sometimes failed to collect their tax from certain departments, supporting once again the relatively weak position of the deans during the 1990s. In subsequent years, when the hospital and the school had no operative affiliation agreement, none of the clinical chairs paid their assessments.[14] Unable to extract more money from the practice plans, Cherniak turned to the hospitals. The 1992 affiliation agreement between the university and University Hospitals of Cleveland included a provision whereby the hospital would give the medical school $1 million per year for five years. The agreement with Metro added $500,000 per year for the school.[21]

Cherniak also talked with Fred Loop and Bernadine Healy, then the director of the Cleveland Clinic's research institute, about an affiliation between CASE and the Clinic, which would enjoy "a co-equal status with University Hospitals and Metro."[21] When a suitable relationship at the Clinic failed to materialize, Cherniak turned to the Henry Ford Hospital in Detroit,[117,156] which "accepted the arrangement I had proposed to the Clinic."[21] Ford, which would give CASE students training in primary care and managed care,[155] an educational experience that the school needed to offer more extensively,[117,157] saw the arrangement adding to its academic standing and hoped that some of the students working there would then choose to become house officers at the Ford Hospital after they graduated,[23] although few did.[157] Teachers at Ford were given appointments on the CASE faculty which, according to a senior medical officer at Ford, "were sometimes bestowed with a very liberal interpretation of academic achievement."[157] Neil Cherniak says that this is a point of view with which not all executives at Ford would agree and emphasizes that each appointment "went through the same procedure as for any other member of the faculty."[155] Ford agreed to support the school with $500,000 per year and to route its NIH research grants and contracts through CASE, thereby raising the medical school's ranking compared with that of other medical schools.[21,117,157]

Cherniak anticipated two campuses for his school, one in Cleveland and one in Detroit, with Ford creating a new medical school in close association with CASE, as would later occur at the Cleveland Clinic.[156] "Ford, however," says Vinod ("Vin") Sahney, the senior vice president of planning and strategic development there, "was having financial troubles at the time and didn't want to get involved in the political troubles inherent in creating a school in a state that didn't want more medical schools."[156]

CASE saw the Ford arrangement as a counterweight to pressures from University Hospitals. A Ford affiliation, Pytte thought, would present less of a threat to the University Hospitals medical staff and administration than a similar arrangement with the Cleveland Clinic.[92] Nevertheless, some of the University Hospitals' doctors were angered by the affiliation with Ford and claimed they had not been consulted about it.[23] Preferring that students take their clinical assignments in Cleveland, and particularly at University Hospitals, Farah Walters and Adel Mahmoud, the chairman of medicine, opposed the arrangement.[117] William Anlyan, chairman of the committee retained by the Cleveland Foundation, thought that the school, in linking with Ford, was "looking for an affiliation to save face."[158]

The more than 150 miles around Lake Erie—thirty-five miles in a straight line across the lake[117]—which separated Cleveland from Detroit discouraged many CASE students from working at Ford. By 2003, the affiliation with its annual $500,000 support and NIH routing scheme had ended, and Ford proceeded to build an academic relationship with the nearby Wayne State medical school.[117,157]

Branding

University Hospitals' loyalists fret about the institution's less than outstanding rank in the *U.S. News & World Report* list of what the magazine calls the nation's "best hospitals." In 2004, University Hospitals of Cleveland missed appearing as one of the top fourteen on what the magazine calls its "honor roll," on which the Cleveland Clinic was fourth.[159] The highest-ranked services at University Hospitals of Cleveland are pediatrics (6), geriatrics (14), and cancer (14). In the 20s were pulmonary (20), cardiac care (20), orthopedics (21), neurology and neurosurgery (22), and endocrinology (23).[159]

The principal unit with national as well as regional name recognition is Rainbow Babies and Children's Hospital.[160]* "We were the hospital of choice in pediatrics," says Dr. William Speck, a former chief of pediatrics there.[160] "Rainbow's the only part of University Hospitals of Cleveland that has a specialty image," according to one of the clinical chairs.[53] Rainbow was built, according to Ellis Avner, the most recent former chairman of pediatrics, on superb programs in neonatology, cystic fibrosis, and developmental and behavioral pediatrics—Benjamin Spock was once associated with Rainbow.[14] "Our white coats identify us as members of both University Hospitals of Cleveland and of Rainbow," says Avner.[14]

Some ascribe the less than stellar ranking of University Hospitals of Cleveland by *U.S. News & World Report* partially to its name. Among the top seventeen—each of which, except the Cleveland Clinic, is, functionally, a university hospital—the public associates the medical centers with a specific name, often that of the universities with which they are affiliated. The name *University Hospitals of Cleveland* indicates no connection to CASE's school of medicine. Recognition of the name suffers, many believe, because it only includes the generic word *university* and the name of the city. Confusion with the Cleveland Clinic occurs frequently. Many even think that the Cleveland Clinic is CASE's university hospital.[23]

Accordingly, from time to time, leaders at the hospital and the university have considered changing the hospital's name. One of the most energetic attempts occurred in the fall of 2001, when the university offered to allow University Hospitals to use its name and become "CASE University Hospital." This change would have helped to distinguish the hospital from the other university hospitals throughout the nation and reverse the perception that the Cleveland Clinic was the principal specialty hospital in the city. The University Hospitals would accede to CASE's affiliating with the Clinic so long as a new and more equitable arrangement would be instituted for distribution of the overheads with a formula based on the location of the facilities in which the funded research was being conducted. The

---

*Farah Walters adds that the Ireland Cancer Center, the only cancer center in northern Ohio to have been designated a comprehensive cancer center by the NIH,[9] and the department of orthopedics have similar reputations.[66]

agreement also included provisions about distribution of credit for the research and how intellectual property, such as patents and royalties, would be shared.[91]

Farah Walters and her board accepted this arrangement,[91] including changing the name of the University Hospitals.[45] James Wagner, the interim president, and Charles Bolton, then chairman of the CASE trustees, supported the change as part of the proposed new agreement.[45] However, at its meeting in December 2001, the CASE board rejected it, the majority not wanting to share the CASE name and concluding that the university was acceding too much to the hospital.[57,161] Furthermore, the CASE trustees didn't want the university to even appear to own the hospital, a responsibility that they and their predecessors had continuously rejected, since ownership would require assuming such duties as liability and fundraising.[45] "What would happen if our name was on the hospital and we didn't control it?" one of the joint trustees asked, expressing what he believed many of his colleagues were thinking.[98]

By 2004, the new administration of the university, medical school, and health system reconsidered how to incorporate the name of the university into that of the medical enterprise without eliminating the name of University Hospitals of Cleveland, which has significant meaning to local citizens who have come to the hospital for treatment and given support to its activities since the middle of the nineteenth century. One possibility being considered was to name the medical campus the "CASE Medical Center," a structure that would include three entities, the university's medical and other schools involved in health care, University Hospitals of Cleveland, and a unified practice plan for the faculty. The hospital would retain its familiar name.[100,135]

MetroHealth System

When Farah Walters came to Cleveland, people would ask her whether she lived on the East Side or the West Side. "They almost seemed like two cities," she thought. "The East Side was more diverse with more professionals and senior businesspeople and a larger Jewish and African-American population. The West Side had more descendents of Eastern Europeans, was more Midwestern in outlook and more conservative."[2]

The geographical dividing line between East and West is the Cuyahoga River, which also separates Cleveland's major health care institutions.[5] On the East, almost adjacent to each other, are the Cleveland Clinic and University Hospitals of Cleveland, and on the West, the campus of the former municipal hospital, originally called City Hospital, Cleveland's first hospital, founded in 1837 and built with public funds.[162]

In 1958, the city transferred ownership of the hospital to Cuyahoga County, and in ensuing decades, the hospital added the Twin Towers and the Core and South buildings, which now house the patients and facilities needed for their care. In 1989, the institution became the MetroHealth System, which now includes the hospital with its 600 acute beds on the campus and 500 long-term beds elsewhere plus twelve primary care sites throughout the city, not in the suburbs where the Cleveland Clinic and University Hospitals have placed their peripheral outpatient facilities.[5] "They don't need me in the suburbs," explains Terry White, the former president and CEO.* A comprehensive outpatient building on the main campus opened three years later. The [Dr. Charles H.] Rammelkamp [Jr.] Center for Education and Research, a seven-storey facility completed in 1994, honors an early developer of antibiotic therapy and a much-admired physician at the hospital.[164]

Only 16 percent of Metro's patients have no insurance. Thirty-six percent have Medicaid, 30 percent private insurance, and 24 percent Medicare. Metro relies on public funding for less than 5 percent of its operating expenses.[5] Rather than create its own cardiac surgery program, Metro contracts with the Cleveland Clinic, whose surgeons perform these operations at the County Hospital.[47,165] "I'm not taking on the Clinic," says White. "I'm putting my resources elsewhere," as in trauma, neonatology, and emergency services.[5] The Clinic hired the director of the emergency department at Metro to also run its new emergency service.[5,47] "Terry versus Farah helped to drive this business to the Clinic," says Richard Olds, former chairman of medicine at Metro.[47]†

By the beginning of the twenty-first century, the medical staff at Metro consisted of 300 full-time physicians, each a member of the faculty of the

*White retired from Metro in December 2003.[163]

†Olds is now chairman of the department of medicine at The Medical College of Wisconsin in Milwaukee.[47]

CASE medical school with which the County Hospital, now Metro, affiliated in 1914.* Unlike at University Hospitals, the physicians at Metro belong to a consolidated practice plan.[16] Currently, the staff at Metro, the favorite site of many of the medical students for training,[47,167] provides 40 percent of the clinical teaching for CASE.[5]

Metro and the university now function under an affiliation agreement of January 11, 1993, which designated Metro as "a principal hospital affiliation for education and research activities associated with CASE's academic programs."[168] The agreement provides, among other features, that the dean of the school of medicine appoints the directors of the clinical departments at Metro who report for educational programs to the academic chairmen based at University Hospitals.[168]

This agreement angered many of the faculty at University Hospitals of Cleveland[11,92,169–171] and was one of the reasons that the chairs prepared the letter of no confidence in Pytte.† In addition to objecting to the independence from the chairs at the medical school that the agreement appeared to guarantee to the Metro chairs, they didn't like the use of the word *principal* in referring to the affiliation with Metro;[23] the union with University Hospitals was the *primary* affiliation.[21] To Dean Cherniak it seemed that "the same thing had been promised to both hospitals."[21] He concluded that Pytte, while favoring a multihospital system, didn't really want formal relationships between CASE and University Hospitals.[21] Pytte explained to a reporter for *The Plain Dealer*, "We obviously want to work with more than one hospital, but UH is the closest historically and geographically. It's also important for the [medical] school to have additional venues to offer the students."[171]

Just as the 1993 agreement with Metro irritated the clinical chairs at University Hospitals, CASE's 1992 agreement with University Hospitals perturbed leaders at Metro, who wanted more recognition and equality for the faculty working there and a greater portion of the overheads from grants to flow through Metro rather than the university.[166] The displeasure between Metro and University Hospital was even more intense, according to Farah Walters. Based on her experience working at Metro during the 1970s and

---

*In the spring of 2005, the full-time clinical staff of the CASE medical school at University Hospitals of Cleveland, Metro, and the Veterans Administration Hospital numbered 1,339.[166,166a]

†See chapter 3.

1980s, "Metro hated UH but loved the Clinic. The docs at Metro felt the docs at University lorded it over them. The hostilities were unbelievable."[2] At one point, Walters considering merging Metro with UH. This would have presented considerable difficulties if only because Metro was a governmental hospital and University a private institution.

Cardiac Services

In December 1995, a for-profit company based in Philadelphia bought Mt. Sinai Hospital in Cleveland,[172] "a fine community hospital long affiliated with CASE's medical school," as described by Dr. Richard Aach, former director of the department of medicine there.[11] The purchaser pledged to maintain the level of service for which the hospital had become known. Soon after the new owner took over the hospital, however, a group of cardiologists there concluded that the pledge would not be honored and started looking for a new home.*

They met with Fred Loop, Eric Topol, and Alan London at the Cleveland Clinic and with Farah Walters and Adel Mahmoud at University Hospitals and CASE. Mahmoud needed to "buy market share in cardiology in Cleveland,"[44] and Adler and his group could bring a well-insured group of patients to University Hospitals. Mahmoud had concluded that UH "couldn't build a clinical practice from below against the Cleveland Clinic."[44]

The Mt. Sinai cardiologists decided to join CASE[176] because, as Dale Adler, the leader of the seven-member group, explains, "At University Hospitals, we could shape the division."[182] At the Clinic, Topol was running the de-

---

*The for-profit company that bought Mt. Sinai and so distressed many of the doctors there filed for bankruptcy in March 1999[173] and closed the hospital a year later.[174] The sequence of events leading to this dénouement, as thoroughly detailed in an article in *The Plain Dealer* on March 20, 2000, makes lamentable reading.[175] Meanwhile, several doctors, in addition to Adler and his group, moved to University Hospitals.[176,177]

University Hospitals wanted to buy Mt. Sinai—in part to obtain Sinai's ambulatory care facility in one of the upscale suburbs, which the Clinic would later acquire[54]—and might have done so had Farah Walters and her trustees been able to convince the Sinai board to include a more substantial part of the hospital's endowment in the deal.[72] The Sinai trustees, however, insisted on converting a larger amount into an independent charity than was acceptable to University Hospitals.[8] Walters and her trustees were also concerned that buying Mt. Sinai, which was having financial problems, would jeopardize the bond rating of University Hospitals.[54] In 2001, CASE bought the Mt. Sinai real estate,[11,178–180] which the university is now developing for medical research, biotechnical commercialization, and public health.[181]

partment, and the group would have had less influence as a part of that large cardiology program.

So on November 1, 1997, Adler and his colleagues brought their size-able practice to the University Hospitals of Cleveland. One of the terms on which Adler insisted was that he become chief of cardiology. Accordingly, Mahmoud informed Dr. Marc Thames, then the division chief, that he would be replaced,[58] citing, as his reason, Thames's difficulty in recruiting clinicians and investigators.[137] As consolation, he was offered the leadership of a new research institute, for which, Thames said, no additional funding was supplied.[58]

Thames says that Adler treated the faculty whom Thames had led "as if they were turkeys," a characterization of their qualities that the former chief specifically refutes.[58] Thames thought the group from Mt. Sinai mediocre and "not at the cutting edge."[58] Furthermore, Thames said, Adler's unit "came in with guaranteed salaries significantly higher than my colleagues were making. After the guarantees ended, their compensation would depend on the success of their practices."[58] By 2003, when their salary guarantees were concluding, five of the seven original recruits who had come with Adler from Sinai had left, three entering private practice and two moving to the Cleveland Clinic.[58]

One of the five who left was Joel Holland, for reasons similar to those of his colleague Michael Rocco.* The department of medicine's recruitment of the Mt. Sinai cardiology group was greeted by "enormous hostility. The place wasn't ready for us, and we were marginalized," Holland remembers. "They were the worst two years of my professional life. As soon as my contract was up, I took some time off, then called Eric [Topol], joined the group practice, and moved to the Clinic,"[183] where Holland contentedly practices general cardiology in the Beachwood ambulatory site and admits his patients to and attends at the main campus.

Deeply dissatisfied with how he and his colleagues had been treated, Thames departed to become chief of cardiology at Temple University in Philadelphia.[58]

Academic veterans will recognize that the changes in cardiology did not follow the usual pattern for the recruitment of the head of one of the largest

---

*See chapter 2.

divisions in the department of medicine at a school with a scholarly tradition. No search was conducted, and the new chief was a clinician, not an investigator. Such a choice, however, does not surprise close observers of the current state of academic cardiology in many medical schools.

For several decades, cardiology divisions generated sizeable surpluses, thanks to the generous amounts that insurers paid for the tests and procedures that these specialists perform. Departments of medicine taxed the clinical income of cardiology divisions to support less financially productive specialties. As the amounts insurers—and particularly Medicare starting in 1997—paid to these doctors dropped, the surpluses decreased, and, in some cases vanished. In the business jargon adopted by medical school leaders, cardiology divisions that were formerly "profit centers" became "cost centers," now requiring support from the department or the hospital. The pressure on chairmen and deans to assure that these divisions succeed financially became so overpowering that, in more than one school, the traditional recruitment of a chief with a distinguished research career gave way to the appointment of a clinician who could assure the admission of a continuing flow of patients to keep the beds full, the laboratories of the university hospital busy, and the surgeons gainfully employed.

By spring of 2005, cardiology at CASE had grown to include thirty-two full-time faculty members working at the University Hospitals, the Veterans Administration Hospital, and the community hospitals affiliated with the system.[12] The primary care physicians employed by University Hospitals and working in surrounding communities refer many of the patients for whom the University Hospitals cardiologists provide care.[12] The cardiologists perform almost 4,000 procedures per year in the cardiac catheterization laboratories at several sites, a respectable number for any medical school although only half as many as are performed at the Cleveland Clinic. Adler believes that he and his colleagues provide their patients with a complete service—"we're very patient oriented. The Clinic is more encounter-driven" since so many are sent to the Clinic for procedures.[12] In addition to his responsibility to lead a major division in a research-oriented medical center, Adler maintains a large personal practice and sees patients from 2:00 p.m. to 8:30 p.m. three or four days per week.[12]

As for cardiac surgery "in this town and in the United States," says James Schulak, Jerry Shuck's immediate successor as chairman of the department of surgery, "it's the Clinic."[53] As expected, the Clinic's dominance in this high-volume, high-profile, high-paying specialty distressed Farah Walters. University Hospitals had developed a program in cardiovascular surgery that was delivering fine care to its patients, but the volume was low, and Walters wanted to compete more successfully in this work with the Clinic. So she took the lead.

"One day," says Schulak—the date was January 10, 1998—"we learned that Farah had recruited Bob Stewart to head cardiac transplant and Tom Kirby to lead lung transplants."[53] Stewart and Kirby were then directing these activities at the Cleveland Clinic and would become co-chiefs of a newly created cardiothoracic surgery department at University Hospitals of Cleveland on February 15.[184] As with Adler in medical cardiology, the surgeons were not selected through the usual academic process of a search committee. "These appointments were opportunistic," says Walters, explaining that speed was essential. Several senior members of the faculty, including surgery chair Jerry Shuck, hospital chief of staff Robert Daroff,* and the dean, Nathan Berger, Walters says, interviewed them and "gave them their blessings."[68]

Since cities the size of Cleveland tend to have only one large cardiac transplant program—the Clinic had performed ninety-one transplants during the previous year, Stewart operating on half of the patients—University Hospitals engaged in some spinning in *The Plain Dealer* to explain why they needed such a program. "We think it's offering an alternative," the newspaper quoted a hospital spokesman, who denied that another transplant program would duplicate services at the Clinic.[184]

Meanwhile, to make way for Stewart and Kirby, who had been hired at very generous salaries,[185] it was necessary to dislodge Dr. Alexander Geha, the chief of cardiac surgery since 1986.[29] Geha says that he never received an official letter relieving him.[29] He remembers Shuck telling him, "What can we do? This is what Farah wants."[29] Dean Berger couldn't help either, saying to Geha, "We have to go along."[29] Geha then appealed to university president Pytte, who told him that although "he couldn't interfere with division director's appointments, he would not approve the creation of a department of cardiothoracic surgery under the direction of Walters's re-

---

*In 2004, Daroff's term as chief of staff at University Hospitals of Cleveland ended, and he was then appointed interim vice dean for education and academic affairs in the medical school.[24]

cruits."[29] A few months later Geha left University Hospitals to direct cardiothoracic surgery at the University of Illinois at Chicago.[29]

Geha was not the only cardiac surgeon to leave. Pediatric surgeons Philip Smith, the chief of the specialty, since 1998, and Michael Spector, decamped from Rainbow for the Akron Children's Hospital, thirty miles away. "I left because there was no leadership in our division. The whole place was a shambles," Spector said. "Kirby was hiring his friends and forcing everybody else out. Every one had special deals with the administration, and it was no longer a cohesive, directed group as it was under Dr. Geha."[186] Several pediatric cardiologists and members of their supporting staff, including the perfusionists who operate the heart-lung machines, departed with them.[185]

Thus, the same sequence of events had occurred in both medical and surgical cardiology. The relevant departments had recruited clinicians from elsewhere in town and displaced those then leading the programs at University Hospitals. This effort to build a strong cardiac surgery program failed. Early in 2001, Walters removed Kirby as co-chief of the division and head of the lung transplant program. Of the few patients operated upon, the results had been disappointing. Then on April 26, 2002, the hospital suspended Kirby "for unspecified charges," as *The Plain Dealer* reported, "relating to the hospital's code of conduct and policies."[187]* Kirby asked a court to order his reinstatement and compensate him for loss of income.[189] The hospital responded by upholding the suspension and listing his alleged transgressions.[190] Criticizing an article in the newspaper that detailed the turmoil among the cardiothoracic surgeons at the hospital,[191] Walters accused Kirby of recruiting friends and unqualified candidates and wrote that he "was demoted for his managerial incompetence."[192] The newspaper countered with an editorial stating, "it is clear that the hospital's top management is far from blameless."[193] Walters acknowledges that hiring Kirby was "the biggest mistake I made."[68]

Walters then named Dr. Alan Markowitz as Kirby's successor with the title of co-chief of cardiothoracic surgery. Markowitz had come from Mt. Sinai Hospital with cardiologist Dale Adler and his group to University Hospitals,

---

*Another cardiac surgeon, whom Kirby had recruited for one of the community hospitals in the health system, was fired at about this time after what the newspaper called "months of contentious discussions about his compensation." The surgeon had been hired with a guaranteed annual salary of $750,000.[188]

where he had trained in cardiac surgery. Kirby sued Markowitz for defama-
tion. In 2003, Kirby withdrew the suit,[87] but several others related to the
hospital's cardiac surgery problems continued in litigation.[187,194]

By February 2002, the hospital had volunteered to stop its cardiac transplant service after a series of unexpected deaths among the patients.[187] After
a comprehensive independent review, the cardiac transplant program was
reinstated.[66] The department, which had lost its accreditation for training
residents in cardiothoracic surgery in the fall of that year, regained this
right by July 1, 2004.[87,195]

Markowitz's cardiac surgical practice is relatively busy—about 300 cases
per year—and is heavily supported by referrals from his colleagues in the
cardiology division who moved with him from Mt. Sinai to University
Hospitals. Stewart's practice is smaller, developed from individual referrals from community physicians. He receives little business from the Sinai
group and, according to Geha, never brought patients from the Cleveland
Clinic as Walters had expected him to do.[29] Nevertheless, says Stewart, who
practiced at the Cleveland Clinic for years, "I'd rather practice at University Hospitals than at the Clinic. I'm a better doctor here, able to spend
more time with the patients and their families."[196] Stewart believes that the
"overwhelming force" at University Hospitals is patient and family satisfaction.* "Patients want to spend more time with their surgeons than is possible with the busy Clinic schedule, where we mostly first saw them when
they were asleep in the OR."[196] Patients whom other University Hospitals
physicians had referred to the Clinic for surgery sometimes reported that,
although their operations had been very successful, they found the place
impersonal and that they seldom, if ever, saw their surgeons.[58]

Emergency Services

Unlike the Cleveland Clinic, which until the 1990s, did not cater to
community patients with little or no insurance, University Hospitals of
Cleveland's emergency department had long provided service for such patients through its primitive but busy emergency ward. For decades, those
directing the hospital withheld investing in emergency services and left the

---

*The Cleveland Health Quality Choice Report and the Ohio Hospital Association cited Univer-
sity Hospitals of Cleveland as the highest-ranked institution in northeast Ohio in patient satisfaction[9] and consequently superior in this respect to the Cleveland Clinic.

professional care there to groups of private practitioners, few of whom were formally trained in the growing specialty of emergency medicine.[197]

"I always pushed hard for a better emergency department," said Farah Walters, "but this was politically tough to do. Finally, I realized that the band-aids wouldn't work any longer."[10] The hospital wanted to develop a first-class emergency department that could attract well-insured patients, many of whom would require admission for well-paying clinical services, and not only the Medicaid and uninsured patients then occupying beds better filled financially by those with better-paying forms of health insurance. That half of the beds in University Hospitals were filled with patients transferred from the emergency department—which admits about 18 percent of those who visit there—attests to its importance as a source of patients for the hospital.[197] Walters convinced her board to renovate the department and specialize the care there with a full cadre of emergency medicine physicians. Many trustees had observed the inadequacies of University Hospitals' emergency care through their own experiences and that of their relatives and friends.

Accordingly, University Hospitals of Cleveland recruited a leader of the emergency department fully trained in emergency medicine to replace the nonspecialists there, create a training program in the specialty, and convert the unit from a community to an academic program. The hospital hired Dr. Edward Michelson as the first full-time director of the emergency department in March 2002.[197] Michelson, most recently the director of the residency training program at Northwestern, would now manage the emergency department in the last of the teaching hospitals in the professional organization known as the Council of Teaching Hospitals (COTH) to conduct its emergency care with specialists and train doctors to become emergency physicians.[197]

Michelson hopes that the hospital will soon approve the construction of a building adjacent to the hospital complex to house a new emergency department. "We have a 'challenged' emergency department now," the new director describes his unit, "which does not afford privacy or the level of service expected by suburban, insured patients."[197] Michelson is lobbying for adequate parking space and all appropriate amenities to attract the class of patients all hospitals need to succeed.

CHAPTER FIVE

University Hospitals of Cleveland
New Leaders

A Psychiatrist-President

On January 17, 2002, the trustees of CASE University elected Dr. Edward Hundert, dean of the school of medicine at the University of Rochester, to become president of the university.[1] Hundert would thereby become CASE's third president in eighteen months.[2]

The new CASE president had received his bachelor's degree (summa cum laude, Phi Beta Kappa in his junior year) in mathematics and the history of science and medicine from Yale* and then attended Oxford University as a Marshall Scholar, receiving his degree with first-class honors in the School of Philosophy, Politics, and Economics. Hundert earned his medical degree from Harvard, trained in psychiatry at the Harvard-affiliated Belmont Hospital, and then became a faculty member and associate dean at Harvard. Though Hundert became the first medical doctor to be president of CASE,[5] this possibility had been previously considered. The dean of the College of

---

*A new president from Yale fits with Western Reserve's once calling itself "the Yale of the West."[3] Yale had long been a favorite college for the sons of leading Cleveland citizens, reflecting historically that the region had once been part of the Connecticut Western Reserve.[4]

Physicians and Surgeons at Columbia University, Herbert Pardes, who had been offered but rejected the CASE presidency before David Auston accepted the job, is, like Hundert, a psychiatrist.*

Described as "a breath of fresh air,"[7] "bright and personable,"[8] "having extraordinary vision,"[9] "easy to work with, someone who takes action and gets things done,"[10] able to "energize people to achieve his goals,"[9] and "committed to education," Hundert teaches undergraduates,[8] an activity not typical of many university presidents. Terry White, the CEO at Metro when Hundert took over, lauded the president's visiting his hospital several times and his willingness to take the initiative,[11] a characteristic that has helped to resolve many of the troubles afflicting CASE's medical center. Considering Metro's experiences with his immediate predecessors, CASE would benefit from Hundert's "expertise as a teacher bringing people together."[12]

Like Pytte before him, Hundert believed that CASE had to strengthen its undergraduate body, which was relatively uncompetitive at the time when compared with the universities that Hundert had attended. CASE suffered in the national rankings because of the large number of acceptances required to fill its classes.[13]†

Despite his exceptional scholarly credentials, observers wondered why CASE had chosen someone with so little administrative experience. Hundert had only been dean of a medical school for two years and had not filled the typical pre-presidential roles of provost at a research university or president of a smaller university or college. One answer is that Hundert is a doctor—CASE's first physician-president[5]—and thus, everyone hoped, should be more able to resolve the longstanding, festering problems with the medical school and its affiliated hospitals.[15,16]‡ And this is what happened, and surprisingly quickly.[18]

"We chose Ed Hundert primarily because of his outstanding qualifica-

*Pardes, former chairman of the department of psychiatry at Columbia, is now CEO of New York–Presbyterian Hospital. Another physician, radiologist William Brody, was chosen president of the Johns Hopkins University, partly to resolve a ruinous conflict afflicting its medical center in the mid-1990s.[6]

† *U.S. News & World Report* ranked CASE thirty-fifth among the nation's national universities offering doctoral programs, just one place below the University of Rochester, Hundert's previous institution. (Yale, where he received his bachelor's degree, is number three, and Harvard, with its medical school he attended, number one.[14])

‡ One of the university trustees, Richard Watson, wondered if Hundert's being a psychiatrist wasn't "more important than his just being a physician."[17]

tions," one of the trustees explained, "but we were also thinking that we would be pilloried if we 'settled' for an insider."[19] A leading candidate to succeed Auston was the acting president, James Wagner, the provost. In 2003, Wagner became president of Emory University.

Some wonder if Hundert, described by one of the deans in the medical school as "something of a wizard,"[20] has his eye on leading a more prestigious university someday. "He told me," said Dr. Ralph Horwitz, the new dean of the medical school, "that he is committed to his children's graduating from Shaker High," a process requiring ten years.[9]

Walters Leaves

On April 11, 2002, Farah Walters announced her retirement in June after completing ten years as CEO of University Hospitals of Cleveland and its health system.[21]* The community was beginning to suspect that Walters's tenure would end when *The Plain Dealer* reported in late February, "There are discussions with UH's board members about Farah's longevity" and that "the affiliation is being drawn up with the idea that she'll be gone."[23]†

Longtime hospital trustee Catharine Lewis, who is the wife of former CASE board chairman John Lewis, said, "I was on the search committee to select Farah, and I still think we made the right choice. She understood medical economics and accomplished great things for us by starting and developing the system and the primary care group. But she's a fighter and was perceived to be one. The people in the hospital were telling me horror stories about the culture of fear that was developing. Farah cared so much, but style can make such a difference."[25] Lewis advised banker Henry Meyer, Dick Pogue's successor as chairman of the hospital and health system boards, that it was time for Farah to leave. "There comes a time for a different person to integrate and collaborate," she said. "Farah couldn't do this."[25]

"Farah had survived for eight years because she was an outstanding CEO," says Meyer. "Farah's style of management worked for University

---

*When she left, according to *The Plain Dealer,* the hospital agreed to pay Walters her 2002 salary of $744,662 for three years and $3.8 million in retirement benefits paid out over seven years.[22]

†Edward Hundert denies the rumor that he had insisted that Walters leave before he would accept the university presidency.[24]

Hospitals when we were smaller but didn't work as well as we got bigger."[26] The more troubled finances of delivering medical care beginning in the late 1990s meant that the surpluses that the trustees had become accustomed to receive under the Walters administration were disappearing. "If Farah's personality had been more reasonable," said one of the trustees, "the dollars alone wouldn't have driven her out."

Faculty members speculate whether Walters voluntarily resigned or was forced out. Huntington Willard, the first director of the research institute, said that she was not fired and that the board was "trying to keep her on. But the affiliation discussions were building up, and it was time."[2] The medical school dean Nathan Berger surmised that "her board felt that a durable agreement could never come about with her in the job."[27] "She overplayed her hand," said one of the joint trustees.[3]

Henry Meyer, the man empowered as chairman of the hospital board to relieve her, said, "I didn't fire her, and I would not have been proud if I had done so, but I was probing what she was doing. I had told the board in executive session that I would meet with her in July and discuss her leaving early. While the situation was deteriorating, Farah made the first move."[26] She resigned but not before advising the board to review Meyer's performance, according to Meyer. Walters denies that she said this. "What I did do was to recommend setting up a governance committee of the board, regardless of who was the chair."[28] Meyer says, "I became Farah's enemy. She told people, 'Henry's doing my job.' She didn't like the board interfering."[26]

Despite Dick Pogue's role, while chairman of the University Hospitals board, in sustaining Walters's job over the years, their relationship did not survive her leaving. "I believe I saw her only once after the one-year affiliation agreement was signed," he said in 2004.[29]* In trying to explain how she stayed in her job so long despite the opposition Walters engendered, a senior faculty member said, "She had a board that backed her and a dean who wouldn't fight her."

Although Walters's leaving was received with relief by some, most of the staff and employees with whom she had worked praised her for her many accomplishments. "I received more than 1,500 letters," she remembers.

---

*Compared with Pogue, Walters says, "I had a much better working relationship and received better advice, insights, and support from Bill Reynolds and Henry Meyer."[30] Reynolds was chairman of the hospital board before Pogue and Meyer afterward.

"There was a huge hospital-wide party; thousands showed up. Some of the staff had tears in their eyes as they said good-bye."[28] The staff prepared a videotape in which several of her leading colleagues praised her work.

New System and Hospital Directors

The hospital trustees decided that Walters's job should be divided into two parts, the structure that Pogue had tried unsuccessfully to convince her to accept several years previously.[31] The board would select a CEO of the University Hospitals Health System who would appoint a director of University Hospitals of Cleveland.[32] It was said that the selection committee was encountering difficulty convincing some particularly qualified candidates to apply or to accept the position if offered because of the turmoil.*

In December, the board appointed Thomas Zenty[34] as CEO of the University Hospitals Health System, effective March 1, 2003.[35] Catharine Lewis, who had participated as a trustee on the selection committees that chose both Walters and Zenty, felt the candidates were much better qualified in 2002 than in 1992. "They were more knowledgeable, more experienced at other systems, and had a greater awareness of the needs of the doctors and how to deal with them. In just ten years, medicine had become a very different world to function in."[25] Lewis remembers that many members of the selection committee initially wanted a doctor for the job. "We then moved away when we found in Tom the skills and experience we needed in someone with a proper style of operation. He was our first choice."[25] One of the senior faculty described him as having "a very different style from Farah. He's engaging, clear when he speaks, and uses crisp words—a no nonsense guy."

Zenty came to Cleveland from Cedars-Sinai Hospital in Los Angeles, where he had been chief operating officer. "My responsibilities were to function as the business unit leader since there was only one CEO for the system. Tom Priselac, my boss, had responsibility for the entire Cedars-Sinai Health System."[36] In selecting a CEO from outside Cleveland, the

---

*Despite their efforts to keep the search committee's deliberations private, officials at University Hospital could not have been pleased to read in a *Plain Dealer* column: "University Hospitals is down to finalists for its top job: an outside candidate . . . and Dr. Fred Rothstein, the interim chief executive appointed when Farah Walters left in June. . . . If the board can't strike a deal with that [outside] candidate, then Rothstein—who has been praised as a 'good listener,' in contrast to the headstrong Walters—will become CEO of University Hospitals Health System."[33]

health system trustees were taking the risk of giving the job to someone unfamiliar with the local scene. John Morley, the chairman of the search committee, saw this as an advantage, telling a reporter for *Crain's Cleveland Business* that Zenty's appointment will bring an outsider's perspective to University Hospitals. "We pretty much have been doing our own thing in northeast Ohio for a long time."[5]

At the Cleveland Clinic, however, some anticipate problems with University Hospitals' choice. "Cleveland's quite provincial in many ways, certainly different from LA," said one of the staff there. "Tom will have to learn the hard way." Zenty acknowledges that the Los Angeles market "is much different from Cleveland. It's a very competitive environment . . . which has not yet consolidated."[37]

Zenty's priorities would be different from those required of Farah Walters when she took over the hospitals and created the health system during the 1990s.[38] While she was CEO, the system expanded its assets of $400 million to $2 billion. More attention was paid during these years to size than to profitability. Emphasis would shift to assimilating the different entities— the last purchase had occurred in 2000.[39] Needed now was what trustee John Morley described as "integration, consolidation, team building, and planning rather than acquisition."[40]

To reverse the financial losses ($100 million on operations during just the two years from 2001 to 2003) Zenty arranged, in December 2003, to close St. Michael's Hospital, which had consistently lost money—more than $6 million that year[41]—and whose beds were increasingly empty.[42] As has accompanied the threat of other hospital closings,[43] Zenty's decision brought objections from members of the public, including congressman Dennis Kucinich, the former mayor of Cleveland who was then a presidential candidate.[42*] The St. Michael's episode introduced the new CEO from Los Angeles to the political complications of working in Cleveland.[46]

To stanch the operating losses and eventually repair the downgrading of University Hospitals Health System's bond rating,[47] Zenty retained Navi-

---

*When the bankrupt Pennsylvania firm that had formerly owned St. Michael's threatened to close it in 2000, Kucinich "brokered a deal," as an article in *The Plain Dealer* reported,[44] that led to its purchase at public auction by University Hospitals Health System.[42,45] Farah Walters had bought St. Michaels[45] after it became known that the Cleveland Clinic, if it had purchased St. Michael's, would close it. Adding the hospital to the University Hospitals Health System proved very expensive since St. Michael's, both when purchased and afterward, consistently lost money.

gant Consulting* for a twelve-week assignment.[36] Zenty insisted, reporter Diane Solov wrote in *The Plain Dealer,* that the group had not been brought to Cleveland "for crisis management," but rather "to compare costs, expenses and staffing levels with similar health systems across the country," a process known as "benchmarking."[41] "We want them to save us money," he explained.[36]

As Zenty went about consolidating rather than expanding the health system, he proceeded, unlike his predecessor, to appoint a director of University Hospitals of Cleveland, thereby splitting the two positions of CEO of the health system from president of the hospital as the trustees desired. With the strong support of the hospital and health system boards and the senior faculty, Zenty chose Dr. Fred Rothstein, acting CEO of the health system since the resignation of Walters, to direct University Hospitals of Cleveland.[26,50]

Walters had brought Rothstein, the former chief of pediatric gastroenterology at Rainbow[51] and then chief of pediatrics and vice president for medical affairs at Mt. Sinai Hospital in Cleveland, to be a senior vice president of the hospitals in 1996.[50] "Farah recruited Fred away from us," remembers Robert Shakno, the Sinai CEO at the time. "A real blessing for University Hospitals."[52] Described by a colleague in pediatrics as "an excellent specialist and a decent, capable administrator,"[51] and by a former senior university leader as "terrific,"[53] Rothstein had won the support of the search committee members,[54] which, in the words of its chairman, "felt it was highly desirable that a doctor should lead the hospital."[55] Trustee Catharine Lewis added, "We needed an M.D. in one of the top positions to heal, and Fred had started the healing process. We insisted that we wanted to keep him."[25]

A New Dean

Farah Walters having left, Nathan Berger departed from the deanship at the end of the 2002 academic year.[15] "It seemed clear to me," Berger explained, "that the community felt new leadership would usher in a new

---

*Navigant now includes what was formerly called "The Hunter Group," consultants whom CEOs and hospital trustees often engage when hospitals are generating red ink. Among the clients who have retained the Hunter Group are UCSF Stanford Health Care, the short-lived merger of the University of California, San Francisco Medical Center, the Stanford University hospitals,[48] and the University of Pennsylvania.[49]

era."[27]* With the exodus of the leaders of the medical school and health system, the university and its principal teaching hospital were prepared for significant change under CASE's new physician-president. Most agree that the presence of Edward Hundert was essential for resolving the most pressing controversies afflicting the medical school and University Hospitals.[16] His influence was thought so important that he has been called the "architect" of what followed.[56]

In January 2003, CASE University announced that Ralph Horwitz, an internist and epidemiologist and chairman of the department of medicine at Yale, would become the next dean of the school of medicine.[57]† Horwitz, in a break from the pattern in recent decades of selecting the dean from among members of the faculty,[58] would also become the first director of the restructured research institute that Farah Walters had founded at the end of the troubled 1990s.[59] Acquiring complete control over research at CASE and the hospital[24,60,61] raised his status within the medical school beyond that of his immediate predecessors.[18]

The hospitals agreed not to pursue Walters's plan of separately administering NIH grants for research conducted there. "It did not make sense for us to duplicate infrastructure activity," says Rothstein, who adds, "the school should be in charge of research, the hospitals in charge of clinical care."[10] University Hospitals of Cleveland continues to administer grants supported by industry for clinical research conducted in the hospitals.[10] The dean would now, in Hundert's words, "be in charge of all research and [laboratory] space."[24]‡

Since he is not a "wet-lab" scientist,[62] Horwitz will appoint a vice dean for research, a basic investigator to assist him in developing this part of the school's program.[63] Jonathan Karn, chairman of the department of molecular biology and microbiology since August 2002,[64] finds that the new dean has "an intense curiosity about basic science and respect for those who do it."[63] "Ralph wants what we want," says Lynn Landmesser, chair of the department of neurosciences. "He'll be an articulate, strong spokesman for

---

*Berger became director of the Center for Science, Health & Society, a unit within the medical school with the goals of making Cleveland a healthier city, educating citizens to help them become better health care consumers, and stimulating more people to enter health careers.[27]

†Another CASE leader from Yale.

‡If Agnar Pytte had given such strong support to his medical school deans as Hundert now demonstrated toward Horwitz, several faculty members suggested, Cherniak and Berger could have been more successful in overcoming Walters's dominance of the medical center.

the school."[65] Improving the research productivity of the school, however, would require significant investment in programs and faculty.

Horwitz decided to eliminate the requirement that 60 percent of the medical students be residents of Ohio and instructed the admissions committee to ignore this factor as a criterion for admitting the class.[66–68] This change would allow the school to recruit more outstanding students from throughout the country.[66–68] Horwitz brought this about by "executing a brilliant strategy," as president Edward Hundert describes the effort.[69] The dean convinced members of the state's board of regents and officials from the governor's office that bringing outstanding students from throughout the country to Cleveland and instituting curricular changes linking research to public health and population medicine—two topics of particular interest to Horwitz[70]—would help to reverse the unfortunate "brain drain" of talent from Cleveland and Ohio.[69] The school would regularly report to the state on the progress of this program.[71]

As for the complaint that too much of the wealth of the medical enterprise flows from the hospital and school to the university, Horwitz responds, "That's a constant grievance at most schools" but may now be changing at CASE. The university and the University Hospitals have each pledged to invest $5 million per year for five years to recruit new faculty members.[9,72] "We have an unfortunate legacy of skepticism and cynicism," Horwitz acknowledges. "What's needed is not a patching over of the wounds and infighting but deeds that will prove to the faculty that we can change."[9]

One of the wounds needing attention was the multiple practice plans operated by each of the clinical departments. By 2004, several were losing money, and the new leadership of both the hospital and the medical school knew that they must deal with this vexing, longstanding anomaly. The health system, in particular, needing to reduce its costs, wanted the practices to prosper so that it could decrease its subsidies to the departments. Accordingly, the new leaders, dean Ralph Horwitz and hospital president Fred Rothstein, asked the clinical chairmen to form a committee—it is being led by neurology chairman Dennis Landis—to evaluate models and then recommend how a single practice plan could be instituted.[10,73]

The chairmen, at last, seemed resigned to participating in a uniform plan. When asked why they were now willing to relinquish personal direction of the departmental plans, Landis explained, "It's financial."[60] In addition to the decreasing reimbursements for clinical services, malpractice insurance premiums in Ohio have increased greatly.* "Since most of the plans now lose rather than make money,[60,74] independence is a less important issue."[74]

Politics, as usual, influenced one of the committee's most important decisions. As one of the chairmen explained, "There's a tug of war between UH and the school about the practice plans. Zenty wants all the practicing docs to be hospital employees like at the Clinic. Ralph doesn't like this."

An Affiliation Agreement, at Last

By December 2002, the University Hospitals of Cleveland and CASE University finally adopted an affiliation agreement, a fifty-year official relationship[75,76] in which the flow of funds between the institutions would be open to renegotiation every five years.[69] The accord, it was hoped, would resolve part of the angst that had roiled the medical school and its primary teaching hospital for decades.

Despite the high-sounding language—"to promote innovative biomedical education, research and clinical care as the nucleus around which to bring together available resources to develop one of the top academic medical centers in the world"[75]—the agreement's principal immediate accomplishment was resolving the governance of the University Hospital Research Institute and of research in general throughout the University Hospitals and school. All medical research on the campus would now be conducted under the aegis of the CASE Research Institute, the new hospital–medical school joint venture directed by the dean of the school of medicine. All federal indirects would be channeled through the university.

The new agreement also prescribed that the university would acquire a 50 percent interest in the $115 million research building from the University Hospitals Health System,[76,77] and the building would no longer be restricted to use by clinical researchers working in University Hospitals, as Farah Walters had planned.[60] By 2004, the university, using borrowed money and philanthropy, had bought the hospital's portion and became the sole owner of the building. CASE also agreed to support eighty new research faculty during the next five years. With the conflicts of the recent

---

*Cleveland joins Chicago and Philadelphia in having some of the highest rates for malpractice insurance among American cities.[10]

past resolved, Iris S. and Bert L. Wolstein donated $25 million for the building, which would be named for them.[69,78,79]

The founders hoped that the "Partnership," as the institutions described the relationship, would provide a basis for many forms of academic and administrative cooperation not possible because of the previous quarrels. The dominance of the chairmen at University Hospitals of Cleveland decreased slightly under the new agreement. Nominations for faculty recruitments and promotions from Metro and the other affiliated hospitals would flow directly from the chairmen there to the dean's office, thereby bypassing the chairmen at University Circle.[51]

After years of controversy, the Clinic and the university agreed to establish a new medical college program at the Cleveland Clinic whose students would receive their M.D. degrees from CASE.[80,81]* CASE would also award master's and doctoral degrees for research conducted in the research facilities of the Clinic under the supervision of Clinic investigators.[82] In addition, the university would bring the Clinic's cancer center under the umbrella of CASE's Comprehensive Cancer Center grant from the NIH.[82]

In describing how he wanted the medical school and University Hospitals to relate to each other, Hundert said, "We'll operate under a 'declaration of interdependence.' "[24] To facilitate this new relationship, Hundert and Rothstein, then the interim CEO of University Hospitals Health System and president of University Hospitals of Cleveland, visited another well-known academic medical center with a governance structure similar to that in Cleveland and spent much time together developing the details of the new relationship.

Among these activities, Hundert and Rothstein spent a whole day together at a club reviewing the problems that had alienated their two institutions from each other during the past decade and a half. They invited the chief financial officers from the university and the University Hospitals to join them for lunch. "You are now a team," the president and CEO assured them.[24] The team then gave the same PowerPoint presentation separately to the two boards, Rothstein to the health system trustees and Hundert to the university trustees. The boards quickly approved the new partnership. Their work together convinced Hundert that Rothstein understood well "what a great teaching hospital is."[69]

---

*See chapter 6.

As Frank Linsalata, then vice chairman and later chairman of the university board, remembers, "Ed took control. We finally had someone who had real knowledge of the NIH, overheads, practice plans, house officers, medical students—all the things we amateurs were trying to understand and deal with. Hundert and Rothstein were now the point guards."[61]

The mood at the medical center had brightened. As James Schulak, the former chairman of surgery said, "We're hopeful and optimistic now."[83] The prediction of Jerold Goldberg, dean of the dental school and acting dean of the school of medicine during the last half of 2002 and the first months of 2003, now seemed possible: "If the hospitals and the university could only get together, how competitive this place would be."[84]*

*By the spring of 2005, it appeared that the hospital and medical school had resolved the controversy over the practice plans. The provisional arrangement calls for the practice plans to be based in the hospital, rather than the school. The hospital will conduct all negotiating for contracts with payers on behalf of both the hospital and the doctors. This should please the insurance companies, which will have to deal with only one entity at the medical center, as they now do at the Cleveland Clinic. With the hospital doing all the billing, more can be collected for procedures than is possible when the billing is conducted by physician practices. The school and the hospital will participate equally in the governance of the new plan.[85]

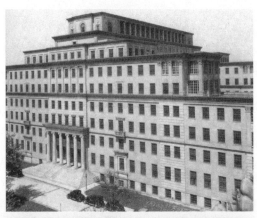

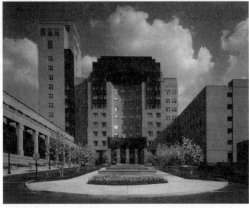

University Hospitals of Cleveland. Lakeside Hospital when it opened in the early 1930s (*top*). Most adult patient beds are now located in the Mather and Lerner buildings (*bottom*). *Courtesy of University Hospitals Health System*

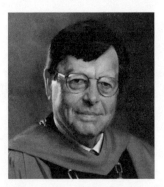

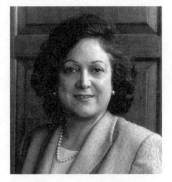

Two presidents: Agnar Pytte (*left*) of Case Western Reserve University (1987–99) and Farah Walters (*right*) of University Hospitals of Cleveland and its health system (1992–2002). Leading separate corporations with different boards of trustees, Pytte and Walters differed over several policies of importance to the medical center. *Photo of Agnar Pytte courtesy of John Howard Sanden; photo of Farah Walters courtesy of University Hospitals Health System*

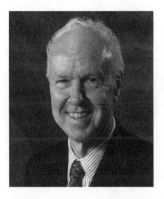 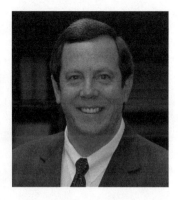

David Auston (*left*) led the university for only twenty-two months (1999–2001). Conflict over a new affiliation agreement with University Hospitals contributed to his early resignation from the presidency. Dr. Edward Hundert (*right*), the academic psychiatrist who became president of CASE in 2002, calmed many of the conflicts roiling the medical school and hospital and encouraged the development of the Cleveland Clinic's medical college. *Photo of David Auston courtesy of Herbert Ascherman; photo of Edward Hundert courtesy of Michael Sands*

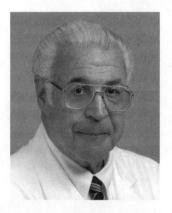 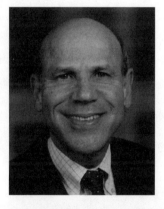

Dr. Nathan Berger (*left*), dean of the medical school from 1996 to 2002. Receiving little financial or moral backing from the university, Berger and his predecessors depended upon University Hospitals for support of the clinical departments. Dr. Ralph Horwitz (*right*), who was imported from Yale as Berger's successor in 2003, was the first dean in decades who had not been a member of the CASE faculty when appointed. *Courtesy of Michael Sands*

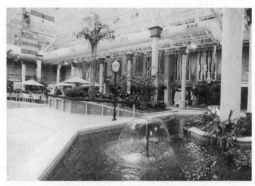

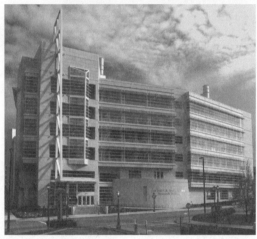

Dr. James Block, when president of University Hospitals, transformed the patio connecting the buildings in the center of the complex into a covered atrium (*top*). This busy space includes restaurants, shops, tables, and chairs. Farah Walters led the construction of a laboratory building (*bottom*) as part of her effort to establish a research program based at University Hospitals that would be separate from the university. After she left, the medical school bought the building. *Courtesy of University Hospitals Health System*

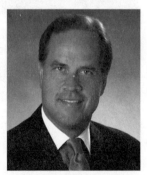 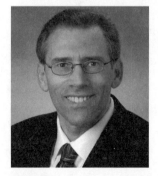

Two executives succeeded Farah Walters. Thomas Zenty (*left*) became president of the University Hospitals Health System and Dr. Fred Rothstein, (*right*) president of University Hospitals. Walters resisted splitting her job when requested to do so by the chairman of the hospital and health system trustees. *Courtesy of University Hospitals Health System*

CHAPTER SIX

The New Medical School

"What was missing was a medical school,"[1] declares Dr. Eric Topol, provost and chief academic officer of the Clinic and responsible, in this role, for the gestating mouthful, "Cleveland Clinic Lerner College of Medicine of Case Western Reserve University School of Medicine."[2] Although leaders at the Clinic had long considered developing a medical school, by the second half of the 1990s the desire for doing so had become quite strong. Al Lerner, the Clinic's great financial supporter for whom the new college would be named, insisted that "to become number one and consistently hire the best people, a medical school was needed."[3]

Creating a New Medical School

Establishing a new medical school in the United States is a daunting proposition. Before admitting any students, the new school must obtain approval from the Liaison Committee on Medical Education (LCME), the organization that accredits medical education programs leading to the M.D. degree in the United States and Canada.[1,4] The accreditation process, which every school must undergo periodically, involves preparation of data by the school and one or more visits from representatives of the committee. Gaining accreditation for a new school is a formidable task,[5,6] and even if the plans for the new school satisfy the LCME, it can only receive provisional status and will be reviewed annually until the committee is satisfied that it can accredit it for several years. Leaders from the Clinic visited the LCME office in Washington and discussed what was needed for the proposed school to become accredited. An LCME delegation came to Cleveland, but warned the Clinic that approval of an application would take time and might be unsuccessful. An application in Florida had recently failed.[7]

Furthermore, to award degrees, the Clinic would need to petition the state of Ohio.[1] In all likelihood at least some of the six other schools in the state would object, concerned about competition for students and funding for the Clinic's new school. One can imagine the attendant political machinations. CASE president Edward Hundert, himself an academic physician and former member of the LCME, predicts, "Starting a new independent medical school in Ohio, now or in the future, is impossible."[8]

Despite these problems, the Clinic persevered, and several of its members, including Andrew Fishleder, chairman of the division of education, and Topol, visited schools to learn more about what the Clinic would have to do to realize this dream. One of these schools was the University of Rochester School of Medicine and Dentistry,* where they met Dr. Lindsey Henson, an anesthesiologist who was senior associate dean for medical education and then deeply involved in developing and instituting a new curriculum there. Impressed by her, the Clinic team asked whether she would be interested in becoming a candidate as the first dean of the Clinic's new medical school.[9] Initially, she thought not, "but Eric persisted and I agreed to visit them."[9] At the Clinic's request, she wrote a document describing what needed to be done. "Wow, just what we're looking for," Topol e-mailed her.[9]

Undiscouraged by the problems inherent in the course they were following, Topol, Fred Loop, the CEO, and Fishleder came to believe that a relationship with Case Western Reserve University (CASE) would best serve

---

*The dialogue between Rochester and the Clinic began when Topol received a congratulatory letter as a distinguished alumnus from Edward Hundert, then dean of the medical school there. In responding, Topol praised Rochester's new curriculum, which he had been reading about, and wondered if it would be applicable to the Clinic's new medical school.[8]

the interests of the new school.[10] "Coming in under CASE would certainly speed the process," says Nathan Berger, then dean of the school of medicine there.[7] However, at this point, the two parties could not resolve their differences about financial issues, faculty participation, fundraising, and how to deal with the endowments. The Clinic did not think having CASE's name attached to the school would help the Clinic even though CASE's research programs were significantly stronger.

A formal link between the Clinic and CASE was not a new idea. Agnar Pytte, when president of CASE, had favored the presence of two medical schools in Cleveland with one based at the Clinic but associated in some way with CASE.[11]* Duncan Neuhauser† remembers, when he arrived at CASE in 1979, "they had on the table the Harvard approach."[12] Under this system, the Clinic, as well as the current CASE teaching hospitals, would operate independently, and the chairs of the usual departments (divisions at the Clinic) would collaborate through committees to resolve educational and other academic issues. But it was not to be. Members of the Clinic "didn't want to be treated only as an affiliate, a secondary partner," according to longtime staff member Donald Vidt. At University Circle, "the clinical faculty at UH viewed us as competition."[13]

When David Auston suddenly resigned as CASE president in the spring of 2000 and was followed in the office by an interim president, Alfred Lerner, president of the Clinic board, rejected the arrangement because of the lack of permanent leadership at CASE. "I never do a deal with someone I've never met," he told Charles Bolton, then chairman of the CASE trustees.[14] Lerner had favored the Clinic's developing its school independent of CASE because, according to Malachai ("Mal") Mixon, chairman of the Clinic board, "he didn't trust Farah."[15] Mixon believes that the Clinic could have created an independent school, and says, "I'm a born optimist." Mixon and Lerner did not, however, try to impose this structure even though, in Mixon's words, "We have powerful people on the board. It was Fred's [Loop] and the docs' choice."[15]

---

*Pytte, who had been provost at Dartmouth College, suggested that Cleveland could follow the example there, where medical students could enter a four-year course solely at the Dartmouth Medical School or an alternative course in which they studied basic science at Dartmouth and took their clinical training during the third and fourth years at Brown University.[11]

†Neuhauser is professor of epidemiology and biostatistics at CASE.

The nature of the school's governance would be resolved with the election of Dr. Edward Hundert as the university's new president and the departure of Farah Walters in 2002. Fred Loop believes that Walters's leaving was the fundamental change required to allow the new relationship to flourish. "The atmosphere has totally changed," he says.[16] Not having inherited University Hospitals' antagonism toward its principal competitor for medical care in Cleveland, Hundert thought a connection between the university and the Clinic, whose reputation he was aware of, had merit.

Lindsey Henson was, in many ways, the ideal person to act as mediator between the university and Clinic for matters concerning "the college program," as the Clinic's school is called to distinguish it from "the university program" based at CASE. She had worked for the new CASE president at Rochester and was by now well known to the leaders at the Clinic. She would be accountable to Topol for those resources and programs relevant to the college.[9]* As executive dean of the college, Fishleder would report to Topol and to the board of governors, as well as to Henson and Ralph Horwitz, the new dean at CASE.[18]

The arrangement that the negotiators at the Clinic and university developed specified that the college operate as part of the CASE school of medicine, which will accredit the program and award the degrees. The dean at CASE will have charge of both programs, a unique administrative arrangement among American medical schools.[7] Consequently, the CASE admissions committee must approve the nomination of every student to be admitted to the Clinic's college. So far, none has been rejected.[6]†

The Clinic agreed to fold its research funding into CASE's total. This deal—"99 percent of their reason to agree," according to Topol[2]—would significantly raise CASE's position in the NIH rankings, increasing it the year after the Cleveland Clinic's college opened.[9,20] Some at CASE don't

---

*A graduate of the CASE medical school who had trained at the Clinic observed that Henson's working for both institutions would have been "unheard of ten years ago."[17]

†Hundert points out the similarities of the new programs to that of the Harvard-MIT Division of Health Sciences and Technology,[8] which is designed to train medical students for careers in which they will seek to create, in the words of the program's Web site, "cost-effective preventive, diagnostic and therapeutic innovations."[19] The Harvard-MIT program admits about thirty students each year, as does the Clinic program. Candidates prepare only one application to apply for the Harvard-MIT program or the standard program at the Harvard Medical School and one application when applying for the university program based at CASE or the college program at the Clinic.[8]

think much of the arrangement. "It's a contrivance," says John Nilson, former chairman of the department of pharmacology. "We're too preoccupied with the NIH listings."[21]

Despite being administratively part of CASE's school of medicine, the Clinic's college will operate separately with its own curriculum for much of the program. The staff physicians at the Clinic and the scientists in the Lerner Research Institute will teach most of the preclinical basic science courses,* but the students will also study with the CASE students a half day per week.[23] The clinical curriculum for the two M.D. programs will be very similar, according to Henson. "College students will have clinical experiences at the Clinic, in its regional practices, and at the other hospitals affiliated with CASE. CASE students in the university program will rotate to the Clinic for required and elective clerkships in the third and fourth years of their program."[24] Those physicians who teach will supervise the students' clinical experiences in the Clinic's hospital and outpatient departments.[25]

The size of the classes will be small, thirty-two students at the beginning.[2,25–27]† A minimum of five years will be required to receive the M.D. degree, the extra year designed to better prepare students for careers in clinical research, a special aim of the college.[24] The students can obtain a master's degree in molecular medicine or clinical investigation within the five-year curriculum. Some will be encouraged to train longer and earn Ph.D. degrees in addition to the M.D. The required five-year course, it was thought when the concept was first introduced, would reduce the expected competition between CASE's university program and the program based at the Clinic.[24] Subsequently, this distinction appeared to disappear. The new dean at CASE, Ralph Horwitz, announced that he would introduce a required thesis for all students in the university program and that many of these students would want to take a fifth year.‡

---

*Initially, the college had planned that the first two basic science years would be taught at CASE.[22]

†Determined, Fishleder explains, by the number of students accommodated in the four conference rooms designed for the problem-based learning (PBL) technique that the school will employ.[28]

‡These are longtime features of the Yale University medical school program which Horwitz, the former chairman of internal medicine there, is transplanting from New Haven to Cleveland. The purpose of the thesis, Horwitz explains, is "to make students better doctors. They will learn new ways of thinking by immersing themselves intensively in a research project. It's easy to go through medical school without knowing something in depth. The student will also develop an intimate academic relationship with a faculty member, which is less likely to happen in the standard curriculum."[29] Nevertheless, when asked whether the thesis program accounts for more of Yale's graduates choosing

A unique feature of the Clinic's college is a ten-week "immersion in research," started when the first year class entered on July 6, 2004, about two months before classes at most medical schools begin. During this period, students will visit laboratories as clinical and basic science investigators define just what research is and, in describing their work, try to interest students in working in their laboratories or with their clinical projects. A course in the ethics of medical practice and research will be given.

"We're trying to create a graduate school atmosphere," says Jeffery Hutzler, a Clinic psychiatrist who is associate dean for admissions and student affairs. "We want to take the students out of the competitive mold characteristic of most medical students into learning how to work together co-operatively."[23] In keeping with this orientation, half of the students' time during the first two years will be free for independent study.

The students will become involved with patients early in their training. During the first year, they will spend a half day per week working in one of the clinic's suburban outpatient practice sites and, on alternate weeks, practicing physical examinations. In the second year, they will spend a half day each week in an outpatient office. By the end of the first two years, each student will have seen about a hundred patients.[23] The clinical-teachers at the sites will know what the students are studying at the college and select relevant cases for review.[23]

Two advisors will work with each student, one for laboratory science and the other for clinical work. The students will take self-learning tests on interactive computers, the results of which will be discussed with them by their advisors. The college does not plan to grade or rank the students.[23]

Students in the college will pay the same fees as do those in the CASE's medical school but will have to pay for only four of the five years.[26] CASE will retain 10 to 15 percent of the tuition collected.[30*] The Clinic hopes to attract particularly competitive candidates by offering liberal scholarships and forgiving loans its students may acquire to pay for their tuition. The Clinic will need to counteract the lower tuition charged at the state schools,† which is less than half as much for Ohio residents as at CASE.[32] To

---

academic careers than at many other medical schools, Horwitz is not sure. "It does attract more students with a scholarly bent."[29]

*This amount was being negotiated between the Clinic and CASE in the spring of 2004.[30]

†The state of Ohio operates five medical schools and one osteopathic school: The Medical College of Ohio in Toledo, Northeastern Ohio Universities College of Medicine in Rootstown (near

encourage students to apply, faculty plan to contact premedical advisors at colleges to tell them about the new college.[26]

The new college's finances got an extraordinary start by receiving a large gift from Clinic board president Alfred ("Al") Lerner (1933–2002), the former CEO of MBNA, the second-largest issuer of credit cards, owner of the Cleveland Browns,[33] and a longtime supporter of the Clinic, where he received much of his medical care. Lerner donated $100 million to endow the new college, which was then named for him and his family.[1*] Lerner had previously partially funded the construction of the handsome research and education building where the basic scientists and Fishleder have their laboratories and offices. Clinic officials estimate that the college will cost $8 to $10 million per year when all the classes are filled.[26]

Unlike at many academic medical centers, where governance of school and hospital is often separate, the Cleveland Clinic's new medical college will be led by a single organization, the board of governors, which is the policy-making body of the group practice.[34,35] This should, many hope, "mean fewer politics"[36] than in most medical schools and teaching hospitals that are not under unified doctor-led governance.

Education at the Cleveland Clinic

The Clinic believes it is prepared to provide an outstanding education to train potential doctors because of its decades teaching graduate physicians, more recent experience with medical students in their clinical years, and the presence of highly competent investigators and well-equipped laboratories. In 2004, the Clinic had fifty-two training programs and 750 fellows and residents.[37]

Although the Clinic trained postgraduates since 1921, medical students seldom worked in the Clinic until the 1970s.[25] Since then, the Clinic estab-

---

Akron, south of Cleveland), Ohio State University College of Medicine in Columbus, University of Cincinnati College of Medicine, and Wright State University School of Medicine in Dayton. The osteopathic school is in Athens. Case Western Reserve University School of Medicine is the only private medical school in the state.[31] Even with the Clinic's college now open, CASE remains Ohio's sole private school since the new college is part of the university. As a leader in medical research, CASE has more support from the NIH than all the other medical schools in Ohio combined.[8]

*Although Lerner had planned to transfer the entire amount to the Clinic, the family, after he died in the fall of 2002, spread the gift over ten years.[16] The Clinic plans to spend only from the income and not invade the principal of the gift itself. The change will, as Loop says, "put a crimp in the scholarship fund."[16]

lished educational relationships with such medical schools as Case Western Reserve, Morehouse, Ohio State, and Pennsylvania State University at Hershey. Students from these and other schools initially trained at the Clinic during clinical electives in their fourth or final year.[38] Beginning in 1992, the Clinic accepted, on a full-time basis, a cadre of students from Ohio State University, who, in their third and fourth years, took most of their clinical training in Cleveland.[25] The Cleveland Clinic received no tuition for this and fully funded the program.[39]

Meanwhile, the Cleveland Foundation, which was trying to develop a coordinated hub for medical care, research, and education within the city of Cleveland, was not so pleased. As Robert Eckardt, now the vice president for programs at the Foundation observed, "Why Ohio State, which is 140 miles away [in Columbus], when CASE is only a stone's throw away?"[40]*

Eckardt and his colleagues needn't have worried. The success of the Ohio State program heightened the enthusiasm at the Clinic to develop its own school.[39] Before doing so, the Clinic tried unsuccessfully to interest Ohio State in establishing a four-year program based in Cleveland.[39,41] Clinic leaders then began to think, "Since we were doing it for another school" and receiving no support from Ohio State for teaching their students, "why not do it ourselves and create a curriculum based on our strength in translational research?"[23] When the Clinic decided to establish its college, the relationship with Ohio State was terminated in accordance with their signed agreement.[42]

The clinical divisions and departments of the Cleveland Clinic have long trained interns, residents, and fellows[38] and given courses for doctors. The Clinic has also, for many years, welcomed trained physicians to work in Cleveland for various periods of time to learn about recent advances and techniques and perfect their ability to perform new procedures. By 1964, a building specifically designed for education opened on the campus. A division of education replaced former units devoted to administering the programs in 1983.

For decades, the Clinic's specialty orientation has impeded its ability to attract interns and residents, particularly in internal medicine.[43] Until fairly

---

*The Clinic's affiliation with Ohio State worked in part because they are 140 miles apart, which prevented much competition for clinical practice.[13] However, the Ohio State faculty disapproved the Clinic's becoming a campus of Ohio State because of the money the university would have had to invest in the arrangement.[13]

recently, relatively few of the more competitive American-trained medical graduates have come to the Clinic for this phase of their training. Consequently, many who hold these positions have trained at foreign medical schools.* "We're known as a specialty place, and it's difficult to get potential medical residents to get out of this pattern of thinking," acknowledges Andrew Fishleder.[25] "Interns and residents feel it's a fellows' hospital," says cardiologist Gary Francis. Many potential candidates, yearning for direct responsibility for patient care once they have obtained their M.D.s, had heard that the method for training at the Clinic was "watch me and you'll learn."[37] Another misconception among intern applicants held that "the bottom line comes first," leading to reduced teaching opportunities for young doctors.[44] "It's not really true," says Francis. "It's the perception, not reality. However, many of the patients are very sick and require much fellow and attending attention. So we must stay close to them."[45]†

Nevertheless, believes pediatrics chairman Michael Levine, "we're still not an intern's hospital." Levine had previously worked at the Johns Hopkins Hospital, where interns have traditionally enjoyed a large amount of responsibility. "Our clinicians are real clinicians, and they want to manage their patients, so the staff exercises much closer supervision than at many teaching hospitals."[47] Accordingly, says Levine, "the Cleveland Clinic's continuity clinics, where house officers care for 'their own' outpatients, are supervised by staff members to a much greater degree than occurs at more typical academic medical centers."[47]

Despite these features, Clinic leaders deny that an internship or residency at the Cleveland Clinic deprives its trainees of the opportunities they need to learn their profession.[25,43,48] "Our program is clearly better than its reputation," says Dr. Susan Rehm,‡ "and is improving every year," adds Loop.[35] The amount of clinical material is matchless, and we encourage the house staff to participate actively in managing the patients."[43]

*Current parlance dictates that they be called "international medical graduates."

†The necessity for attending physicians and surgeons to personally care for all patients, even in teaching hospitals, has decreased the ability of interns and residents to decide the diagnostic and therapeutic plans for patients assigned to them. Several changes account for this. The insurance carriers will no longer pay faculty members for "supervising" care; they must actually deliver it. Furthermore, the increasing severity of illness of many patients admitted to hospitals often requires immediate care by experienced physicians and surgeons. Finally, the pressure to shorten the length of time patients spend in hospitals has reduced the opportunities for interns, residents, and medical students to work up patients, a process that takes more time and is less efficient than when rendered by experienced doctors.[46]

‡Rehm directed the training program in internal medicine from 1994 to 1997.

"Education is a division that provides a central resource to enhance our academic programs," claims Fishleder in explaining the central position education has held in the Clinic since its founding.[25] With so many leading physicians and surgeons at the Clinic to learn from and such varied clinical experience from the many patients the Clinic attracts,[43,44] those involved in education continue to wonder why the internships and residencies don't attract more competitive American graduates. "We're not a university hospital and people think our residency is not academic," Byron Hoogwerf, who currently directs the training program in internal medicine, explains. "The first is true, the second is not."[48] And then the city of Cleveland isn't most fourth-year students' first choice of a place to live.

Hoogwerf, who is never pressured to accept applicants with questionable qualifications whose candidacy has been touted by alumni or contributors, sees the quality of his interns and residents, both American and international, constantly improving. As proof of this, he draws attention to the fact that almost all the residents passed their certifying examinations in internal medicine for the past three years, and, increasingly, more Clinic residents who want to become specialists are being admitted to competitive fellowship programs.[48] Many of the fellowships the Clinic offers have become very popular and draw residents from the best-known academic medical centers for advanced training in the specialties.[25]

The Clinic also presents continuing medical education courses throughout the year in Cleveland, Florida, and elsewhere. To a great extent, these courses will be brought back to Cleveland to be presented in the conference center of the new Clinic-owned hotel.[49]

As for the financial basis of the education division, Fishleder explains, "We're a net cost center and depend upon a substantial subsidy from Clinic operations to function."[25]

Research at the Cleveland Clinic

The third traditional mission of medical schools is the advancement of knowledge, and, despite the Clinic's emphasis on clinical care, the institution has long supported research, an enthusiasm of the founders, particularly George Crile.[50] Nevertheless, compared with clinical care, research at the Cleveland Clinic, until fairly recently, held a lower priority, and less investigative productivity was expected of the staff than was typical of leading medical schools.[51] As Michael Levine has observed, "Despite the tremendous growth of the Lerner Research Institute, research still occurs tangential to clinical work."[47] However, Levine says, "developing criteria to measure the success of investigators here will be much easier than deciding how to promote clinicians at Hopkins."[47]

In 1945, the Clinic officially organized the research into a new division directed by Dr. Irvine Page, a leader in hypertension studies.[52] In 1985, when Dr. Bernadine Healy became its director, she renamed it the Cleveland Clinic Research Institute,[53] later to become the Lerner Research Institute in response to the donation from the Lerner family.

Healy liked the atmosphere she found at the Clinic and in the research institute. "There was a strong sense of group, team work, and collegiality."[39] However, when she arrived at the Clinic, Healy saw much of the research emphasizing physiological subjects and little infrastructure or support for protein chemistry or molecular biology.[39] Nevertheless, Healy found it relatively easy to recruit investigators. The Clinic had decided to allocate sufficient money to do this as well as building new laboratories as research at the Cleveland Clinic, in Healy's words, "stopped being a stepchild."[39] Since 75 percent of the members of the research institute held the Ph.D. degree, there were few physicians to be distracted from their basic laboratories by clinical responsibilities. When George Stark,* chairman of the Lerner Research Institute from 1992 to 2002, succeeded Healy, about sixty principal investigators worked in the research institute. The number had doubled during Healy's administration and would double again under Stark.[54]

Although the intense clinical competition between the Clinic and University Hospitals has prevented the creation, until recently, of patient-oriented ties between the Clinic, University Hospitals, and CASE, individual investigators, particularly basic scientists, have developed productive academic relationships with investigators at CASE when collaboration benefits both parties.[55] In the absence of the Cleveland Clinic's having university status, several of the investigators hold faculty positions at CASE, Cleveland State, Ohio State, or Kent State universities, where they teach part-time. These affiliations also allow the staff to train Ph.D. students registered at one of the universities. Convincing excellent Ph.D. candidates to take their training at the Clinic, however, has been difficult. The leaders hope that

---

*Stark is the Clinic's only current member of the National Academy of Sciences. He is also a Fellow of the Royal Society, Britain's honorary scientific institute.

with the medical college, some of the students will take the combined M.D./Ph.D. program and train in the Lerner Research Institute.[53] In common with many laboratories elsewhere, most of the postdoctoral fellows who work at the research institute are not American, with a large proportion coming from Asia.[54]

The Clinic recently assigned overall direction of research at the Clinic to Eric Topol, the chief of cardiology who has become, in preparation for the opening of the medical college, provost in charge of research and education. An academic council of chairmen, led by Topol, has formulated a new policy for clinical research favoring disease-specific programs to coordinate research between the clinical departments and the research institute.[54,56] "We've cut down on useless research," Loop says.[56] Much of the research now conducted in the clinical departments is "translational," interpreting and applying the discoveries in basic laboratories to clinical problems.[57]

One of the most productive clinical investigators in Topol's shop is Dr. Michael Lauer, an unlikely recruit to the Clinic. Lauer had trained at two of Harvard's renowned teaching hospitals, the Massachusetts General (MGH) in medicine and the Beth Israel in cardiology. His interest in cardiac epidemiology had led him to a post at the Leahy Clinic and the Harvard Medical School. Lauer came to Cleveland because his wife, also trained at the MGH, had been offered a particularly attractive position at the Clinic in her field of infectious diseases. "I was the trailing spouse," he explains.[58]

"The first year, I thought I'd made a big mistake," Lauer says.[58] Despite wanting to emphasize clinical research in his career, Lauer, like most newcomers to the Clinic, spent most of his time taking care of patients. For one day per week, Topol relieved him of these duties to develop his research program. "Each year I got more time off," Lauer describes his progress to nearly full-time investigator.[58] Receipt of a grant from the American Heart Association brought him another day. A grant from the NIH and an administrative job as director of the exercise lab earned him more protected time. Eventually his clinical responsibilities became limited to seeing outpatients one day per week and caring for inpatients for no more than two months per year. Without his grants and the income generated by his work in the exercise laboratory, where much of his research is generated, the Clinic would not have allowed such a schedule.

"I used to think the MGH was a large hospital until I came here. It's nothing like we have here," says Lauer. The great volume of clinical experience in his specialty plus the Clinic's sophisticated computer technology gives him and his colleagues access to extraordinarily large clinical databases. "The surgical material goes back to the 1970s. The sample size is close to 30,000."[58]

Lauer no longer has reservations about working at the Clinic as he did when he first arrived. "It's not an accident that we have innovative people. People do feel free to try things out. Our leaders don't micromanage us."[58] Lauer likes that each member of the Clinic is salaried. "We're all part of the same practice. None of us is a threat to the other."[58] Lauer describes the Cleveland Clinic as a "Mom and Pop shop in a technically advanced place." He and his secretaries know each of their patients. "Many of us give patients copies of our office notes. They love this, and it helps to make them partners in what we do here." Finally, Lauer adds, "this is a place where you can do your academic work without a lot of academic baggage."[58]

The large clinical services attract investigators, like Lauer, to the Clinic who want to concentrate on studying clinical problems. A good example is Dr. Brian Bolwell, the director of the bone marrow transplant program in the Taussig Cancer Center. Bolwell, a graduate of Harvard College and the CASE medical school who received his specialty training at the Dana-Farber Cancer Institute in Boston, came to the Clinic "for a reason." At many academic medical centers, Bolwell has found, clinicians are "second-class citizens" compared with researchers. Furthermore, in his opinion, many consider clinical research, compared with more basic studies, "unintellectual and pedestrian, unworthy of praise despite its ability to save lives. I wanted to be at a place that emphasizes clinical care."[59]*

Clinical Research

Clinical research at the Clinic is coordinated by neurologist Richard Rudick, who came to the Clinic from the University of Rochester in 1987 to conduct investigations in neurology. He was appointed director of the Mellen Center for Multiple Sclerosis Treatment and Research, which had been established with a gift of $2 million from a local family. Since 2001, Rudick has also led the Clinic's center for clinical research, and, in this role, reports to Eric Topol. With associates who feel similarly, Rudick hopes to con-

*Brian Bolwell is the son of Harry Bolwell, the chairman of the University Hospitals board of trustees in the 1970s and 1980s.

vince the executive management at the Clinic to invest more resources in clinical research. He finds that doctors on the board of governors are supportive, but, perhaps not unexpectedly, "the hospital administrators are less so."[60]

Rudick is trying to standardize many aspects of clinical research, including the amount of indirect costs paid by corporate sponsors at 30 percent of direct costs. Before the clinical research center was established, many projects generated less than 10 percent.[60]

For highly qualified applicants, Rudick's unit awards $50,000 toward salary and $25,000 for expenses to young staff members who wish to develop careers as clinical investigators. The support is contingent on a department's guarantee that at least half of the staff's time will be protected from clinical responsibilities for research.[60]

The research center also sponsors courses in clinical research and has arranged that interested members of the staff can work toward master's degrees in investigation and health science research at Case Western Reserve University, a project that Rudick describes as "important for our medical college."[60] Finally, Rudick is trying to improve the infrastructure for clinical research at the Clinic by consolidating computer databases and coordinating compliance with the provisions of the Food and Drug Administration.

Responding to lobbying by Rudick and Eric Topol, the board of governors awarded divisional status to the Center for Clinical Research in December 2002. The new division of clinical research succeeded in attracting a large grant from the NIH to establish a general clinical research center in April 2003, and has established clinical coordinating centers in neurology, the cancer center, and ophthalmology to complement a similar coordinating center in cardiology.

Rudick is regularly "pushing for increasingly academic departments," an activity that is not without controversy. "Opinions about what I do vary," he says. Some clinical departments are threatened by his challenges to do more research, others are "counting on me to help them."[60]

Basic Science

All basic science research remains the administrative responsibility of the Lerner Research Institute, now directed by Paul DiCorleto, who was appointed George Stark's successor in 2002. DiCorleto, like Stark before him, is a member of the Clinic's division heads committee, a group of the most senior leaders that is chaired by Kay as the Clinic's chief of staff.

Bernadine Healy began the process of integrating into the research institute the occasional basic scientist who had been recruited by a clinical department but whose work had not prospered. Many such individuals have benefited from working in the collegial and supportive environment of the institute.[53] Prompted by unimpressive research produced in laboratories in some of the clinical departments, Loop has insisted on the present policy.[61] Currently, only in the eye and neurological institutes and in the cancer center is basic research performed outside the Lerner laboratories. "We won't do that again," says Robert Kay, referring to the basic science laboratories in the eye institute, which were insisted upon by Hilel Lewis when he was being recruited to direct the institute. "Some islands of basic research may remain in the divisions, but most will be centered in the Lerner Research Institute. It's an interesting challenge," Kay adds, "outside recruitees wanting their own researchers."[62] The policy of performing all basic research in the research institute, however, is not universally acclaimed. "I would prefer having basic research in my department," says Hans Lüders, chairman of the department of neurology. "It produces a schism away in the Lerner."[61]

When the Clinic hired DiCorleto (Ph.D., Cornell) in 1981 from his postdoctoral fellowship at the University of Washington, he saw the place as having "much 'Herr Professor' style." People were brought to the research division, DiCorleto remembers, "to fill niches, not because they were so good."[53] Bernadine Healy recruited increasingly competent investigators and "raised the idea that people could be independent."[53] Accordingly, by 1989, DiCorleto's laboratory had become a separate department of cell biology within the research institute.

Recruiting investigators to work in an organization that does not offer the type of tenure characteristic of universities presents a challenge to the leaders of the research institute. "We must sell other things," says DiCorleto. " 'We'll support you,' we tell them and will cover 60 percent of their salaries from Clinic funds." Many private medical research universities expect senior faculty to raise more of their expenses. "We offer environment, and you won't have to teach courses if you don't want to."[53] Clinic leaders hope that the new medical college will increase the attraction of working at the Cleveland Clinic to able investigators and academically oriented physicians whom Loop wants to recruit and retain.[63]

Although formerly surpluses from the clinical practice funded many of the research programs,[54] now grants from the usual governmental and industrial sources support most, although not all, of the expenses of the institute. Increasingly, the Clinic is recruiting physicians who are interested in performing research as well as investigators holding the Ph.D. degree. "The word is out," says DiCorleto. "Loop and now Topol want all departments to do more research."[53]

In the spring of 2005, according to Clinic sources,[64] the Cleveland Clinic Foundation received for research, during the most recent twelve-month period, $78 million from the federal government, of which 90 percent was from the NIH and $36 million from corporate sources. Nevertheless, the total research budget pales in comparison with the $4.5 billion spent annually in operating the entire Cleveland Clinic Foundation. Richard Rudick, one of the most vocal supporters of research at the Clinic and for its new medical college, says, "The small percentage of the total spent on research makes it almost a sideline, a hobby of the Clinic. As focus in the Clinic shifts to research, more of the Clinic's staff are realizing that we have enormous potential."[60] So far, the Clinic has avoided the traditional conflict between hospital and medical school on how to spend resources by centralizing decision making where the founders placed it and where many members of the Clinic think it should remain.

The Clinic has long published its own medical journal, currently edited by Dr. John Clough, the Clinic's resident historian. The board of governors has now taken on the additional responsibility of establishing the Cleveland Clinic Foundation Press, which will publish books for both the professional and lay markets with Clough as its first director. Like the medical college, the leaders hope that the Press will increase recognition of the Cleveland Clinic as a comprehensive academic center.[63]

Collaborative Clinical Centers

The recent administrative changes at the CASE medical school and University Hospitals have raised the probability that research will, in the future, become increasingly coordinated between the institutions at University Circle and the Cleveland Clinic. As one example, CASE has designated the Lerner Research Institute as its "department of molecular research." Accordingly, the university appointed Paul DiCorleto, director of the institute at the Clinic, to be chairman of this new department at the university. DiCorleto has become equal administratively to the other basic science chairs at CASE and meets and works with them as if he were based at CASE.[8]

The Clinic, in keeping with one of the missions of its new medical college and the university medical school, has applied to the NIH for a grant to train doctors and medical scientists to perform clinical research.[8,66] The principal investigator is Richard Rudick from the Clinic, and the co-principal investigators are Dr. Pedro Delgado, chairman of the department of psychiatry at the university, and Dr. Randall Cebul, director of the Center for Health Care Research and Policy at MetroHealth Medical Center. All the CASE health-related schools and teaching hospitals—University, Metro, and the Veterans Administration—and more than seventy well-funded investigators who have agreed to act as mentors for the trainees participated.[66] Rudick reported that the NIH has given the grant "an outstanding priority score," and added, "this is a key part of the NIH plan to reengineer the clinical research enterprise."[66] Hundert, enthusiastic as usual, believes the grant "will help our institutions to become the country's leading place to train in clinical research."[8]

With the creation of the new medical college and the link with CASE, George Stark, the Clinic's distinguished basic scientist and former director of the Lerner Research Institute, established a laboratory at the university for the basic science portion of his genetics program. Half of his time is now assigned to CASE and half to the Clinic.[8]

The Clinic had tried unsuccessfully to convince the NIH to designate it as a comprehensive cancer center. Whereas basic and clinical research in cancer are both performed in the Ireland Cancer Center at University Hospitals, cancer research at the Clinic is split between the Lerner Research Institute, where scientists perform basic research studies, and the Taussig Cancer Center, where physicians carry out clinical research supported, for the most part, by industry rather than the NIH.[67]

Concluding that a further independent effort to obtain comprehensive cancer center status might also fail, the Clinic's leaders looked to CASE, which has such a center. Dr. James Willson, the director of the Ireland Cancer Center at University Hospitals, agreed to apply to the NIH for extension of its designation as a comprehensive cancer center to include work being done at the Clinic.[68,69] "Not being part of an NIH unit prevents our working effectively with novel drugs being administered through the NIH," says Ronald Bukowski, the acting chairman of the department in 2003, who then adds, "we'll be able to participate in clinical trials easier also."[68] The NIH accepted the proposal in 2004.[70] Hundert reports that the CASE comprehensive cancer center will rank fifth in grants from the National

Cancer Institute in 2004. Such a cooperative endeavor would never have been possible during the administration of Farah Walters, whose animus toward the Clinic was legendary.

The union has, however, raised concerns among some of the oncologists at the Clinic. "Cooperation sounds great," says Brian Bolwell, "but we must maintain our independence. There's fear here that we will be integrated into Ireland. People at the top think some sort of 'non-merger merger' will occur. We'll see."[59] Bukowski emphasizes that the combination with CASE will only apply to research, both clinical and basic science. The patient-care activities and the financial management of the Clinic's Taussig Cancer Center will remain separate from the University Hospitals Ireland Cancer Center.[68]

Criticism and Concerns

Although most of the CASE faculty, according to dean Ralph Horwitz, support the creation of the college,[71] some at both University Circle and the Clinic criticize the concept.

"I think the deal with the Clinic is an unmitigated disaster," declares Dr. Adel Mahmoud, a twenty-six-year CASE veteran and chairman of the department of medicine from 1987 to 1998. "A medical school is the last piece the Clinic needs to compete with CASE in every way."[72] Speaking from the point of view of a CASE loyalist, Mahmoud worries that the new college will attract good students that might otherwise go to CASE's medical school. "The Clinic can legitimately say about its own college, 'come to a CASE medical school,' and they'd be right. If the schools were separate, I wouldn't be so upset."[72]

Jerry Shuck, the longtime chairman of the department of surgery at CASE and one-time acting vice president of the university, says, "I buy into CASE's need for the college as I buy into Cleveland's weather in January and February."[73]

Few of the CASE faculty had any influence on the creation of the college,[74,75] and some object to not being allowed to read the agreement between CASE and the Clinic that established the college.[74,75] "I should have known more about it," says former pharmacology department chair John Nilson, "but it was all done 'way up there' and everyone is expected to support it." Nilson predicts that the Clinic will become "the tail wagging the dog. They will want to run it, and they have the resources to do it."[21]

Nilson calls the proposed program of training students to become clinical investigators in five years "laughable. They need deep not superficial training, something analogous to the M.D./Ph.D. program."[21] Some who wish the school well are skeptical about the emphasis on clinical research. Medical students, most of whom apply in their early twenties, don't even know what research is really like.[6] However, they know what to tell admissions committees even though research careers may not be what they have in mind when they apply. Will this new school have greater success generating physician-investigators when most medical students, even at the most competitive schools, become practitioners, and few choose academic careers? CASE president Edward Hundert believes that the college is bound to help relieve the national need for more doctors performing clinical research. "If only half do it [enter careers in clinical research], we'll be in the vanguard compared with other schools."[8]

CASE faculty fear that the university program will lose potential students if the Clinic's college program offers its applicants advantageous financial arrangements like forgiving tuition and other expenses, remissions that the university program based at CASE cannot afford.[76,77] "They'll pay students to get good ones," fears Dr. Antonio Scarpa, chairman of CASE's distinguished department of physiology.[77] "The Clinic has developed a school not for education but for competition. Once you've got a school—small or large, doesn't matter—you've got a school."[77] CASE neurology department chairman Dennis Landis adds, "With a medical school, the Clinic can advertise itself as a research incubator. The Clinic can now market its affiliation with CASE. This really angers people here."[76]

Many members of the CASE faculty believe that eventually the Cleveland Clinic will separate the college from CASE.[75,76] "Both the closeness and the durability of the relationship of the Clinic with the school of medicine is yet to be proven," says Pamela Davis, the director of the pulmonary division in the department of pediatrics at CASE and an authority on cystic fibrosis. "The Clinic wants to be the Clinic. They really don't want to be with us. They'll use us as long as is necessary and then split off."[74]

"We're just training the people at the Clinic how to run a medical school," Albert Kirby, the senior admissions officer at CASE, has heard some of his colleagues say.[6] Other faculty members at CASE also fear that the college will eventually become independent[78] and that autonomy is what the Clinic really wants. "The conventional wisdom," says Landis, "is that the Clinic is doing a school because Mayo has a school." Landis is not alone in believing that eventually the Cleveland Clinic will do what the Mayo Clinic did in breaking from its relationship with the University of Minnesota and operating its own school.[76] "Not true," says Eric Topol. "We have no intention whatsoever of ever disconnecting from CASE."[79]

Not everyone at CASE opposes the solution the institutions have chosen. Dr. Jerold Goldberg, dean of the CASE school of dentistry who was interim dean of the school of medicine from July 2002 to March 2003, believes "the new college has great potential."[80] Ralph Horwitz calls the college "an exciting experiment in medical education" and predicts that it will enrich the university's program.[81] Former CASE provost James Wagner says, "Given time, the people at the Clinic may fall in love with us."[82] The affiliation agreement keeps them together until 2014.[8] "If the combination hasn't proven mutually beneficial to everyone by then," university president Edward Hundert says, "we failed."[8]

Patrick Walsh, the Hopkins urologist and Case Western Reserve alumnus and trustee, thinks that the new college's link with CASE is a better solution than operating independently. "Strengthening one will help the other," he believes. Walsh sees a similarity between the Cleveland Clinic college with its emphasis on training clinical investigators and the combined program that the Harvard Medical School operates with the Massachusetts Institute of Technology. He is concerned, however, about whether the Clinic's comprehensive method of caring for patients—"You go there, and they take care of everything"—will mesh with the more typical customs of medical school teaching hospitals, where house officers and students order tests and consultations.[83] "Many people here at CASE see the Clinic organized along corporate, almost military lines," says Albert Kirby. "Education doesn't work that way."[6]

As the date for opening the college approached, it became clear to the dean at CASE and the officials at the Clinic that a full-time director of the new college was needed.[70] For this position Loop and Topol turned to Lindsey Henson, their earlier choice for dean before the relationship with CASE developed.[84] "She's the intellectual force behind the curriculum and its evaluation," said Horwitz. "The college is her baby."[29] "Our baby," adds Topol. "We had done considerable work both before and after Lindsey arrived to design a unique, innovative curriculum and take full advantage of starting with a clean slate."[79]

Henson, as CASE's vice dean for the Cleveland Clinic Lerner College of

Medicine, works most of the time at the Clinic and retains her clinical role as a staff anesthesiologist there and her faculty appointment at the college.[24] To fill her position in the university program, Horwitz appointed Robert Daroff, former chairman of the department of neurology and, more recently, chief of staff at University Hospitals, to become interim vice dean for education at CASE.[29] Both vice deans, one for the university program and one for the Clinic's college program, report to the dean of the CASE school of medicine. This arrangement eliminates "another level of management" if Daroff and Henson were to report to a senior associate dean over both schools, explains Edward Hundert.[70]

Although few members of the Clinic strongly object to starting the college, some remain unconvinced that it serves the long-term interests of the Foundation. Despite the endowment, will funds that would have been spent on clinical programs now be diverted to feed the interests of the scientists in the medical college's basic science programs?[85,86] Already, the Clinic had been supporting the research enterprise strongly. During Fred Loop's tenure, investment in research had increased from $12 to $30 million per year.[87] Pediatrics chairman Levine has heard some of his colleagues express the concern that, as the Clinic recruits clinician-investigators for the school, the full-time clinicians may feel threatened.[47]

Most believe that the college will raise the prestige of the Clinic, providing, of course, that it becomes a distinguished one, "but it's risky," says John Clough, the Clinic's historian. "We don't understand the opportunity costs for people who will have to work in it."[50] Joseph Iannotti, the chairman of orthopedics, agrees. "A medical school," he reflects from his experience at the University of Pennsylvania, "has many missions, many roles. How will we get people to see patients as they always have with the school requiring their time? There'll be an interesting change of culture."[88]

Clinic leaders[89] as well as observers at CASE[90] share Clough and Iannotti's concern about the amount of time and work the college will require from the Clinic's busy practitioners and suspect that incentives may need to be modified to assure that clinical teaching becomes a priority.[90] Because of the Clinic's traditional emphasis on clinical practice, there is a sense around the place that those who do not concentrate on providing clinical care are "not quite equal."[50] Consequently, some observers wonder how this mystique will blend with the academic demands to teach and administer educational programs required of a group practice that has acquired a medical school.[50] "Not having to politic with a medical school has been one of the Clinic's great strengths," says Brian Bolwell. "Here we're all under one roof. Our model's great for the practice of medicine."[59]

Others, however, believe that the college, as Hans Lüders, the chairman of neurology puts it, "won't make that much difference. We're used to medical students. I think it'll have little impact on our large staff."[61] Ernest Borden, a senior oncologist in the cancer center and a veteran member of the faculties at several academic medical centers, favors the new school, which should provide "a base for future faculty who know the Clinic."[91] The last word administratively comes from Toby Cosgrove, the new CEO and former chairman of cardiothoracic surgery, who feels that a small medical school "can only help us and won't get in the way."[92]

CHAPTER SEVEN

Conclusions

Surviving, let alone prospering, in the era of managed care drove the leaders of teaching hospitals to consider solutions seldom thought necessary before the 1990s. Without effective action, could their institutions continue to fulfill the traditional missions of academic medical centers: educating the physicians and medical scientists of the future, delivering exemplary medical care, and advancing knowledge in the life sciences? As insurers forced hospitals to reduce expenses by limiting the amount of time patients spend in the hospital and emphasizing outpatient care, hospital executives like Fred Loop and Farah Walters sought means to keep their beds filled and their bottom lines black.

Networks of Hospitals

Institutions like the Cleveland Clinic and University Hospitals of Cleveland have attempted to solve their problems by linking with community hospitals and physicians, by either purchase or affiliation. Many community hospitals welcomed such arrangements[1] because of the increasingly risky economics of health care. Becoming part of large medical centers might, the community hospital executives and trustees hoped, assure the continued success, if not the survival of, their institutions.

Many of these leaders preferred associating with not-for-profit academic institutions like the Clinic and University Hospitals rather than for-profit corporations, with their tighter administrative and economic control and greater risk to jobs. Fortunately for this preference, the attempts of for-profit corporations to enter the Cleveland market failed, and companies like Columbia-HCA decided to withdraw. Others, such as the purchaser of Mt. Sinai Hospital, couldn't prevent the hospital from going bankrupt and closing. These efforts, particularly the Columbia-HCA attempt, accelerated the desire of community hospitals to affiliate with the medical centers and contributed to the current status of Cleveland as what has been called a "two-system town"[2] as far as hospital care is concerned.

Thirty-six hospitals were operating in 1980[3] and 27 in 1990[4] during a decade when 9 general hospitals in Cleveland and the immediate surrounding region closed. Of the 27 still open in 1990, 6 were components of consolidated groups—4 within the Meridia Health System and 2 within Health Cleveland—leaving 23 independently operating general hospitals or hospital holding companies in 1990. Following further consolidations and closures during the next 14 years, the city and region retained only 9 independently operating general hospitals or hospital holding companies by 2004. Of the 23 general hospitals operating in the region that year, the Cleveland Clinic Foundation owned 9* and University Hospitals Health System wholly owned 8.† The number of hospitals in the Cleveland area had decreased 36 percent and the number of independent entities 75 percent from 1980 to 2004.‡

Networks of Doctors

Tying community physicians more closely to the medical centers to assure their referrals forms the second major effort to keep the beds filled. The two Cleveland institutions went about this somewhat differently as befits the fundamental dissimilarity in their organization. The Clinic decided to bring community doctors fully into the group practice by employing them

---

*Including the Cleveland Clinic's main hospital.

†Counting the components on the University Circle campus as one hospital. University Hospitals Health System also owned 50 percent of each of four other hospitals.

‡See appendix 2.

in the same manner as the doctors working at the downtown campus.* Similarly, the Clinic bought or built outpatient centers where these doctors would see their patients and made certain that these facilities would provide the same attractive appearance and high level of service as at the main campus.

In developing a network of employed primary care physicians, the Cleveland Clinic changed one of its basic tenets. Previously, the Clinic had studiously avoided competing directly with the doctors who referred to it.[6] "Now managed care plans could compel the Clinic's traditional referrers to use other designated specialty care and not send their patients to the Clinic, no matter how satisfied these community doctors were with the Clinic's care," explains Duncan Neuhauser of CASE.† "To counter this trend the Clinic needed its own network of primary care physicians whose insurance agreements would allow their referred patients' care to be paid for at the Clinic. This decision to compete with some of their referrers was a major strategic change for the Clinic with far-reaching consequences."[7]

It might be useful to compare the Clinic's approach with that undertaken by the University of Pennsylvania Health System in Philadelphia, an academic medical center recently studied by the author.[8] At Penn, the leaders also brought community physicians into the organization by creating an organization called Clinical Care Associates (CCA), which purchased their practices, costing Penn more than $100,000 per doctor. CCA then directly employed the doctors, paying all their professional expenses and benefits and collecting the revenue produced by their services.

The leaders of many academic medical centers, including Penn, had less experience than the Clinic's administration in operating a comprehensive group practice of physicians. Managing such a venture differs in many ways from running academic practice plans such as the one that employed the full-time physicians at the Hospital of the University of Pennsylvania (HUP).[9] The HUP doctors are mostly specialists. Many also have research or educational responsibilities or both and can defray some of their expenses with grants.‡

---

*The Clinic does not appear to have experienced the tendency of some private practitioners when entering full-time appointments to decrease their workload, a trend noted elsewhere.[5]

†Neuhauser is professor of epidemiology and biostatistics at Case Western Reserve University.

‡Such vertical and horizontal integration as applied at Penn, the Cleveland Clinic Foundation, University Hospitals of Cleveland, and other academic medical centers runs "counter to current business theory of focusing on what you do best . . . and getting rid of everything else," suggests Neuhauser. He wonders whether "this business theory may predict the future of" the Cleveland Clinic and University Hospitals.[6]

With little experience in this kind of work, Penn also had to devise financial and medical systems to service the primary care, off-campus practices. The Cleveland Clinic had had decades of experience with this type of administration and could more easily extend it to the external sites. The Clinic was, in effect, expanding its proven method of employing clinicians, the only difference being that they worked outside the main campus.

Consequently, CCA at Penn lost money, and, as best can be determined, did not produce sufficient "downstream revenue" in the form of referrals to HUP and use of centralized services to justify the losses. These results led to shedding of some of the practices as the physicians' contracts ran out—the capital costs remained, of course—and adjustment of the terms of employment to emphasize greater responsibility by the doctors in running their practices.

The Cleveland Clinic regional health network of employed doctors also does not by itself make money. It's a loss leader with, on average, each doctor costing more than he or she earns from his or her professional services. But when one adds the income produced by the laboratory tests the network physicians order and the value of the referrals to the physicians and surgeons at the Clinic's owned hospitals and main campus, the losses disappear. The Clinic considers its regional network critical to the continuing success of the Cleveland Clinic Foundation.[2]

In addition to the members of the group practice working in the suburban centers, the Clinic has also been able to attract the allegiance of privately practicing physicians, many of whom admit patients to the community hospitals owned by the Clinic by, among other attractions, participating in the Cleveland Clinic Health Network, which obtains contracts from health care insurers.

At University Hospitals' Primary Care Practices, the physicians are employed by University Hospitals Health System but encouraged to conduct their practices as they think best. The scheme is similar to how Clinical Care Associates at Penn's health system now operates, with significant incentives to encourage the physicians to practice efficiently.

As did several academic medical centers, University Hospitals created its own third-party administrator and provider-owned health plan. The purpose of establishing QualChoice, of course, was to contract with a group of patients who would be admitted to University Hospitals or, after the expansion of University Hospitals Health System, to those admitted to one of the system's community hospitals.

An Instructive Suit

With the Cleveland Clinic, University Hospitals, and their networks the dominant providers of private hospital services in the Cleveland region, competition between them for medical business is intense. Sometimes, the rivalry has reached the courts. For example, nine doctors from the Cleveland Clinic who were practicing in a West Side suburb sued a nearby community hospital in the University Hospitals system for privileges to admit their patients there. The Clinic doctors wanted privileges at the University Hospitals facility because that hospital, where ambulances often took their patients, was closer to the doctors' offices than the nearest hospital affiliated with the Cleveland Clinic. Denying the Clinic doctors privileges prevented them from caring for their patients in the University Hospitals facility and then referring them for further treatment to Clinic hospitals, rather than to University Hospitals and its specialists. Furthermore, pleased by the services where they had been hospitalized, patients might switch their future care to University Hospitals doctors and facilities.

In June 2003, a Common Pleas Court judge ruled against the Clinic doctors by supporting the authority of nonprofit hospitals to limit staff privileges to doctors who admit patients to them.[10] In explaining its disapproval of the decision, the Clinic asserted that the ruling "will severely restrict a patient's right to choose their [sic] own physician," according to an article about the suit in *The Plain Dealer*.[10] University Hospitals officials told the newspaper's reporter that "its privileged policy had nothing to do with hospital rivalry" and described its approach as a "focused strategy of trying to control quality and have a dedicated medical staff that develops and improves the hospital and patient care."[10] Despite these explanations, the fundamental theme was competition and its economic consequences in this highly competitive environment.

Rule by Doctors versus Rule by Trustees and a Lay Executive

"Everyone needs a Cleveland Clinic down the block," said James Block[11] in referring to the medical center toward which he and his successor Farah Walters looked—with respect by Block, with obsessive concern by Walters.

Both Block's respect and Walters's concern are appropriate. The Clinic, a twentieth-century creation without a medical school or the traditions of the older Lakeside Hospital and Western Reserve University, was, by the beginning of the twenty-first century, larger, more widely known, and higher-ranked among hospitals in general and for many of its clinical services in particular. What accounts for the success of this offspring of its principal competitor?

From its founding by doctors, the Cleveland Clinic had been run by doctors for the primary purpose of providing them, as members of a group practice, with the means of practicing their profession under the most professional and convenient circumstances. The nine elected members of the board of governors, each of whom is a doctor, represent the interests of the doctors in the group practice, and together with the CEO, also a doctor, and the administrative staff decide how the Clinic should operate and develop.

During the 1990s, as the Clinic and University Hospitals of Cleveland competed to dominate the region by linking to community hospitals and incorporating physician practices, the Clinic's efficient corporate structure allowed decisions to be reached rapidly and, once made, instituted expeditiously. Loop, however, was not free to carry out his plans before justifying them to an elected group of his colleagues.

For example, even though it is unlikely that a savvy cardiac surgeon like Fred Loop would make such a mistake, the governors would have been available to evaluate and advise against such decisions as the disastrous recruitment and administrative assignment of the cardiac surgeons at University Hospitals.* The recruiting process is difficult enough. Even with the advice of knowledgeable colleagues, the appointing authority can never be sure that even the most attractive candidate will succeed. In contrast to most academic medical centers, where the faculty and dean lead the recruiting of the professional staff, Walters participated actively in the recruitment of doctors, and the only group to which she was responsible was her board. The trustees, the board's executive committee, and the chairmen, under the force of her commanding presence and persuasive arguments, participated much less intimately in her decisions than did the members of the board of governors at the Clinic in the actions proposed by Loop. As one would

---

*It was rumored that Loop, knowing that their work would, to put it gently, disappoint their new employers, deliberately encouraged the recruitment of the surgeons by University Hospitals.[12]

expect, medical school faculty fault the recruiting of clinicians and investigators by lay hospital directors. As one senior member of the faculty at University Hospitals said, "When nonprofessionals intrude into things like selecting professionals, organizations can deteriorate."[13]*

Although members of the administrative staff at the Clinic were clearly Loop's and now Cosgrove's to hire and fire, the members of the board of governors are elected by the members of the group practice—albeit from a slate of candidates proposed by the governors—not appointed by the CEO. Loop's predecessor as CEO sees the three principal centers of power there— the governors, the CEO, and the trustees—"watching each other; thus, checks and balances."[15] University Hospitals of Cleveland, like many academic medical centers, has no group like the Clinic's board of governors to influence, and when necessary, control the actions of the CEO. Management at the Cleveland Clinic Foundation during the 1990s—a decade of "halcyon years" for the Clinic, according to a leading trustee at CASE[16]—was clearly less hierarchical and more collaborative than at its less successful neighbor.

Notwithstanding the usually efficient governance shared by the CEO with the board of governors, the Cleveland Clinic Foundation has made decisions of questionable value. Although the Clinic now seems committed to continuing the venture, for many years its leaders considered closing the Florida satellite, which had brought much political turmoil and serious financial losses since its founding.[17]

Application of the Cleveland Clinic Model to Other Medical Centers

Is the Cleveland Clinic's structure applicable at most academic medical centers? This seems doubtful. The most likely prospects are those institutions that are governed by one entity. This includes medical schools and teaching hospitals that are ruled by one executive at the twelve state-owned centers such as the University of California, San Francisco,[18] or at the twenty-nine privately owned centers such as the University of Pennsylvania.[19]

---

*Walters insists that she did not undertake recruitments without consulting and involving the appropriate members of the faculty.[14] Many members of the University Hospitals staff with whom I spoke think otherwise.

History and tradition are the biggest stumbling blocks. The Clinic was founded for the ambulatory care of the patients of its founders and their colleagues. A hospital, the teaching of medical students, training of house officers and fellows, and research were added in subsequent years. The Clinic only had a medical school it could call its own eighty-five years after its beginning.

Medical schools began specifically to train students to become doctors. At first, the faculty, who charged personal fees for the students to attend their lectures, often considered the schools their private fiefdoms. Gradually, the doctors lost their direct control, to be replaced by universities, which set the curriculum and collected tuition to pay either fully or partially employed faculty. The need for places to train their students led, in some cases, to the universities' either founding or acquiring one or more hospitals.

The clinicians at most medical schools and, for most of the time American schools have existed, were independent practitioners who joined the faculty for the advantages this brought them. These included admitting privileges to the university's hospital, the prestige associated with such an affiliation, the opportunity to teach and supervise students and trainees, and the scholarly benefit of association with other like-minded doctors and the basic scientists that the school employed. Only during the second half of the twentieth century did medical academic medical centers begin to consolidate their practitioners into full-time employees of the school or the hospital. In some centers, an important group of faculty members continued to practice independently, their value to the hospital measured in how many patients they admitted and to the school by the time they devoted to teaching students and supervising the care provided by the house officers and fellows.

Despite the apparent consolidation of the clinicians within the corporate structure, the primary criterion for promotion at most of the older schools was, and continues to be, academic productivity—the university's sense of what constitutes a successful senior faculty member. At the Clinic, the constant theme remains, "Are you a good clinician?" So far, it does not appear that Loop's recruitment of academic leaders from other institutions as departmental chairmen has substantially changed this basic concept.

A constant feature of most academic medical centers continues to be the competition, sometimes the conflict, between hospital, medical school, and doctors. At the Clinic, at least until now, this tension has been muted since, from the beginning, the leading activity has been clinical care, provided by a unified group of clinicians who have chosen to work together for their joint and individual benefit. The CEO, usually a doctor,* typically a surgeon, heads the entire organization subject to the gentle advice of the board of trustees. Although he has an administrative staff to help him, it is the board of governors, who, with the CEO, operate the Clinic. So far, the addition of a growing basic research program has not interfered with the dominance of the group practice. How the presence of the medical college will affect the practice remains to be seen and troubles some of the more traditionally minded doctors.

Bringing the Clinic's operation to some of the nation's medical schools is, however, an attractive thought. Although obviously biased by their affiliation, current and past members of the staff believe that some features of their unique institution must be exportable. Doing so, however, will be difficult. "Our coordinated system would interfere with the different interests those in the hospital and medical school have," acknowledges the new Clinic CEO Toby Cosgrove, who has worked at and observed several of the country's most respected traditional academic medical centers.[21]

Transitions

One is struck by the differences between how changes of leadership occur at the executive level and for more routine jobs. A paper trail of criticism, admonitions, and advice on how to improve performance must precede the firing of the average employee. Not so at the highest levels. "Executives like chief operating officer, chief financial officer, and my position serve at the pleasure of senior authority," explains Robert Ivancic, the director of human relations at the Cleveland Clinic.[22] "These jobs depend more on whether the executive fits with the boss in style, philosophy, and attitude and less on questions of job performance," says Ivancic, "and explains why the arrival of a new boss can lead to changes." In nonexecutive jobs, "the main question is whether the employee is doing what is expected from the job description."[22]

How well do leaders of academic medical centers handle senior person-

---

*Laymen were the senior executives of the Clinic from 1940, when George Crile, the last of the founding doctors retired, until 1969 when the board of governors, created fourteen years previously, asserted its control and chose the Clinic's first physician-manager.[20]

nel matters? "Most docs don't have managerial experience," says Robert Coulton, the director of professional staff affairs at the Cleveland Clinic, "and think that managing is a simple thing to do."[23] Lacking such knowledge, "they're thrown into new responsibilities."[23]

Many physicians in managerial positions find communicating criticism difficult.[23] Consequently, the subordinate—and this seems to apply more to administrative than professional staff—may find himself relieved of his job without knowing where he failed or how his boss wanted him to improve his performance. This seems to have happened to some of those nonphysician executives recently relieved or retired at the Clinic.

Part of the problem probably lies in the inability of the boss to articulate what he wants in language that the manager can understand. He just knows he's unhappy with the associate's performance, but can't quantify it partly because he hasn't grown up in the management business. The severity of the problem can probably be reduced by putting criticisms in writing and sharing them with the person being evaluated. This will reduce the misunderstandings that can result when criticisms are buried in compliments, as in, "I wish you could improve your performance in this area, but, I must tell you, you're doing a terrific job." Which part of this sentence will the employee remember? Despite the realization, as the director of human relations at the Clinic was heard to say, that "these jobs are so vulnerable,"[24] managers want, or should want, to know about their deficiencies so that they can improve their performances whether or not they remain in their current jobs.

Although evaluating the administrative skills of physician- or lay managers can challenge physician-executives, appraising clinical abilities presents fewer difficulties. Many, though regrettably not all, doctors know when it's time to retire, and if not, their decreasing clinical skills become relatively easy to document if the institution incorporates the type of review process followed by the Clinic. The criteria—operative deaths for a surgeon, to take an extreme example, or repeatedly missed diagnoses and inappropriate treatment for an internist—are well understood and accepted. Physicians, unlike most professional managers, are an independent lot, not given to marching to an organization's tune. Although many of the doctors at the Cleveland Clinic see themselves as cogs in a large group practice, they know, so long as they maintain their professional skills, no one will interfere with what they have been trained and hired to do—caring for patients.

Trustees

Despite the clout of CEOs like Fred Loop and Farah Walters, the ultimate authority at both the Cleveland Clinic and University Hospitals of Cleveland resides in their boards of trustees. "Although Cleveland is a large city, it is, in many ways, rather like a small town," in the opinion of Karen Horn, who chaired the CASE board in the 1990s but was not a Cleveland native or perpetual resident.[25] Consequently, the number of community leaders suitable to join these groups is not large,[26,27] and is even too small in the opinion of one leading Clinic trustee "to have separate boards for CASE and University Hospitals."[27] Accordingly, several influential leaders serve on more than one board. This overlap has raised concerns,[28,29] particularly for trustees on the boards of both the CASE and University Hospitals, institutions with recurrent conflicts about affiliation agreements.

The members of hospital boards tend to be local residents since hospitals, for the most part, are community resources supplying medical care to the trustees' fellow citizens, and not incidentally, to the trustees themselves and their families. Consequently, the members of the University Hospitals board, in the opinion of one of the CASE board chairs, "felt closer to the hospital, which was smaller and had more connection to the institution [than did the average university trustee to CASE]."[25] The relationship of University Hospitals trustees to their academic partner could be fairly distant. Although, until recently, few members of the CASE board have been alumni,* the number of University Hospitals trustees who held degrees from CASE was even smaller.[31]

Many trustees accept positions on hospital as well as university boards primarily for the prestige such membership brings, according to Malvin Bank, a leading Cleveland attorney and himself a member of, and advisor to, many charitable boards, including CASE. "Most don't intend to spend a substantial amount of time," Bank has observed, "and not all fully understand the fiduciary responsibilities they have assumed in joining boards,"[32] a point of view shared by others who criticize hospital trustees for their lack of knowledge of specific hospital and medical issues.[33] Although trustees

---

*Edward Hundert has changed this. By the summer of 2004, 75 percent of the board were alumni.[30] Frank Linsalata, the current chairman of the board of trustees of Case Western Reserve University, received his undergraduate degree in mechanical engineering from what was then the Case Institute of Technology.

understand that they will be asked to make financial contributions, many, according to Bank, donate from the resources of their corporations, where they tend to hold one of the top positions, or from foundations they control or influence. Relatively few are sufficiently rich to give substantial amounts from their own wealth.[32]

Bank has seen how many trustees, CEOs, in many cases, who have used their political skills to help them reach their positions, may think twice before taking strong positions on charitable boards. "Most trustees," his experience has taught him, "are reluctant to become involved in bitter fights to relieve chief executives since it takes significant effort to get people out and can cause a great deal of friction among friends."[32] Trustees of charitable boards, in Karen Horn's experience, "often prefer to avoid controversy. Besides, everybody in the business community knows each other."[25] Accordingly, it is not surprising to learn that the CASE trustees rejected the effort of the clinical chairmen to replace the university president,[25] just as the University Hospitals board long resisted taking action against its CEO. "They don't want to use up their credits with the other trustees," Bank has said,[32] or "say 'no' to their golf partners" in the words of one of the CASE medical school chairmen.[34] The city fathers "simply don't like conflict or contention or being in the spotlight," according to another chairman, which, he concluded, "is how Walters influenced her trustees."[35] This pattern helps to explain how Farah Walters kept her job particularly during the last two years of her administration when many from the hospital and the university strongly opposed her decisions and methods of operating. One of the longtime members of the board found the trustees to be "the usual cadre of volunteer leaders who can't give the amount of attention needed to their volunteer jobs." One observer went so far as to say that "the board should be blamed as much as Farah."

During the 1990s and earlier, most members of the board of Case Western Reserve University were, like the hospital trustees, from Cleveland.[16,25,31,36,37] Recently, more alumni, a few of whom are doctors[38] and most of whom live in other cities, have become trustees of CASE.[16,31,38] The university and hospital boards, however, have historically included more members of "Cleveland's first families"* than has the Cleveland Clinic board.[15,31] "Their families had all gone to UH," said one of the Clinic

---

*Observers of the local scene believe that the influence of Cleveland's first families on the CASE and University Hospitals boards has decreased in recent years.[37,39]

trustees in describing the loyalty of many University Hospitals board members, "and they still do."[40] Of the trustees with personal affluence, those on the board of the University Hospitals of Cleveland were more likely, at least in the past though less so now,[41] to have "old money" when compared with the Cleveland Clinic trustees, the wealth of many, as a general rule, having been acquired more recently.[15,31,37,40,42-44] Perhaps in accord with these observations, the Clinic board has been more successful in raising money than the University Hospitals trustees.[45]

In addition to supplying valuable financial advice, the Clinic trustees tend to take the long view on strategic topics, while the governors plan and conduct day-to-day operations.[46] "We're ambassadors for the Clinic in the community and elsewhere," explains trustee William MacDonald III.[43] "The meetings are mostly for information sharing and education. One of the doctors usually describes the latest medical advances." Art Model* adds, "It's a contributing board. They'll put in time for the institution,"[44] but, adds MacDonald, "we don't micromanage."[43]

In keeping with the Clinic's greater national and international reputation, Loop had arranged that several non-Cleveland residents be appointed to the Clinic board, more than are trustees of University Hospitals. Loop had become widely known within the profession for his surgical work before he became CEO, and the people he tends to associate with are not the "old Cleveland types."

Many of the CASE trustees, when Karen Horn was serving as a member and then as chair in the 1990s, seemed, in her words, "less than fully informed about what was going on."[25] Others also believe that many of the CASE trustees did not have much knowledge of medical school and hospital affairs and "had to learn during a period of stress."[31] Local members were often chosen more for the jobs they held, their personal financial resources,

---

*One of the most loyal Clinic trustees, Modell suffered the fate of prominent people whose actions arouse the enmity of sports fans. Arthur ("Art") Modell bought the Cleveland Browns football team in 1961; in 1996, he moved the franchise to Baltimore, where the team became the Ravens.[47] Though the Browns name stayed in Cleveland, which acquired a new stadium and an expansion team, local fans never forgave him.[44,48]

In recognition of Modell's many contributions, including being president of the board for nine years—which he describes as "a labor of love for me"—the Clinic dedicated the large cardiac waiting area to Modell, who had had bypass surgery at the Clinic.[44] His decision to move the team so aroused the public that a large bronze plaque erected in the atrium to honor him had to be removed.[40] Feeling that he would not be welcome in Cleveland, where he has many friends, Modell has never visited there since he left.[40,44]

or, in a few cases, social standing than from a desire to serve their alma mater with their expertise and judgment since few held CASE degrees anyway. It was these local members who tended to think that the university and medical school were "okay."[25] The business members who had been imported to jobs in Cleveland from elsewhere felt that both could be better.[25]

Anthony Kovner,* who has specialized in studying not-for-profit hospitals, feels strongly that the inadequacies of hospital boards need to be better recognized. "The members of all too many nonprofit hospital boards don't understand what their function should be. They don't really comprehend the business of hospitals, which isn't helped when the executives feed them bad information, and, finally, they're not accountable to anyone."[49] Kovner adds that on for-profit boards many of the trustees are executives in similar companies, which is not the case for most hospital trustees. "It would help if hospital boards included CEOs from other similar institutions," he advises.[49]

"Trustees are the great strength and the great weakness of such places," says Bradford Gray.† "You go to a nonprofit in trouble, and you find the boards asleep at the switch."[50] Gray disapproves of the unlimited terms of trustees on many nonprofit boards‡ and questions the lengthy service of many CEOs.[50]

Loyalty to their institutions, however, is not the problem on boards that lead such centers as the Cleveland Clinic Foundation. When interviewed, trustees there couldn't say enough good things about their charge:

- "It's deeply dedicated to continuous improvement. Don't know of any other institution in Cleveland that is such a shining star raising the reputation of the city."[17]
- "It's so good because of its ability to attract great medical people."[43]
- "A doc-centered institution with the ability to attract talent and good leadership. The leading institution of its kind in Cleveland."[51]
- "Truly an amazing place."[27]
- "A legacy unmatched anywhere."[44]

---

*Kovner is professor and director of the program in health policy and management at New York University's Wagner Graduate School of Public Service.

†Gray is director of the division of health and science policy at the New York Academy of Sciences.

‡At the Clinic, the trustees' terms are not limited. "But," says trustee Patrick McCarten, "we're talking about that."[51]

As Kevin Roberts, who worked at the Cleveland Clinic before he became chief financial officer at University Hospitals Health System, ruefully admits, "their trustees are marketing the place all the time."[52]

Choosing the CEO

It is often said that the principal role of trustees in the type of organizations studied here is to hire or fire the chief executive. But how meaningful is this power at the Cleveland Clinic and University Hospitals of Cleveland?

Although a joint committee of governors and trustees participated in the search for a CEO at the Cleveland Clinic in 1989, the doctors on the board of governors dominated the choice and the trustees authorized it. At University Hospitals of Cleveland, a search committee of four trustees and three members of the medical faculty* nominated the current CEO.[53] Each of the faculty members was a respected physician or scientist, but each had been appointed to the committee by the trustees, not elected to this responsibility by the medical staff. In the end, the committee recommended, and the trustees selected, a hospital administrator, not a clinician, as the CEO of the University Hospitals Health System. The new CEO, strongly advised to do so by the trustees and leading doctors, then selected a physician as director of University Hospitals. Although he had practiced pediatrics and directed clinical departments earlier in his career, the new hospital director had assumed primarily administrative duties as senior vice president under Walters from 1996 and acting CEO of the health system after she resigned.

Although its search committee considered hiring a nonphysician as CEO in 1989,[40] the Cleveland Clinic followed its custom and chose a doctor. It seems highly unlikely that the Clinic would have appointed someone like James Block or Farah Walters. Although a pediatrician, Block had practiced little during his career, and Farah Walters was not a doctor. Furthermore, the style of leadership exercised by Farah Walters at University Hospitals of Cleveland would not have been accepted by the members of the Cleveland

---

*The faculty members were Dennis Landis, chairman of the department of neurology and president of the council of clinical chairmen (a temporary post elected by his chairmen of the clinical departments); Huntington Willard, a geneticist but not a physician whom Walters had appointed director of the University Hospitals Research Institute and who would soon leave for Duke University; and Hermann Menges, one of the founders of University Suburban Health Center.[53,54] The trustees, and especially the chairman of the committee, trustee John Morley, kept them fully involved and informed during the search process, according to one of the physician members.[54]

Clinic. Although few would describe Fred Loop as docile, he has led the Clinic by collaborating closely with the doctors on the board of governors and the senior leaders of the divisions and departments and the administration. So it appears that in choosing recent CEOs at both institutions, the doctors, through their board of governors, dominated the choice at the Cleveland Clinic Foundation, whereas at University Hospitals Health System, the trustees made the appointment.

Trustees of teaching hospitals, few of whom are members of the medical or academic professions, will favor as leaders those with the organizational, motivational, and financial skills they have emphasized in their careers. And in institutions that are independently ruled and not subsidiaries of universities—the most common form of governance at American teaching hospitals[8]—such nonacademic and nonmedical criteria may become paramount in the selection of who will lead the hospital and health system. To facilitate the process, advises attorney and former CASE trustee Malvin Bank, "boards should spend more time on developing well-thought-out, detailed job descriptions for hospital CEOs. They must make sure that successful candidates have the most important of the characteristics sought, and they must check references in person. If they do all of that, they will avoid making mistakes."[55]

Does the appointment of a professional hospital administrator as CEO at an academic medical center necessarily bode ill for accomplishing the complex missions of such institutions while at the same time achieving financial success? The answer is no in some cases and regrettably yes in others, but the same can be said for the presence of a doctor in the big corner office of the hospital executive suite.

Conflict of Interest

On May 29, 2001, an article appeared in *The Plain Dealer* pointing out the problems inherent when trustees serve on the boards of both CASE and University Hospitals of Cleveland.[29] "If an individual serves on more than one board, it clearly is a duality of interest, and probably a conflict," a consultant on nonprofit health care governance was quoted as saying, "especially in periods of market crisis and in situations of intense competition or sensitive negotiations."[29]

When reporter Diane Solov wrote the piece, four trustees were members of both boards, and the wife of the CASE board chairman was a longtime trustee of University Hospitals. The article appeared only one month after David Auston had suddenly resigned from the presidency of the university partly because he felt that some of his trustees were pushing him to oblige the university to accept an affiliation agreement with University Hospitals of Cleveland, the terms of which he thought detrimental to CASE.[56] It was clear that Auston had less control over his board than did Farah Walters over hers, giving her the ability, in the word of one consultant, to "neutralize" the university president.[56]

The criticism particularly applies when trustees or their spouses simultaneously serve on the boards of directly competing institutions such as the Cleveland Clinic and University Hospitals of Cleveland. No example of this combination existed in Cleveland, except in the case of the wife of one of the officers of the Clinic board who was a trustee of University Hospitals.[57]*

What complicated the situation at University Circle was the conflict agitating the relationship of CASE with its principal hospital affiliate. Former university president Agnar Pytte attributed some of his difficulty resolving the differences between the university and hospitals during his term to joint membership on the university and hospital boards by some of the trustees. "Clearly a conflict of interest," he believed.[58] What should have been solved with an arrangement advantageous to both was complicated by the specific aims of the leaders. In the face of such disharmony, trustees who owed allegiance to both institutions through membership on both boards could not fulfill the purpose of their dual service to seek collaboration for the benefit of both institutions.[56] As an attorney who is a member of the CASE and several other for-profit and nonprofit boards said, "They get so involved personally that they ignore their fiduciary responsibilities."[57] With new administrations at both the university and the hospital, perhaps the two institutions can now relate to each other more as partners than as antagonists.

Although some board members defend overlapping trusteeships and argue that they do not produce conflicting interests,[59,60] there can be little doubt that the potential for these exist when hospitals contract with business organizations that are led by trustees in such businesses as ac-

---

*Hundert has dealt with this problem as follows: "CASE trustees who are members of boards of any of the hospitals with which the university is affiliated, or if their spouses are on such boards, now recuse themselves from discussion or voting on any matters relating to hospital affiliations."[30]

counting, banking, hospital services, law, and public relations.[61] Administrators and CEOs, whose jobs depend on maintaining good relations with leading trustees, may respond to perceived pressures and allow personal considerations to affect business decisions.

Conflict among Leaders

Conflict between the chief executives of University Hospitals of Cleveland and Case Western Reserve University has affected the academic and clinical missions of the medical school and hospital. The difficulty was not limited to the 1990s. Harry Bolwell, chairman of the hospital board from 1978 to 1987 and the dominant leader for much of that time, didn't believe that a medical school was necessary for a hospital to be great and was so anti-CASE that he wouldn't read mail on university stationery.

When James Block became president of the hospital in 1986, and Agnar Pytte president of the university a year later, the quarrel continued. They soon fell out with each other, and it was this tradition of discord that Farah Walters inherited when she succeeded Block in 1992. Both highly able with strong personalities, neither Pytte nor Walters reported to the other but to separate boards of trustees, which, despite some overlapping members, acted quite independently of each other. Caught in the midst of their struggle were the deans of the CASE medical school, not well supported or appreciated by Pytte and subservient to Walters because of their dependence on the hospital for financial support to the clinical departments.

Personal conflict between executives at academic medical centers can so roil medical institutions that changes in governance may result.[8] This happened at the University of Pennsylvania and the Johns Hopkins University. At Penn the conflict between the leader of the medical enterprise and the university president resulted in the dean/executive vice president of the academic medical center losing his job. The university then undertook a comprehensive study of the governance linking the medical center to the university, which had historically owned the principal teaching hospital and, of course, the medical school. Eventually, the trustees, strongly influenced by the medical faculty and the new dean, decided not to change the governance.

At Hopkins, the controversy between the dean of the medical school and the president of the hospital—the two enterprises have always been separate corporations—led to the creation of one comprehensive entity, Johns Hopkins Medicine, directed by one man with the titles of dean of the medical school and CEO of the Johns Hopkins Health System, which included the famous Johns Hopkins Hospital. At University Hospitals of Cleveland and Case Western Reserve University, the governance remained the same although changes had frequently been considered.

Penn, Hopkins, and the medical institutions at University Circle suffered primarily because of the conflicts between their leaders. In Cleveland, the arrival of a new university president, an academic physician and psychiatrist, and new leaders of the health system, hospital, and medical school suggested that the problems of past decades will not recur.

As the leaders of the institutions at University Circle struggled with each other, their neighbor one mile west on Euclid Avenue grew and flourished. Untroubled by divided governance, the Cleveland Clinic concentrated on its primary purpose of delivering high-quality clinical care, with education and research clearly secondary missions. The Clinic's unusual method of conducting its business through a board of physician governors and a single CEO accounted, as much as any single factor, for its stability and growth.

Cleveland Clinic and University Hospitals of Cleveland Are Different, but How Different?

Despite its success, not all doctors want to work for the Cleveland Clinic. "The corporate culture is not for me," said Alan Markowitz, the cardiac surgeon at University Hospitals. However, he admits, for University Hospitals to compete successfully with the Clinic, "the same model may be needed here. It's too expensive for a private practice to succeed in a university hospital."[62] Markowitz recommends adopting at least one part of the Clinic's organization. "We need a board of governors."[62]

Markowitz is expressing a point of view shared by other doctors working at University Hospitals. "Our place," says John Haaga, the chairman of radiology who formerly worked at the Clinic, "has more individuality, permits more inventiveness, and has more free spirits. We're not all marching in step. Our setup better brings out individual strengths."[63] Haaga remembers having to submit a book he wanted to publish to a committee for approval at the Clinic, a restriction not required at the university. "The downside here at UH is that there's more strife." Haaga acknowledges that "the Clinic has better esprit de corps. 'We're the one,' they feel. 'Let's pull together.' The culture perceived outside is correct. The Clinic's monolithic, but it's also less chaotic."[63]

Despite its renowned bureaucratic approach, "there's more 'out-of-the-box' thinking at the Clinic," believes Scott Cowen, who was dean of the CASE business school before becoming president of Tulane University.[64]

The doctors and investigators working at University Hospitals of Cleveland and the CASE medical school perform significantly more funded clinical and basic medical research than do those at the Clinic, which is consistent with research being one of the fundamental missions of the institutions at University Circle. Data from the NIH, whose grants are considered to be among the most competitive to receive, support this contention. For the fiscal year ending September 30, 2003, Case Western Reserve University School of Medicine stood eighteenth out of 121 schools with $203,512,407 in total awards, just below such respected research medical schools as those at the University of Alabama and Vanderbilt University.[65] Among research institutes, which is where the NIH places it, the Cleveland Clinic received $46,875,052 in fiscal 2003, ninth in that group.[66] Higher on the list are several other well-known research institutions. If the Clinic, with this amount of NIH support, was ranked among medical schools, it would have stood sixty-seventh in 2003.[66a]

Another method used by those interested in such matters to rank academic medical centers counts the number of faculty who are members of the honor societies that elect academic physicians and surgeons to membership.[67–70]

- Institute of Medicine—CASE 8, Clinic 1
- American Society for Clinic Investigation (which honors physician scientists—most of whom are members of departments of medicine—who have achieved success in research relatively early in their careers)—CASE 22, Clinic 7
- Association of American Physicians (the senior society of, for the most part, distinguished members of departments of medicine)—CASE 8, Clinic 2
- American Surgical Association (the senior society of distinguished surgeons)—CASE 4, Clinic 6.

- And in the most competitive of them all, the National Academy of Sciences, CASE has 2 members from the medical school and the Clinic 1

These data confirm the superior academic accomplishments of the medical faculty at CASE and University Hospitals when compared with members of the Clinic staff. Clinic loyalists explain this difference by emphasizing that the primary purpose of the Clinic has been to deliver clinical care and that an energetic research enterprise is a development of recent years. The greater number of Clinic doctors in the American Surgical Association supports this premise and emphasizes the Clinic's traditional leadership in surgery.

In recent years, the differences between the two institutions have tended to decrease. Emphasis on clinical work at University Hospitals has grown as the Clinic has become more academic.[71] The Clinic is acquiring many of the attributes of academic medical centers with growing strength in basic research and a tradition of graduate and postgraduate education and, more recently, medical student training. Only its own medical school had been missing—until now.

Founded by doctors for doctors, the Cleveland Clinic has fulfilled its mission of delivering large-scale, first-class medical care because it has concentrated on the practice of medicine and in doing so has paid continuous attention to supplying the facilities and services the patients and their doctors require. A practicing doctor as CEO represents the ultimate expression of the dominance of the group practice as the basis of the Cleveland Clinic's operation. The Cleveland Clinic succeeds as a unique medical institution, uniquely organized. There are few others like it.

The New Medical College

Although the leaders and many of their colleagues have long thought that the Cleveland Clinic needs a medical school, one could ask whether the nation needs another one.[72] Manpower studies, a controversial topic subject to limited predictability, suggested in the 1990s that the United States had more physicians than it required, and that the addition of more doctors would increase the cost of medical care while not providing additional care for underserved populations. One commission recommended that, by 2005, the country should reduce the size of its graduating classes from the current 16,000 to about 13,500 and that one-quarter of the medical schools should close.[73] Recent studies suggest that the country will need more, not fewer, doctors in the next two decades.[74]

In deciding to join Case Western Reserve rather than forming a completely separate medical school, Cleveland Clinic leaders may have realized that lobbyists for the other state-supported medical schools might use the manpower argument to impede certifying the Clinic to award degrees. Similar reasoning may explain why the Clinic does not intend to request state support such as the other private medical school in the state at Case Western Reserve receives, the price of which required, until recently, that CASE admit more than half of its students from Ohio.

Of course, the effect of adding thirty-two more graduates each year—an increase of only 0.2 percent per year, or 0.24 students if spread among all the nation's medical schools—will change very little the total number of new physicians working in the United States. If most of the Cleveland Clinic students choose a career in clinical research, as the founders hope they will, the pool of practicing physicians will rise even less. CASE president Edward Hundert emphasizes the national need for more doctors performing clinical research. "If only half do it [enter careers in clinical research], we'll be in the vanguard compared with other schools."[75]

What many thoughtful observers of the Clinic's history and traditions are also asking is whether the development of a medical school will so change the Clinic model that it will begin to experience some of the turmoil that afflicts many academic medical centers, as Clinic leaders could observe in its neighbor during the 1990s. The unified governance at the Clinic should help to limit these potential problems.

The leaders and members of the nation's other medical schools will be watching with interest to see whether the Clinic's unique form of governance will lend itself to the successful conversion of one of the nation's leading clinical providers into a successful comprehensive academic medical center with its medical school tightly linked to a university, an arrangement which is associated with the Clinic's principal clinical competitor. As the CASE doctor-president Edward Hundert puts it, "Can competition for national leadership collectively replace competition between themselves?"[30]

Interviewees

Past and present titles at the Cleveland Clinic, University Hospitals, or CASE are listed first. Titles without dates are those held when this appendix was prepared in the spring of 2004. Locations are in Cleveland, unless otherwise indicated.

CASE = Case Western Reserve University; CC = Cleveland Clinic; CCF = Cleveland Clinic Foundation; CEO = chief executive officer; College = Cleveland Clinic Lerner College of Medicine of Case Western Reserve University School of Medicine; Ireland = Ireland Cancer Center; LRI = Lerner Research Institute; MacDonald = MacDonald Hospital for Women; P & S = Columbia University College of Physicians and Surgeons, New York; Rainbow = Rainbow Babies & Children's Hospital; SOM = Case Western Reserve University School of Medicine; UMDNJ = University of Medicine and Dentistry of New Jersey–New Jersey Medical School, Newark; UHC = University Hospitals of Cleveland; UHHS = University Hospitals Health System.

Name	Position
Aach, Richard D., M.D.	Associate Dean & Director, Residency & Career Planning, SOM
Abbey, Charles R.	Executive Director, University Suburban Health Center
Abzug, Rikki, Ph.D.	Assistant Professor, Nonprofit Management Program, Milano Graduate School of Management and Urban Policy, New School University, New York City
Adler, Dale, M.D.	Chief, Division of Cardiology, UHC
Ahmad, Muzaffar, M.D.	Chairman, Division of Medicine (1991–2003), CC
Altus, Gene	Administrator, Board of Governors, CC
Anker, Daniel E., Ph.D.	Associate Dean for Faculty & Institutional Affairs, SOM
Anlyan, William G., M.D.	Chairman, Cleveland Foundation Study Commission on Medical Research & Education (1991–92); Chancellor for Health Affairs, Duke University (1964–89)

Name	*Position*
Avner, Ellis D., M.D.	Director, Children's Research Institute at Children's Hospital & Health System & Associate Dean for Research, Medical College of Wisconsin, Milwaukee; Chairman, Department of Pediatrics, SOM (1995–2003)
Balke, C. William, M.D.	Senior Associate Dean for Clinical Research & Director, Institute of Molecular Medicine, University of Kentucky School of Medicine, Lexington; Head, Division of Cardiology, University of Maryland School of Medicine (2000–2004)
Bank, Malvin E.	Trustee, CASE; Senior Partner, Thompson Hine LLP
Baznik, Richard E.	Director, Institute for the Study of the University in Society, CASE
Behrman, Richard E., M.D.	Dean, SOM (1980–89); Executive Chair, Federation of Pediatric Organizations
Berger, Nathan A., M.D.	Director, Center for Science, Health & Society, CASE; Dean, SOM (1996–2002)
Bickers, David R., M.D.	Chairman, Department of Dermatology, P & S; Chairman, Department of Dermatology, SOM (1979–93)
Blazar, James M.	Chief Marketing Officer, CC
Block, James A., M.D.	President & CEO, UHC (1986–92)
Bloomfield, Daniel K., M.D.	Author, *Keys to the Asylum,* Champaign, IL, New Medical Press, 2000
Bolton, Charles P.	Trustee, Chairman, Board of Trustees (2001–4), CASE
Bolwell, Brian J., M.D.	Director, Bone-Marrow Transplantation Program, CC
Bolwell, Harry J.	Chairman, Board of Trustees, UHC (1978–87)
Bond, Meredith, Ph.D.	Member of the staff, LRI (1986–2003); Chairman, Department of Physiology, University of Maryland School of Medicine, Baltimore
Borden, Ernest C., M.D.	Department of Hematology & Medical Oncology, CC
Brieger, Gert H., M.D., Ph.D.	Director, Department of History of Science, Medicine & Technology, Johns Hopkins University & Johns Hopkins University School of Medicine (1984–2002)
Bronson, David L., M.D.	Chairman, Division of Regional Medical Practice, CC
Burry, John, Jr.	Chairman & CEO, Blue Cross/Blue Shield of Ohio & Medical Mutual (1982–97)
Calman, Angela	Chief Communications Officer, CC

Name	Position
Carpenter, Charles	Professor of Medicine, Brown University; Physician-in Chief, The Miriam Hospital, Providence, RI; Chairman, Department of Medicine, SOM (1973–86)
Cascorbi, Helmut F., M.D.	Professor of Anesthesiology, SOM; Chairman, Department of Anesthesiology, SOM (1980–2000)
Cherniak, Neil S., M.D.	Professor of Medicine & Physiology, UMDNJ; Dean, SOM (1990–95)
Chrencik, Robert A.	Executive Vice President & Chief Financial Officer, University of Maryland Medical System, Baltimore
Christianson, Jon B., Ph.D.	James A. Hamilton Chair in Health Policy & Management, Carlson School of Management, University of Minnesota
Clough, John D., M.D.	Executive Director, Cleveland Clinic Foundation Press; Editor-in-Chief, Cleveland Clinic Journal of Medicine
Coleman, Keith T.	President, University Hospitals Faculty Services
Colten, Harvey R., M.D.	Vice President & Senior Associate Dean, Translational Research, P & S
Cooper, Kevin D., M.D.	Chairman, Department of Dermatology, SOM
Copeland, Ronald L., M.D.	Executive Medical Director, Ohio Permanente Medical Group
Cosgrove, Delos M., M.D.	Chairman, Department of Thoracic & Cardiovascular Surgery, CC
Coulton, Robert W., Jr.	Administrator, Professional Staff Affairs, CC
Cowen, Scott S.	President, Tulane University
Cronin, Gina	Administrator, Department of Thoracic & Cardiovascular Surgery, CC
Crowe, Joseph P., M.D.	Director, Breast Center, Department of General Surgery, CC
Daroff, Robert B., M.D.	Interim Vice Dean for Education, SOM; Chief of Staff & Senior Vice President for Medical (later Academic) Affairs, UHC (1994–2003)
Davis, Pamela B., M.D., Ph.D.	Chief, Pulmonary Division, Department of Pediatrics, UHC & Associate Dean for Research, SOM
Devereaux, Michael W., M.D.	Professor of Neurology, SOM & Vice President, Clinical Integration, UHHS
DiCorleto, Paul E., Ph.D.	Chairman, LRI
Duda, Rick	Director of Sales & Marketing, Intercontinental Hotels

Name	*Position*
Eckardt, Robert E.	Vice President for Programs & Evaluation, The Cleveland Foundation
Egan, Michele M.	Vice President of Corporate Communications, Center for Health Affairs
Ellner, Jerrold J., M.D.	Chairman, Department of Medicine, UMDNJ; Acting Chairman, Department of Medicine, SOM (1997–98)
Emerman, Charles, M.D.	Chairman, Department of Emergency Medicine, CC
Estes, Melinda (Mindy) L., M.D.	CEO & Chairman, Board of Governors, Cleveland Clinic Florida (2001–3); CEO, Fletcher Allen Medical Center, Burlington, VT
Falcone, Tommaso, M.D.	Chairman, Department of Obstetrics & Gynecology, CC
Fazio, Victor, M.D.	Chairman, Department of Colorectal Surgery, CC
Ferry, John, M.D.	Senior Vice President, The Hunter Group, a unit of Navigant Consulting, Inc.; Senior Vice President & General Manager, UHC (2000–2002, 2003); Acting President & CEO, UHC (2002–3)
Fishleder, Andrew J., M.D.	Chairman, Division of Education, CC; Executive Dean, College
Fishman, Alfred P., M.D.	Senior Associate Dean, University of Pennsylvania School of Medicine, Philadelphia
Fitzpatrick, Joyce, R.N., Ph.D.	Elizabeth Brooks Ford Professor of Nursing, CASE; Dean, School of Nursing, CASE (1982–97)
Ford, Allen H.	Trustee, CASE; Chairman, Board of Trustees, CASE (1987–92)
Francis, Gary, M.D.	Department of Cardiovascular Medicine, CC
Franco, Irving, M.D.	Department of Cardiovascular Medicine, CC
Galaskiewicz, Joseph J., Ph.D.	Professor of Sociology, University of Arizona, Tucson
Geha, Alexander S., M.D.	Chief, Division of Cardiothoracic Surgery, University of Illinois at Chicago; Director, Division of Cardiothoracic Surgery, UHC (1986–98)
Gerson, L. Stanton, M.D.	Director, Center for Stem Cell & Regenerative Medicine, SOM; Associate Chief, Ireland
Gifford, Ray W., M.D.	Chairman, Department of Nephrology & Hypertension, CC (1966–93)
Gillinov, A. Mark, M.D.	Department of Thoracic & Cardiovascular Surgery, CC
Goldberg, Jerold S., D.D.S.	Dean, School of Dentistry, CASE; Interim Dean, SOM (2002–3)
Goldberg, Victor M., M.D.	Professor of Orthopedic Surgery, SOM; Chairman, Department of Orthopedics (1989–2002), SOM

Name	*Position*
Goldfarb, James M., M.D.	Director, Infertility Services, CC
Gotthainer, Jerome	Partner, Oasis: The Center for Mental Health; President & CEO, QualChoice (1991–95)
Gray, Bradford H., Ph.D.	Editor, *The Milbank Quarterly*, & Director, Division of Health & Science Policy, New York Academy of Medicine
Grimberg, William C.	Managing Partner, Consumer Innovation Partners; Chairman, Department of Institutional Advancement, CC (1994–2001)
Gross, Rhonda I.	Vice President for Administration & Chief Financial Officer, Carnegie Museums of Pittsburgh, Carnegie Library of Pittsburgh; Executive Vice President & Chief Operating Officer, CASE (2001–3)
Haaga, John R., M.D.	Chairman, Department of Radiology, SOM
Hadden, Elaine G.	Trustee, CASE
Hahn, Joseph, M.D.	Chairman, Division of Surgery, CC (1987–2003)
Hammack, David C., Ph.D.	Hiram C. Haydn Professor of History, CASE
Hardy, Russell W., Jr., M.D.	Professor of Neurological Surgery, SOM; Co-Director, University Hospitals Spine Center, UHC
Harris, C. Martin, M.D.	Chief Information Officer, CC
Harris, John W., M.D.	Professor of Medicine Emeritus, SOM
Hartwell, Shattock W., Jr.	Director, Professional Staff Affairs, CC (1973–86)
Healy, Bernadine P., M.D.	Director, Research Institute, CC (1985–91)
Henrich, William L., M.D.	Chairman, Department of Medicine, University of Maryland School of Medicine, Baltimore
Henson, Lindsey C., M.D., Ph.D.	Vice Dean for Cleveland Clinic Lerner College of Medicine, CASE
Hermann, Robert E., M.D.	Chairman, Department of General Surgery, CC (1969–89)
Holland, Joel B., M.D.	Department of Cardiovascular Medicine, CC
Hoogwerf, Byron J., M.D.	Director, Internal Medicine Residency Program, CC
Horn, Karen, Ph.D.	Partner, Brock Capital, New York; Trustee, CASE (1983–98); Chairman, Board of Trustees, CASE (1992–95)
Horwitz, Ralph I., M.D.	Dean, SOM
Hundert, Edward M., M.D.	President, CASE
Iannotti, Joseph P., M.D., Ph.D.	Chairman, Department of Orthopedics, CC
Inkley, Scott R., M.D.	President, UHC (1982–86)
Ivancic, Robert	Executive Director, Division of Human Resources, CC

Name	*Position*
Jackson, Brooks	Director (chairman), Department of Pathology, Johns Hopkins University School of Medicine; Director, Clinical Pathology, UHC (1989–96)
Jacobs, M. Orry	Executive Vice President, UHC (1994–2002); Senior Vice President, UHHS & Executive Director, University Hospitals Regional Network (2002–3)
Karn, Jonathan, Ph.D.	Chairman, Department of Molecular Biology & Microbiology, SOM
Kay, Robert, M.D.	Chief of Staff, CC; Vice Chairman, Board of Governors, CC
Kelley, Mark A., M.D.	Executive Vice President, Henry Ford Health System & CEO, Henry Ford Medical Group, Detroit
Kelley, William N., M.D.	Professor of Medicine, University of Pennsylvania School of Medicine
Kiderman, Sam	Director of Finance, Clinic Care, CC
Kirby, Albert C., Ph.D.	Associate Dean for Admissions, SOM
Kiser, William S., M.D.	Chairman, Board of Governors, CC (1977–89)
Korn, David, M.D.	Senior Vice President, Association of American Medical Colleges
Kovner, Anthony R., Ph.D.	Professor & Director, Program in Health Policy & Management, Wagner Graduate School of Public Service, New York University
Lamm, Michael E., M.D.	Joseph R. Kahn Professor of Pathology, SOM; Chairman, Department of Pathology, SOM (1981–2001)
Landis, Dennis M. D., M.D.	Chairman, Department of Neurology, SOM
Landis, Story C., M.D., Ph.D.	Director, National Institute of Neurological Diseases & Stroke, National Institutes of Health; Chairman, Department of Neurosciences, SOM (1990–95)
Landmesser, Lynn T., Ph.D.	Chairman, Department of Neurosciences, SOM
Langenderfer, Randy	Director of Internal Audit, UHHS
Lauer, Michael S., M.D.	Director, Clinical Research, Department of Cardiology, CC
Lenkoski, L. Douglas, M.D.	Professor of Psychiatry Emeritus, SOM
Levine, Michael A., M.D.	Chairman, Division of Pediatrics, CC
Lewis, Catharine M.	Trustee, UHC
Lewis, Hilel, M.D.	Chairman, Division of Ophthalmology, CC; Director, Cole Eye Institute, CC
Lewis, John F.	Trustee, CASE; Chairman, Board of Trustees, CASE (1995–2001); Senior Counsel, Squire Sanders
Linsalata, Frank N.	Chairman, Board of Trustees, CASE

Name	*Position*
Lintz, Robert	Trustee, CC; Plant Manager (retired), General Motors Corporation, Parma, OH
Liu, James, M.D.	Chairman, Department of Obstetrics & Gynecology
Loessin, Bruce	Executive Director of Institutional Advancement, CC
London, Alan E., M.D.	Executive Director, Managed Care, CC
Loop, Floyd D., M.D.	CEO, CC; Chairman, Board of Governors, CC
Lordeman, Frank L.	Chief Operating Officer, CC
Lüders, Hans O., M.D., Ph.D.	Chairman, Department of Neurology, CC
Ludmerer, Kenneth M., M.D.	Professor of Medicine, Professor of History, Washington University in St. Louis
MacDonald, William E., III	Trustee, CC; Vice Chairman, National City Corporation
MacDonald, William E.	Trustee, CC; CEO (retired), Ohio Bell Telephone Company
Markman, Maurie, M.D.	Vice President for Clinical Research, University of Texas M. D. Anderson Cancer Center; Department of Hematology & Medical Oncology, CC (1992–2003)
Mahmoud, Adel A. F., M.D., D.P.H., Ph.D.	President, Merck Vaccines, Whitehouse Station, NJ; Chairman, Department of Medicine, SOM (1987–98)
Mahowald, Anthony P., Ph.D.	Louis Block Professor of Molecular Genetics & Cell Biology Emeritus, University of Chicago; Henry Willson Paine Professor, SOM (1982–90)
Markowitz, Alan H., M.D.	Co-Chief, Division of Cardiothoracic Surgery, UHC
Maurer, Walter G., M.D.	Director, Quality Management, CC
Mayberg, Marc R., M.D.	Chairman, Department of Neurosurgery, CC
McCartan, Patrick F.	Trustee, CC; Senior Partner, Jones Day; Managing Partner, Jones, Day, Reavis & Pogue (1993–2002)
McCarthy, Patrick M., M.D.	Department of Cardiothoracic Surgery, CC (1990–2004); Chief, Cardiac Surgery & Co-Director, Northwestern Cardiovascular Institute, Feinberg School of Medicine, Northwestern University, Chicago
Menges, Hermann, Jr., M.D.	Clinical Professor of Medicine, SOM; Chairman, Board of Trustees, University Suburban Health Center (1985–97)
Meyer, Henry L., III	Chairman, Board of Trustees, UHC & UHHS; Chairman & CEO, KeyCorp
Meyer, Roger E., M.D.	CEO, Best Practice Project Management, Inc., Washington, DC

Name	*Position*
Michelson, Edward A., M.D.	Chairman, Department of Emergency Medicine, UHC
Michener, William M., M.D.	Chairman, Division of Education, CC (1973–91)
Mieyal, John J., Ph.D.	Professor of Pharmacology, SOM
Miller, Carol Poh	Author & historical consultant
Mills, Roger M., M.D.	Department of Cardiovascular Medicine, CC
Miner, Charles B.	Consultant, CCF; President & CEO, Meridia Health System (1994–2003)
Mixon, A. Malachai, III	Chairman, Board of Trustees, CC; Chairman & CEO, Invacare Corporation
Modell, Arthur B.	Chairman Emeritus, CC; Chairman, Executive Committee, Board of Trustees, CC (1991–96)
Modic, Michael T., M.D.	Chairman, Division of Radiology, CC
Moodie, Douglas S., M.D.	Chairman, Division of Pediatrics, CC (1987–2002)
Morley, John C.	Trustee, CASE & UHC; President, Evergreen Ventures, Ltd.
Murad, Ferid, M.D., Ph.D.	Trustee, CASE; Chairman, Department of Integrative Biology, Pharmacology & Physiology, University of Texas, Houston
Neuhauser, Duncan V., Ph.D.	Professor of Epidemiology & Biostatistics, CASE
Nilson, John H., Ph.D.	Director, School of Molecular Biosciences, Washington State University, Pullman; Chairman, Department of Pharmacology, SOM (1997–2003)
Nochomovitz, Michael L., M.D.	President & Chief Medical Officer, University Primary Care Practices, UHHS
Novick, Andrew C., M.D.	Chairman, Urological Institute, CC
O'Boyle, Michael P.	Chief Financial Officer, CC
Olds, G. Richard, M.D.	Chairman, Department of Medicine, Medical College of Wisconsin, Milwaukee; Chairman, Department of Medicine, MetroHealth Medical Center (1993–2000)
Ornt, Daniel B., M.D.	Associate Dean for Clinical Affairs, SOM, CASE
Ouriel, Kenneth, M.D.	Chairman, Division of Surgery, CC
Pardes, Herbert, M.D.	President & CEO, New York–Presbyterian Hospital
Petrovic, Frank	Administrator, Department of Cardiovascular Medicine, CC
Philipson, Elliot, M.D.	Head, Section of Maternal & Fetal Medicine, Department of Obstetrics & Gynecology, CC
Pogue, Richard W.	Trustee, UHC & UHHS; Chairman, Board of Trustees, UHC & UHHS (1994–99); Honorary Trustee, CASE; Advisor, Jones Day, formerly Managing Partner, Jones, Day, Reavis & Pogue

Name	Position
Pohl, Marc, M.D.	Department of Nephrology & Hypertension, CC
Ponsky, Jeffrey, M.D.	Director, Surgical Endoscopy, CC; Director, Graduate Medical Education, CC
Proudfit, William L., M.D.	Chairman, Department of Cardiology, CC (1965–74)
Pytte, Agnar, Ph.D.	President, CASE (1987–99)
Rabovsky, Michael A., M.D.	Medical Director, Beachwood Family Health Center, CC
Ramage, Lisa K.	Executive Director, International Center, CC
Ratcheson, Robert A., M.D.	Chairman, Department of Neurological Surgery, SOM
Rehm, Susan J., M.D.	Department of Infectious Disease, CC; Director, Internal Medicine Residency Program, CC (1994–97)
Relman, Arnold S., M.D.	Professor Emeritus of Medicine & Social Medicine, Harvard Medical School; Editor-in-Chief Emeritus, *New England Journal of Medicine*
Resnick, Martin I., M.D.	Chairman, Department of Urology, SOM
Reynolds, A. William	Chairman, Board of Trustees, UHC & UHHS (1987–94)
Robbins, Frederick C., M.D.	Dean, SOM (1966–80)
Roberts, Kevin V.	Senior Vice President & Chief Financial Officer, UHHS; Treasurer, CCF (1992–2000)
Roberts-Brown, Margaret M.	Administrator, Department of Cardiothoracic Anesthesiology, CC
Rocco, Michael B., M.D.	Department of Cardiovascular Medicine, CC
Rosselli, Virginia	Ombudsman, CC
Rothstein, Fred C., M.D.	President & CEO, UHC
Rottman, Fritz M., Ph.D.	Chairman, Department of Molecular Biology & Microbiology, SOM (1981–99)
Rudick, Richard A., M.D.	Director, Center for Clinical Research, CC
Sahney, Vinod K., Ph.D.	Senior Vice President, Planning & Strategic Development, Henry Ford Health System
Scarpa, Antonio, M.D., Ph.D.	Chairman, Department of Physiology & Biophysics, SOM
Schulak, James A., M.D.	Director, Organ Transplantation, UHC; Chairman, Department of Surgery, SOM (2000–2004)
Seals, Thomas C.	Director, Protective Services, CC (1984–2003)
Shah, Linda A., R.N.	Nurse Manager, General Internal Medicine Ambulatory Clinics, CC

Name	*Position*
Shakno, Robert J.	President & CEO, Jewish Family Service Association of Cleveland; Vice Dean for Administration, SOM & Associate Vice President for Medical Affairs, CASE (1998–2002)
Shine, Kenneth I., M.D.	Executive Vice Chancellor for Health Affairs, University of Texas, Austin
Shirey, Earl K., M.D.	Department of Cardiac Catheterization Laboratory & Cardiovascular Medicine, CC (1957–88)
Sholiton, David, M.D.	Staff ophthalmologist, Cole Eye Institute & Co-Director, Regional Ophthalmology, CC
Shuck, Jerry M., M.D.	Associate Dean of Graduate Medical Education, CASE; Chairman, Department of Surgery, SOM (1980–2000); Interim Vice President for Medical Affairs, CASE (1993–95)
Silvers, J. B., Ph.D.	Associate Dean for Resource Management & Planning, Weatherhead School of Management, CASE
Singer, Lynn T., Ph.D.	Deputy Provost & Vice President for Academic Programs, CASE
Smith, Philip, M.D., Ph.D.	Chief, Division of Cardiovascular Surgery & Clinical Director, Heart Center, Akron Children's Hospital; Chief, Section of Pediatric & Congenital Cardiothoracic Surgery, Rainbow (1998–2001)
Solov, Diane	Medical Reporter, *The Plain Dealer*
Speck, William T., M.D.	Director & CEO, Marine Biological Laboratory, Woods Hole, MA; Chairman, Department of Pediatrics, SOM (1982–92)
Spector, Michael L., M.D.	Associate Chief, Division of Cardiovascular Surgery, Akron Children's Hospital; Division of Cardiothoracic Surgery, Rainbow (1984–2001)
Stark, George R., Ph.D., FRS	Chairman, LRI (1992–2002)
Stewart, Robert W., M.D.	Co-Chief, Division of Cardiothoracic Surgery, UHC
Stranscak, Sandra S.	Executive Director, Alumni Affairs, CC
Sullivan, Thomas A.	President, QualChoice (2000–2004); CEO, United Health Care
Tait, Paul G.	Senior Vice President, Planning, Marketing & Contracting, UHHS
Thames, Marc D., M.D.	Cardiovascular Consultants, Ltd., Phoenix; Chief, Division of Cardiology, UHC (1989–97)
Theofrastous, Theodore C.	Chief, Commercialization Council, CC
Thier, Samuel O., M.D.	Professor of Medicine & Health Care Policy, Harvard Medical School, Boston

Name	*Position*
Topol, Eric J., M.D.	Provost & Chief Academic Officer, CC; Chairman, Department of Cardiovascular Medicine, CC
Traboulsi, Elias I., M.D.	Division of Ophthalmology, Cole Eye Institute, CC
Ulreich, Shawn M., R.N.	Vice President, Patient Care Services, Spectrum Health, Grand Rapids, MI; Chief Nursing Officer & Chairman, Division of Nursing, CC (1998–2003)
Utian, Wulf H., M.B., B.Ch., Ph.D.	Consultant to the Professional Staff in Women's Health, CC; Arthur H. Bill Professor Emeritus, Department of Reproductive Biology, CASE
Vidt, Donald G., M.D.	Chairman, Department of Nephrology & Hypertension, CC (1985–91)
Vehovec, Michael R.	Corporate Controller, UHHS
Wade, Richard H.	Senior Vice President for Communications, American Hospital Association, Washington, DC
Wagner, James W., Ph.D.	President, Emory University, Atlanta; Provost, CASE (2000–2001, 2002–3); Interim President, CASE (2001–2)
Walsh, Patrick C., M.D.	Trustee, CASE; Director (chairman), Department of Urology, Johns Hopkins University & Hospital
Walsh, Richard A., M.D.	Chairman, Department of Medicine, SOM
Walters, Farah M.	President & CEO, UHC & UHHS (1992–2002)
Warden, Gail W.	President & CEO, Henry Ford Health System
Watson, Richard T.	Trustee, CASE
Weimer, Gary W.	Senior Vice President, Department of Development, UHHS
Welch, K. Michael, M.B., Ch.B.	President, Rosalind Franklin University of Medicine & Science (formerly, Finch University of Health Sciences/The Chicago Medical School), North Chicago, IL
Weldon, Virginia, M.D.	Member, The Cleveland Foundation Commission on Medical Research & Education (1991–92)
White, Terry	President & CEO, MetroHealth System (1994–2003); Executive Vice President & Senior Executive Vice President, UHC (1986–91)
Willard, Huntington F., III, Ph.D.	Director, Institute for Genome Sciences & Policy; Vice Chancellor for Genome Sciences, Duke University; Director, Center for Human Genetics, UHC (1992–2002); President, Research Institute, UHC (1999–2002)
Young, Clare M., R.N.	Chief Nursing Officer & Chairman, Division of Nursing, CC

Name	*Position*
Young, James B., M.D.	Chairman, Division of Medicine, CC
Zaccagnino, Joseph A.	President & CEO, Yale–New Haven Health System
Zenty, Thomas F., III	President & CEO, UHHS
Zeroske, Joanne	Administrator, Division of Radiology, CC

Hospitals in Cleveland and Cuyahoga County in 1990 and 2004

1990
Brentwood Hospital, Warrensville Heights
Cleveland Clinic Foundation
Community Hospital of Bedford
Deaconess Hospital, Cleveland
Grace Hospital, Cleveland
Health Cleveland
    Fairview General Hospital
    Lutheran Medical Center, Cleveland
Health Hill Hospital for Children, Cleveland
Lakewood Hospital
Marymount Hospital, Garfield Heights
Meridia Health System
    Meridia Euclid Hospital
    Meridia Hillcrest Hospital, Mayfield Heights
    Meridia Huron Hospital, Cleveland
    Meridia Suburban Hospital, Warrensville Heights
MetroHealth Hospital for Women, Cleveland
MetroHealth Medical Center, Cleveland
Mount Sinai Medical Center, Cleveland
Parma Community General Hospital
Richmond Heights General Hospital
Saint Alexis Hospital Medical Center
Saint John Hospital, Cleveland
Saint John & West Shore Hospital, Westlake
Saint Luke's Hospital Association, Cleveland
Saint Vincent Charity Hospital, Cleveland
Southwest Community Health System & Hospital, Middleburg Heights
University Hospitals of Cleveland
Veterans Administration Medical Center

2004
Cleveland Clinic Foundation
    Cleveland Clinic hospital
    Euclid Hospital
    Fairview Hospital
    Hillcrest Hospital, Mayfield Heights
    Huron Hospital, Cleveland
    Lakewood Hospital
    Lutheran Hospital, Cleveland
    Marymount Hospital, Garfield Heights
    South Pointe Hospital, Warrensville Heights
Grace Hospital, Cleveland
Louis Stokes Cleveland Veteran Affairs Medical Center
MetroHealth Medical Center, Cleveland
Parma Community General Hospital
St. John West Shore Hospital, Westlake
St. Vincent Charity Hospital, Cleveland
Southwest General Health Center, Middleburg Heights
University Hospitals Health System
University Hospitals of Cleveland
    Bedford Medical Center
    Brown Memorial Hospital, Conneaut
    Geauga Regional Hospital, Chardon
    Heather Hill Hospital, Chardon
    Laurelwood Hospital, Willoughby
    Memorial Hospital of Geneva
    Richmond Heights Hospital

Notes

Preface

1. Robinson, JC. *The Corporate Practice of Medicine.* Berkeley: University of California Press, 1999, 120–122.

2. Kastor, JA. *Mergers of Teaching Hospitals in Boston, New York, and Northern California.* Ann Arbor: University of Michigan Press, 2001.

3. Kastor, JA. *Governance of Teaching Hospitals: Turmoil at Penn and Hopkins.* Baltimore: Johns Hopkins University Press, 2004.

ONE: Cleveland and Its Medical Centers

1. Pogue, Richard W., Esq., Cleveland, 3/13/03.

2. Christianson, JB, Lesser, CS, Felland, L, Felt-Lisk, S, Ginsburg, P, Vratil, AK, and Eagan, E. Community report, Cleveland, OH, fall 2000. www.hschange.org/CONTENT/286.

3. Christianson, Jon B., Ph.D., Minneapolis, MN, by telephone 11/8/02.

4. Baznik, Richard E., Cleveland, by telephone 12/8/03.

5. Mahmoud, Adel A. F., M.D., Ph.D., West Point, PA, 1/14/03.

6. Behrman, Richard E., M.D., Palo Alto, CA, by telephone 12/23/02.

7. Colten, Harvey R., M.D., New York, by telephone 2/15/03.

8. Bickers, David A., M.D., New York, by telephone 1/31/03.

9. Ponsky, Jeffrey L., M.D., Hunting Valley, OH, by telephone 12/18/03.

10. Ferry, John J., M.D., Cleveland, by telephone 12/13/02.

11. Eckardt, Robert E., Cleveland, by telephone 3/5/03.

12. Block, James A., M.D., Baltimore, 3/18/03.

13. MacDonald, William E., III, Cleveland, 7/10/03.

14. Topol, Eric J., M.D., Cleveland, by telephone 11/11/02.

15. Kastor JA. UCSF Stanford: Formation. In: *Mergers of Teaching Hospitals in Boston, New York, and Northern California.* Ann Arbor: University of Michigan Press, 2001, chap. 6, 266.

TWO: Cleveland Clinic: The Clinical Factory

1. *U.S. News & World Report,* honor role of best hospitals. www.usnews.com/usnews/health/hosptl/honorroll.htm. 2003

2. Loop, Floyd D., M.D., Cleveland, by mail 4/12/04.

3. Clough, John D., M.D., Cleveland, by e-mail 4/23/04.

4. Clough, JD, editor. *To Act as a Unit: The Story of the Cleveland Clinic,* 3rd ed. Cleveland: Cleveland Clinic Foundation, 1996.

5. The First Years, 1921–1929. In: Clough, *To Act as a Unit,* chap. 2, 15.

6. The Disaster, 1929. In: Clough, *To Act as a Unit,* chap. 3, 27–34.

7. Hartwell, Shattuck W., M.D., Cleveland, by telephone 11/14/03.

8. Michener, William M., M.D., Cleveland, by telephone 10/23/03.

9. Kiser, William S., M.D., Cleveland, 7/10/03.

10. 2001 annual report, the Cleveland Clinic Foundation.

11. MacDonald, William E., Cleveland, 7/11/03.

12. Mixon, A. Malachai, III, Cleveland, 7/10/03.

13. The LeFevre Years, 1955–1968. In: Clough, *To Act as a Unit,* chap. 6, 62.

14. McCartan, Patrick F., Esq., Cleveland, 7/9/03.

15. Lintz, Robert L., Cleveland, 7/11/03.

16. Clough, John D., M.D., Cleveland, 9/11/02.

17. Seals, Thomas L., Cleveland, 11/22/02.

18. Miller, Carol Poh, Cleveland, by telephone 2/20/03.

19. Miller, CP, Wheeler, RA. *Cleveland: A Concise History, 1796–1996,* 2nd ed. Bloomington: Indiana University Press, 1997.

20. Grimberg, William C., Cleveland, by e-mail 4/9/04.

21. Jay Miller. "Many Rode Rockefeller Coattails to Own Riches." *Crain's Cleveland Business,* 9/30/96.

22. Armstrong, F, Klein, R, Armstrong, C. *A Guide to Cleveland's Sacred Landmarks.* Kent, OH: The Kent State University Press, 1992, 36–39.

23. The Kiser Years, 1977–1989. In: Clough, *To Act as a Unit,* chap. 8, 78–81.

24. Loop, Floyd D., M.D., Cleveland, 9/10/02.

25. Vidt, Donald G., M.D., Cleveland, by telephone 3/1/04.

26. Lüders, Hans O., M.D., Ph.D., Cleveland, 10/31/02.

27. Diane Solov. "Dr. CEO." *The Plain Dealer,* 4/18/04.

28. Modell, Arthur B., Baltimore, 9/23/03.

29. Pohl, Marc A., M.D., Cleveland, 9/10/02.

30. Stark, George R., Ph.D., Cleveland, 9/9/02.

31. Ouriel, Kenneth, M.D., Cleveland, by telephone 2/2/04.

32. DiCorleto, Paul E., Ph.D., Cleveland, 9/11/02.

33. Lordeman, Frank L., Cleveland, 10/31/02.

34. Loop, Floyd D., M.D., Cleveland, 7/9/03.

35. Young, Clare, R.N., Cleveland, by telephone 3/19/04.

36. Hoogwerf, Brian, M.D., Cleveland, 11/21/02.

37. Traboulsi, Elias, M.D., Cleveland, by telephone 11/14/03.

38. Rehm, Susan J., M.D., Cleveland, by telephone 11/20/03.

39. Ahmad, Muzaffar, M.D., Cleveland, 7/8/02.

40. Kay, Robert, M.D., Cleveland, 7/8/02.

41. Estes, Melinda L., M.D., Cleveland, 9/9/02.

42. Altus, Gene, Cleveland, 10/30/02.

43. Fishleder, Andrew J., M.D., Cleveland, 10/31/02.

44. Blazar, James M., Cleveland, 9/9/02.

45. Ivancic, Robert, Cleveland, 10/30/02.

46. Lordeman, Frank L., Cleveland, 7/8/02.

47. Roberts, Kevin V., Cleveland, 3/14/03.

48. Lordeman, Frank L., Cleveland, 11/21/02.

49. Ulreich, Shawn M., R.N., Cleveland, 10/31/02.

50. Ulreich, Shawn M., R.N., Cleveland, by telephone 11/24/03.

51. Francis, Gary, M.D., Cleveland, 10/30/02.

52. Mayberg, Marc C., M.D., Cleveland, 11/1/02.

53. Novick, Andrew C., M.D., Cleveland, 7/10/03.

54. Rudick, Richard A., M.D., Cleveland, 11/20/02.

55. Loop, Floyd D., M.D., Cleveland, 7/9/02.

56. Coulton, Robert W., Jr., Cleveland, 11/20/02.

57. Lewis, Hilel, M.D., Cleveland, 11/22/02.

58. Bronson, David L., M.D., Cleveland, by telephone 11/14/02.

59. Moodie, Douglas S., M.D., New Orleans, by telephone 10/20/03.

60. Levine, Michael A., M.D., Cleveland, by telephone 1/7/04.

61. Stewart, Robert W., M.D., Cleveland, 4/18/03.

62. Clapesattle, HB. *The Doctors Mayo.* Garden City, NY: Garden City Publishing Co., 1941, 561.

63. Gottlieb, M. *The Lives of University Hospitals of Cleveland.* Cleveland: Wilson Street Press, 1991, 181–182.

64. Robbins, Frederick C., M.D., Cleveland, 2/13/03.

65. Mills, Roger M., M.D., Cleveland, 9/11/02.

66. Iannotti, Joseph P., M.D., Ph.D., Cleveland, 11/21/02.

67. Fazio, Victor W., M.B., B.S., by telephone 10/24/03.

68. Hahn, Joseph F., M.D., Cleveland, 7/8/02.

69. Cosgrove, Delos M., M.D., Cleveland, 9/10/02.

70. Chernow, BA and Vallasi, GA, editors. *The Columbia Encyclopedia,* 5th ed. New York: Columbia University Press, 1993, 1852.

71. Kay, Robert, M.D., Cleveland, 9/11/02.

72. Young, James B., M.D., Cleveland, by telephone 3/12/04.

73. Rabovsky, Michael A., M.D., Cleveland, by telephone 10/25/03.

74. Borden, Ernest C., M.D., Cleveland, by telephone 11/17/03.

75. Hermann, Robert E., M.D., Cleveland, by telephone 10/24/03.

76. Ahmad, Muzaffar, M.D., Cleveland, by telephone 11/21/03.

77. Ivancic, Robert, Cleveland, by telephone 12/3/03.

78. Hahn, Joseph F., M.D., Cleveland, by telephone 11/24/03.

79. Theofrastous, Theodore C., Esq., Cleveland, by telephone 12/12/03.

80. Cosgrove, Delos M., M.D., Cleveland, by telephone 7/7/04.

81. Coulton, Robert W., Jr., Cleveland, by telephone 11/26/03.

82. Seals, Thomas L., Cleveland, by telephone 11/19/03.

83. Clough, John D., M.D., Cleveland, by telephone 11/26/03.

84. Ulreich, Shawn M., R.N., Cleveland, by e-mail 3/9/04.

85. Diane Solov. "Clinic Lost Millions in Risky Stock Plan." *The Plain Dealer,* 12/8/02.

86. "Report: Cleveland Clinic Lost Millions on Stocks." *The Plain Dealer,* 12/8/02.

87. Alison L. Cowan. "Endowment Losses Hurt Major Cleveland Hospital." *The New York Times,* 3/10/03.

88. O'Boyle, Michael P., Cleveland, 7/10/03.

89. Roger Mezger. "Clinic Will Raise Money, Pay Debts with Bond Sale." *The Plain Dealer*, 3/4/03.

90. John Caniglia. "Clinic Pays $4 Million in Medicare Settlement: U.S. Claimed Improper Billings." *The Plain Dealer*, 1/15/03.

91. Chrencik, Robert A., Baltimore, 11/17/03.

92. Moody's Investor Services, ratings on Cleveland Clinic Health System. www .moodys.com/moodys/cust/qckSearch/qckSearch_search_result.asp?n_id=803618610 &fr_ref=P&PB2_nam=Cleveland+Clinic+Health+System&searchQuery=cleveland+ clinic&search=1&searchIdent=qcksearch&searchresult=named&portid=&frameOf Reference=municipal. 2004.

93. Moody's Investor Services, bond ratings. www.moodys.com/moodys/cust/ staticcontent2000200000265736.asp?section=rdef. 2004.

94. Jeff Stacklin. "Hospitals' Debt Ratings Slip." *The Plain Dealer*, 3/7/03.

95. Kiderman, Sam, Cleveland, by telephone 12/15/03.

96. Cook, Daniel J., Ph.D., Cleveland, by telephone 12/15/03.

97. Aach, Richard D., M.D., Cleveland, 2/13/03.

98. Anker, Daniel E., Ph.D., Cleveland, by telephone 12/13/02.

99. Haaga, John R., M.D., Cleveland, 3/14/03.

100. Duda, Rick, Cleveland, 2/25/04.

101. Stranscak, Sandra S., Cleveland, 11/21/02.

102. McCarthy, Patrick M., M.D., Cleveland, 10/30/02.

103. Anker, Daniel E., Ph.D., Cleveland, by e-mail 1/16/03.

104. Shannon Mortland. "New Hotel Comes at Hard Time." *Crain's Cleveland Business*, 1/13/03.

105. Rosselli, Virginia A., Cleveland, 7/4/03.

106. Harris, C. Martin, M.D., Cleveland, 9/11/02.

107. Shannon Mortland. "Clinic Turns to Tech for Records." *Crain's Cleveland Business*, 12/15/03.

108. Harris, C. Martin, M.D., Cleveland, by telephone 2/6/04.

109. About MyChart. www.mychart.clevelandclinic.org/. 2004.

110. Jeff Stacklin. "Clinic Deal to Offer Saudis Second Opinion via Web." *Crain's Cleveland Business*, 2/10/03.

111. Copeland, Ronald L., M.D., Cleveland, 11/20/02.

112. Philipson, Elliot H., M.D., Cleveland, 7/9/03.

113. Shah, Linda A., R.N., Cleveland, by telephone 10/31/04.

114. Gotthainer, Jerome H., Annapolis, MD, by telephone 12/31/03.

115. Regina McEnery. "Clinic Shirks on Care of Poor, Report Says: Nationwide, Hospitals Score Low on Charity." *The Plain Dealer*, 1/16/03.

116. Calman, Angela, Cleveland, 11/22/02.

117. Emerman, Charles, M.D., Cleveland, 11/21/02, and by telephone 5/27/05.

117a. Copeland, Ronald L., M.D., Cleveland, by telephone 3/18/05.

117b. Kaye Spector. "Clinic Moving Birth Centers to Suburban Hospitals." *The Plain Dealer*, 1/20/05.

117c. Levine, Michael A., M.D., Cleveland, by telephone 2/28/05.

117d. Levine, Michael A., M.D. Cleveland, by telephone 3/15/05.

118. London, Alan E., M.D., Cleveland, 10/31/02.

119. London, Alan E., M.D., Cleveland, by e-mail 7/13/04.

120. Bronson, David L., M.D., Cleveland, 9/10/02, and by e-mail 6/4/05.

121. Neuhauser, Duncan V., Ph.D., Cleveland, by telephone 2/4/04.

121a. Bronson, David L., M.D., Cleveland, by e-mail 1/25/05.

122. Goldfarb, James M., M.D., Cleveland, by telephone 10/20/03.

123. Raquel Santiago. "ObGyns Leaving UH for Clinic." *Crain's Cleveland Business*, 6/19/00.

124. Goldfarb, James M., M.D., Cleveland, by e-mail 5/19/04.

125. Utian, Wulf H., M.B., B.Ch., Ph.D., Cleveland, by telephone 12/18/03.

126. Falcone, Tommaso, M.D., Cleveland, by telephone 10/20/03.

127. Sholiton, David B., M.D., Cleveland, by telephone 11/14/03.

128. Rocco, Michael B., M.D., Cleveland, by telephone 11/5/03.

129. Raquel Santiago. "ColumbiaHCA Market Entry to Turn Up Heat." *Crain's Cleveland Business*, 5/22/95.

130. Pogue, Richard W., Esq., Cleveland, 3/13/03.

131. Diane Solov. "Blue Cross Execs' Plan to Rake in Millions—The Inside Story: Two Years Later, Memos Detail How Officials Hoped to Gain Wealth by Merging with Columbia, HCA, and How the Deal Fell Apart." *The Plain Dealer*, 4/25/99.

132. Diane Solov. "Columbia to Sell Stake in Hospitals." *The Plain Dealer*, 12/30/98.

133. "Hospital Wars' Latest Casualty: Columbia Stayed in the Local Competition Just Long Enough to Reshape the Market." *The Plain Dealer*, 3/4/99.

134. Tait, Paul G., Cleveland, 11/20/02.

135. Jacobs, M. Orry, Cleveland, 4/16/03.

136. Kastor, JA. *Governance of Teaching Hospitals: Turmoil at Penn and Hopkins*. Baltimore: Johns Hopkins University Press, 2004.

137. Raquel Santiago. "Hospitals Will Lose Meridia Name." *Crain's Cleveland Business*, 10/5/98.

137a. Lordeman, Frank L., by e-mail 1/11/05.

138. Mary C. Jaklevic. "Ohio System Spurns For-Profit Bids." *The Plain Dealer*, 7/15/96.

139. Diane Solov. "Health Systems Vie for Meridia." *The Plain Dealer*, 7/13/96.

140. Miner, Charles B., Cleveland, by telephone 10/23/03.

141. Diane Solov. "Clinic Is Winner in Competition for Merger with Meridia System." *The Plain Dealer*, 10/5/96.

142. Raquel Santiago. "Walters: Top Blue Cross Execs Swayed Meridia Vote." *Crain's Cleveland Business*, 10/21/96.

143. Santiago. "Hospital Will Lose Meridia Name."

144. "Cleveland Clinic Heart Surgery Program Oversees Cardiac Surgery at Meridia Hillcrest Hospital." *PR Newswire*, 5/13/98.

145. Cleveland Clinic, Florida. In: Clough, *To Act as a Unit*, chap. 20, 235–243.

146. Loop, Floyd D., M.D., Cleveland, by telephone 7/25/04.

147. Ramage, Lisa K., Cleveland, 11/1/02.

148. Roger Mezger, Diane Solov. "Cleveland Hospitals Feel Mideast Tension: Fewer Foreign Patients Admitted since Sept. 11." *The Plain Dealer*, 12/2/01.

149. Raquel Santiago. "Deal Spreads Clinic's Influence to India." *Crain's Cleveland Business*, 5/1/01.

150. Clough, John D., M.D., Cleveland, by e-mail 1/5/04.

151. Loessin, Bruce A., Cleveland, by telephone 12/8/03.

152. Cleveland Tomorrow. www.nortech.org/tomorrow.html. 2003.

153. Grimberg, William C., Cleveland, by telephone 11/26/03.

154. Zeller, John H., Baltimore, by e-mail 12/9/03.

155. *U.S. News & World Report*, best hospitals: cardiac. www.usnews.com/usnews/health/hosptl/rankings/specihqcard.htm. 2003.

155a. Petrovic, Frank, by e-mail 5/31/05.

156. Healy, Bernadine P., M.D., Washington, DC, by telephone 3/19/04.

157. Proudfit WL. F. Mason Sones, Jr., M.D. (1918–1985): The Man and His Work. *Cleveland Clinical Quarterly* 1986;53:121–124.

158. Loop FD. Classics in Thoracic Surgery. F. Mason Sones, Jr., (1918–1985). *Annals of Thoracic Surgery* 1987;43:237–238.

159. Franco, Irving, M.D., Cleveland, by telephone 12/11/03.

160. Proudfit, William L., M.D., Cleveland, by mail 11/4/03.

161. Division of Medicine. In: Clough, *To Act as a Unit*, chap. 10, 104.

162. Shirey, Earl K., M.D., Cleveland, by e-mail 11/11/03.

163. Division of Surgery. In: Clough, *To Act as a Unit*, chap. 12, 131–132.

164. Markman, Maurie, M.D., Cleveland, 11/1/02.

165. Lerner, BH. *The Breast Cancer Wars: Hope, Fear, and the Pursuit of a Career in Twentieth-Century America*. New York: Oxford University Press, 2001, 104–106.

166. Cronin, Gina, by telephone 9/11/03.

167. Kastor JA. Atrial Fibrillation. In: *Arrhythmias*, 2nd ed. Philadelphia: W. B. Saunders, 2000, chap. 4, 85–86.

168. McCarthy, Patrick M., M.D., Cleveland, by telephone 5/20/04.

169. Gillinov, A. Mark, M.D., Baltimore, 10/30/03.

170. Petrovic, Frank, and Topol, Eric J., by e-mail 11/12/02.

171. Topol, Eric J., M.D., Cleveland, by e-mail 10/16/02.

172. Topol, Eric J., M.D., Cleveland, 7/8/02.

173. Holland, Joel B., M.D., Cleveland, by telephone 2/23/04.

174. Roberts-Brown, Margaret M., by telephone 9/10/03.

175. Zeroske, Joanne, by telephone 9/10/03.

176. *U.S. News & World Report*, best hospitals: urology. www.usnews.com/usnews/health/hosptl/rankings/specihqurol.htm. 2003.

177. Walsh, Patrick C., M.D., Baltimore, 1/16/03.

178. Crowe, Joseph P., M.D., Cleveland, 7/9/03.

179. Donald G. McNeil Jr. "Fixing Aneurysms without Surgery." *The New York Times*, 10/12/02.

180. Lewis, Hilel, M.D., Cleveland, 11/22/02.

181. Lewis, Hilel, M.D,. Cleveland, by e-mail 12/18/02.

182. Byers, Richard J., by e-mail 12/18/02.

183. *U.S. News & World Report*, best hospitals: orthopedics. www.usnews.com/usnews/health/hosptl/rankings/specihqorth.htm. 2003.

184. Levine, Michael A., M.D., Baltimore, 2/4/03.

185. Division of Pediatrics. In: Clough, *To Act as a Unit*, chap. 11, 119–125.

186. Division of Surgery. In: Clough, *To Act as a Unit*, chap. 11, 140.

187. Modic, Michael T., M.D., Cleveland, by telephone 1/26/04.

188. Diane Solov. "Clinic Leader Looking for His Replacement: But Loop Not Planning to Leave Job Soon." *The Plain Dealer*, 1/8/04.

189. Diane Solov. "From C's and D's to Clinic's Helm." *The Plain Dealer*, 6/9/04.

190. Diane Solov. "Cosgrove Is Selected as Clinic's Next Chief Surgeon to Replace CEO Loop This Fall." *The Plain Dealer*, 6/2/04.

191. Bronson, David L., M.D., Cleveland, by telephone 6/28/04.

192. Mixon, A. Malachai, III, Cleveland, by telephone 7/8/04.

193. Fazio, Victor W., M.B., B.S., by telephone 6/7/04.

194. Diane Solov. "Seven Doctors Seeking to Lead Clinic Health System." *The Plain Dealer*, 3/17/04.

195. Bronson, David L., M.D., Cleveland, by e-mail 7/12/04.

196. Lordeman, Frank L., Cleveland, by telephone 6/7/04.

197. Hermann, Robert E., M.D., Cleveland, by telephone 6/7/04.

198. Clough, John D., M.D., Cleveland, by e-mail 6/8/04.

199. Topol, Eric J., M.D., Cleveland, by e-mail 6/8/04.

200. Ponsky, Jeffrey L., M.D., Hunting Valley, OH, by telephone 12/18/03.

THREE: University Hospitals of Cleveland: Turmoil in University Circle

1. History of University Circle. www.universitycircle.org/uc_ab_history.shtml. 2004.

2. Gottlieb, M. *The Lives of University Hospitals of Cleveland*. Cleveland: Wilson Street Press, 1991.

3. Daroff, Robert B., M.D., Cleveland, by telephone 5/3/04.

4. Chernow, R. *Titan: The Life of John D. Rockefeller, Sr.* New York: Random House, 1998.

5. Gottlieb, *The Lives of University Hospitals of Cleveland*, 181–182.

6. Kastor, JA. Partners: Formation. In: *Mergers of Teaching Hospitals in Boston, New York, and Northern California*. Ann Arbor: University of Michigan Press, 2001, chap. 2, 31.

7. Kastor, JA. New York–Presbyterian: Formation. In: *Mergers of Teaching Hospitals in Boston, New York, and Northern California*, chap. 4, 125.

8. Cramer, CH. *Case Western Reserve: A History of the University, 1826–1976.* Boston: Toronto, 1976.

9. Cramer, *Case Western Reserve*.

10. Cramer, *Case Western Reserve*, 85.

11. Cramer, *Case Western Reserve*, 105.

12. Bonner, TN. A Legend Is Born. In: *Iconoclast: Abraham Flexner and a Life in Learning.* Baltimore: Johns Hopkins University Press, 2002, chap. 5, 69–90.

13. Kastor, JA. *Governance of Teaching Hospitals: Turmoil at Penn and Hopkins*. Baltimore: Johns Hopkins University Press, 2004.

14. Bickers, David A., M.D., New York, by telephone 1/31/03.

15. Cramer, *Case Western Reserve*, 300–304.

16. Ludmerer, KM. The Forgotten Medical Student. In: *Time to Heal: American Medical Education from the Turn of the Century to the Era of Managed Care.* New York: Oxford University Press, 1999, chap. 11, 201–203.

17. Mieyal, John J., Ph.D., Cleveland, by telephone 12/23/03.

18. Williams, G. *Western Reserve's Experiment in Medical Education and Its Outcome.* New York: Oxford University Press, 1980.

19. Behrman, Richard E., M.D., Palo Alto, CA, by telephone 12/23/02.

20. Cramer, *Case Western Reserve*, 303.

21. Murad, Ferid, M.D., Ph.D., Houston, by telephone 7/18/03.

22. Lawrence K. Altman. "F. C. Robbins, Virus Researcher, Dies at 86." *The New York Times*, 8/5/03.

23. Robbins, Frederick C., M.D., Cleveland, 2/13/03.

24. Ludmerer, Kenneth M., M.D., St. Louis, by telephone 1/3/03.

25. Williams, Jack Caughey, One-man Admissions Committee. In: *Western Reserve's Experiment in Medical Education and Its Outcome*, chap. 33, 406–409.

26. Colten, Harvey R., M.D., New York, by telephone 2/15/03.

27. Kirby, Albert C., Ph.D., Cleveland, by telephone 12/8/03.

28. Mahmoud, Adel A. F., M.D., Ph.D., West Point, PA, 1/14/03.

29. Carpenter, Charles C. J., M.D., Providence, RI, by telephone 2/19/03.

30. Fishman, Alfred P., M.D., Philadelphia, by telephone 2/11/03.

31. NIH Support to U.S. Medical Schools, Fiscal Years 1970–2000. http://grants1.nih.gov/grants/award/trends/medsup7000.txt. 2002.

32. Anker, Daniel E., Ph.D., Cleveland, by telephone 12/13/02.

33. Eckardt, Robert E., Cleveland, by telephone 3/5/03.

34. Rottman, Fritz M., Ph.D., Grand Rapids, MI, by telephone 5/5/03.

35. Nilson, John H., Ph.D., Cleveland, 2/13/03.

36. Mahowald, Anthony P., Ph.D., Stanford, CA, by telephone 5/7/03.

37. Scarpa, Antonio, M.D., Ph.D., Cleveland, 4/17/03.

38. Fitzpatrick, Joyce J., Ph.D., New York, by telephone 1/29/04.

39. Walsh, Patrick C., M.D., Baltimore, 1/16/03.

40. Ford, Allen H., Cleveland, 6/12/03.

41. Cowen, Scott S., Ph.D., New Orleans, by telephone 7/22/03.

42. Baznik, Richard E., Cleveland, by telephone 12/8/03.

43. Grimberg, William C., Cleveland, by telephone 11/26/03.

44. Olds, G. Richard, M.D., Milwaukee, by telephone 4/7/04.

45. Walters, Farah M., Cleveland, by telephone 3/18/04.

46. Reynolds, A. William, Vero Beach, FL, by telephone 3/29/04.

47. Hadden, Elaine G., Cleveland Heights, OH, by telephone 12/5/03.

48. Lewis, John F., Esq., Cleveland, 4/16/03.

49. Anlyan, William G., M.D., Palm Beach, FL, by telephone 12/18/02.

50. Bank, Malvin E., Esq., Cleveland, 6/11/03.

51. Cascorbi, Helmut F., M.D., Ph.D., Cleveland, 2/14/03.

52. Cherniak, Neil S., M.D., Parsippany, NJ, by telephone 12/31/02.

53. Gerson, Stanton L., M.D., Cleveland, by telephone 1/5/04.

54. Horn, Karen, Ph.D., New York, by telephone 3/20/03.

55. Lamm, Michael E., M.D., Cleveland, 3/14/03.

56. Landis, Story C., Ph.D., Bethesda, MD, by telephone 2/11/03.

57. Lenkoski, L. Douglas, M.D., Cleveland, by telephone 2/8/03.

58. Lewis, Catharine M., Cleveland, 6/11/03.

59. Mahmoud, Adel A. F., M.D., Ph.D., West Point, PA, by telephone 2/27/03.

60. Menges, Hermann, Jr., M.D., South Euclid, OH, 4/17/03.

61. Meyer, Roger E., M.D., Washington, DC, by telephone 2/21/03.

62. Mixon, A. Malachai, III, Cleveland, 7/10/03.

63. Pogue, Richard W., Esq., Cleveland, 3/13/03.

64. Relman, Arnold S., M.D., Boston, by telephone 3/6/03.

65. Shakno, Robert J., Cleveland, by telephone 2/20/04.

66. Warden, Gail L., Detroit, by telephone 2/5/03.

67. Willard, Huntington F., Ph.D., Cleveland, by telephone 11/25/02.

68. Williams, Dynamics of Change—A Strong Dean. In: *Western Reserve's Experiment in Medical Education and Its Outcome*, chap. 2, 28–29.

69. Inkley, Scott R., M.D., 3/13/03.

70. Jackson, J. Brooks, M.D., Baltimore, 4/29/03.

71. Thames, Marc D., M.D., Philadelphia, by telephone 11/7/03.

72. Neuhauser, Duncan V., Ph.D., Cleveland, by telephone 2/4/04.

73. Walters, Farah M., Cleveland, by telephone 7/8/04.

74. Pytte, Agnar, Ph.D., Etna, NH, by telephone 2/3/03.

75. Meyer, Roger E., M.D., Bethesda, MD, by e-mail 10/7/03.

76. Thier, Samuel O., M.D., Boston, by telephone 2/5/03.

77. Berger, Nathan A., M.D., Cleveland, by telephone 12/13/02.

78. Kelley, William N., M.D., Philadelphia, by telephone 12/16/02.

79. The Cleveland Foundation. www.clevelandfoundation.org/page1426.cfm. 2002.

80. The Cleveland Foundation. Study Commission on Medical Research and Education. 1992.

81. Weldon, Virginia, M.D., Crevecoeur, MO, 3/1/03.

82. Case Western Reserve University/University Hospitals of Cleveland report of the joint trustee committee on affiliation. 3/6/92.

83. Diane Solov, John Mangels. "Secret Talks Target City's Medical Future: Clinic, University Hospitals, CWRU Negotiate Partnership." *The Plain Dealer*, 10/26/00.

84. Daroff, Robert B., M.D., Cleveland, by telephone 12/19/02.

85. Bolwell, Harry J., Vero Beach, FL, by telephone 2/5/03.

86. Kastor, Partners: Formation. In: *Mergers of Teaching Hospitals in Boston, New York, and Northern California*, chap. 2, 50–53.

87. Joan M. Mazzolini. "Mediator Easing Tensions: CWRU Medical School, President at Odds over Higher Fees." *The Plain Dealer*, 6/13/93.

88. Ratcheson, Robert A., M.D., Cleveland, 3/12/03.

89. Joan M. Mazzolini. "Hospitals Have Case of Sibling Rivalry." *The Plain Dealer*, 6/13/93.

90. Ford, Allen H., Cleveland, by fax 10/7/03.

91. Morley, John C., Cleveland, 6/12/03.

92. Bank, Malvin E., Esq., Cleveland, by telephone 5/4/04.

93. Bolton, Charles P., Cleveland, 6/13/03.

94. Pogue, Richard W., Esq., Cleveland, by e-mail 5/10/04.

95. Brieger, Gert H., M.D., Baltimore, 7/20/01.

96. Cascorbi, Helmut F., M.D., Ph.D., Cleveland, by telephone 5/13/03.

97. Letter to Karen Horn from A. William Reynolds, 1/15/93.

98. Resolution. University Hospitals of Cleveland and the executive committee of University Hospitals Health System, Inc. board of trustees. 1/23/93.

99. Letter to author from Robert B. Daroff, 12/20/02.

100. Shuck, Jerry M., M.D., Cleveland, 2/14/03.

101. Thier, Samuel O., M.D., Boston, by telephone 10/8/03.

102. Shine, Kenneth I., M.D., Arlington, VA, by telephone 2/21/03.

103. Bickers, David A., M.D., New York, by e-mail 2/9/03.

104. Block, James A., M.D., Baltimore, 3/18/03.

105. Speck, William T., M.D., Woods Hole, MA, by telephone 1/13/03.

106. Burry, John, Jr., Scottsdale, AZ, by telephone 5/7/03.

107. Daroff, Robert B., M.D., Cleveland, speech 1/27/87.

108. Raquel Santiago. "Ahead of the Curve: University Hospitals' Determined CEO Works to Reshape the Face of Health Care." *Crain's Cleveland Business*, 4/3/00.

109. Walters, Farah M., Cleveland, 2/25/04.

110. Resolution to amend agreement with university hospitals. 6/3/76.

111. Kastor, Partners: Formation. In: *Mergers of Teaching Hospitals in Boston, New York, and Northern California,* chap. 2, 20–21.

112. Letter to Daniel E. Anker from Robert B. Daroff, 1/2/03.

113. Letter to Charles B. Womer from Louis A. Toepfer, 6/13/80.

114. Landmesser, Lynn T., Ph.D., Cleveland, 3/12/03.

115. Affiliation agreement between Case Western Reserve University and University Hospitals of Cleveland and University Hospitals Health System, Inc. 5/12/92.

116. Mahmoud, Adel A. F., M.D., Ph.D., West Point, PA, by telephone 10/13/03.

117. Pogue, Richard W., Esq., Cleveland, by e-mail 5/17/04.

118. Letter to John F. Lewis from Henry L. Meyer III, 12/11/99.

119. Daroff, Robert B., M.D., Cleveland, by e-mail 1/6/03.

120. Baznik, Richard E., Cleveland, by telephone 12/17/03.

121. Linsalata, Frank N., Cleveland, 4/15/04.

122. Singer, Lynn T., Ph.D., Cleveland, 6/12/03.

123. Goldberg, Victor M., M.D., Cleveland, by telephone 4/26/04.

124. Meyer, Henry L., III, Cleveland, 6/11/03.

125. Korn, David, M.D., Washington, DC, by telephone 2/10/03.

126. Goldberg, Jerold S., Cleveland, 3/13/03.

127. Diane Solov. "Can Boardroom Who's Who Snarl What's What? CWRU Chief's Departure Raises Issue of 1 Decision-Maker Serving on 2 Boards." *The Plain Dealer*, 5/19/01.

128. John Mangels, Diane Solov. "Interim CWRU Chief Hits Job Running: Wagner Must Smooth Waters Stirred Up by Auston's Departure." *The Plain Dealer*, 5/2/01.

129. Morley, John C., Cleveland, by e-mail 10/7/03.

130. Wagner, James W., Ph.D., Cleveland, 4/17/03.

131. Daroff, Robert B., M.D., Cleveland, by e-mail 5/31/04.

132. Zaccagnino, Joseph A., New Haven, by telephone 6/9/04.

133. Walters FM. Review and rebuttal by Farah M. Walters (with background and some documentation) as to draft of chapters received from Dr. John Kastor. 5/31/04, 30.

134. Henson, Lindsey C., M.D., Ph.D., Cleveland, 11/22/02.

135. Jeff Stacklin. "CWRU-UH Talks Wavering: New Affiliation Pact Still Stalled over Credit for Research Dollars." *Crain's Cleveland Business*, 11/19/01.

136. Diane Solov. "CWRU, University Hospitals Deal Hits Snag." *The Plain Dealer*, 2/26/02.

137. Diane Solov. "Accreditation Looms as Issue: Snag in UH Affiliation Is Potential Hurdle in CWRU Med School Review." *The Plain Dealer*, 3/1/02.

138. Hundert, Edward M., M.D., Cleveland, 4/15/04.

139. Hundert, Edward M., M.D., Cleveland, by telephone 7/13/04.

140. Hundert, Edward M., M.D., Cleveland, by telephone 7/14/04, by e-mail 7/14/04.

FOUR: University Hospitals of Cleveland: The Farah Walters Years

1. Connie Schultz. "Farah the Fearless." *The Plain Dealer*, 6/16/96.
2. Walters, Farah M., Cleveland, 2/25/04.
3. Walters, Farah M., Shaker Heights, OH, by telephone 6/8/04.
4. Block, James A., M.D., Baltimore, 3/18/03.
5. White, Terry R., Cleveland, by telephone 12/23/02.
6. Reynolds, A. William, Vero Beach, FL, by telephone 3/29/04.
7. Mahmoud, Adel A. F., M.D., Ph.D., West Point, PA, by telephone 3/29/04.
8. Pogue, Richard W., Esq., Cleveland, 3/13/03.
9. Walters, Farah M., Cleveland, by fax 7/20/04.
10. Walters, Farah M., Shaker Heights, OH, by telephone 6/10/04.
11. Aach, Richard D., M.D., Cleveland, 2/13/03.
12. Adler, Dale S., M.D., Cleveland, 2/12/03, and by telephone 6/6/05.
13. Anker, Daniel E., Ph.D., Cleveland, by telephone 12/13/02.
14. Avner, Ellis D., M.D., Cleveland, 6/13/03.
15. Bank, Malvin E., Esq., Cleveland, 6/11/03.
16. Berger, Nathan A., M.D., Cleveland, by telephone 12/13/02.
17. Berger, Nathan A., M.D., Cleveland, 2/13/03.
18. Bickers, David A., M.D., New York, by telephone 1/31/03.
19. Bolwell, Harry J., Vero Beach, FL, by telephone 2/5/03.
20. Cascorbi, Helmut F., M.D., Ph.D., Cleveland, 2/14/03.
21. Cherniak, Neil S., M.D., Parsippany, NJ, by telephone 12/31/02.
22. Coulton, Robert W., Jr., Cleveland, 11/20/02.
23. Daroff, Robert B., M.D., Cleveland, by telephone 12/19/02.
24. Daroff, Robert B., M.D., Cleveland, by telephone 3/24/04.
25. Cowen, Scott S., Ph.D., New Orleans, by telephone 7/22/03.
26. Devereaux, Michael W., Ph.D., Cleveland, 4/17/03.
27. Ellner, Jerrold J., M.D., Newark, NJ, by telephone 3/27/03.
28. Ferry, John J., M.D., Cleveland, by telephone 12/13/02.
29. Geha, Alexander S., M.D., Chicago, by telephone 5/17/03.
30. Gerson, Stanton L., M.D., Cleveland, by telephone 1/5/04.
31. Goldberg, Jerold S., Cleveland, 3/13/03.
32. Goldfarb, James M., M.D., Cleveland, by telephone 10/20/03.
33. Gotthainer, Jerome H., Annapolis, MD, by telephone 12/31/03.
34. Jackson, J. Brooks, M.D., Baltimore, 4/29/03.
35. Jacobs, M. Orry, Cleveland, 4/16/03.
36. Kelley, William N., M.D., Philadelphia, by telephone 12/16/02.
37. Kiser, William S., M.D., Cleveland, 7/10/03.
38. Korn, David, M.D., Washington, DC, by telephone 2/10/03.
39. Lamm, Michael E., M.D., Cleveland, 3/14/03.
40. Landis, Dennis M. D., M.D., Cleveland, 4/18/03.
41. Lenkoski, L. Douglas, M.D., Cleveland, by telephone 2/8/03.
42. Lewis, Catharine M., Cleveland, 6/11/03.
43. Lewis, John F., Esq., Cleveland, 4/16/03.

44. Mahmoud, Adel A. F., M.D., Ph.D., West Point, PA, 1/14/03.

45. Meyer, Henry L., III, Cleveland, 6/11/03.

46. Modic, Michael T., M.D., Cleveland, by telephone 1/26/04.

47. Olds, G. Richard, M.D., Milwaukee, by telephone 4/7/04.

48. Ponsky, Jeffrey L., M.D., Hunting Valley, OH, by telephone 12/18/03.

49. Rabovsky, Michael A., M.D., Cleveland, by telephone 10/25/03.

50. Ratcheson, Robert A., M.D., Cleveland, 3/12/03.

51. Robbins, Frederick C., M.D., Cleveland, 2/13/03.

52. Scarpa, Antonio, M.D., Ph.D., Cleveland, 4/17/03.

53. Schulak, James A., M.D., Cleveland, 3/12/03.

54. Shakno, Robert J., Cleveland, by telephone 2/20/04.

55. Shuck, Jerry M., M.D., Cleveland, 2/14/03.

56. Silvers, J. B., Ph.D., Cleveland, 4/16/03.

57. Singer, Lynn T., Ph.D., Cleveland, 6/12/03.

58. Thames, Marc D., M.D., Philadelphia, by telephone 11/7/03.

59. Topol, Eric J., M.D., Cleveland, 7/8/02.

60. Utian, Wulf H., M.B., B.Ch., Ph.D., Cleveland, by telephone 12/18/03.

61. Walsh, Patrick C., M.D., Baltimore, 1/16/03.

62. Walsh, Richard A., M.D., Cleveland, by telephone 1/20/03.

63. Willard, Huntington F., Ph.D., Cleveland, by telephone 11/25/02.

64. Walters FM. Review and rebuttal by Farah M. Walters (with background and some documentation) as to draft of chapters received from Dr. John Kastor. 5/31/04.

65. Ruthann Robinson. "Farah Says Farewell: Issues Remain for Women." *Crain's Cleveland Business,* 4/15/02.

66. Walters, Farah M., Shaker Heights, OH, by telephone 7/15/04.

67. Walters FM. Review and rebuttal by Farah M. Walters (with background and some documentation) as to draft of chapters received from Dr. John Kastor. 5/31/04, 30.

68. Walters, Farah M., Cleveland, by telephone 3/18/04.

69. Kastor, JA. University of Pennsylvania: Kelley the Builder. In: *Governance of Teaching Hospitals: Turmoil at Penn and Hopkins.* Baltimore: Johns Hopkins University Press, 2004, chap. 3, 75.

70. Raquel Santiago. "Ahead of the Curve: University Hospitals' Determined CEO Works to Reshape the Face of Health Care." *Crain's Cleveland Business,* 4/3/00.

71. Tait, Paul G., Cleveland, 11/20/02.

72. Pogue, Richard W., Esq., Shaker Heights, OH, by e-mail 5/10/04.

73. Walters, Farah M., Cleveland, by telephone 7/8/04.

74. Moody's Investor Services, ratings on University Hospitals Health System. www .moodys.com/moodys/cust/qckSearch/qckSearch_search_result.asp?n_id=803618610 &fr_ref=P&PB2_nam=Cleveland+Clinic+Health+System&searchQuery=cleveland+ clinic&search=1&searchIdent=qcksearch&searchresult=named&portid= &frameOf Reference= municipal. 2004.

75. Jeff Stacklin. "Hospitals' Debt Ratings Slip." *The Plain Dealer,* 3/7/03.

76. Bank, Malvin E., Esq., Cleveland, by telephone 5/4/04.

77. Chrencik, Robert A., Baltimore, 6/26/03.

78. Morley, John C., Cleveland, 6/12/03.

79. Raquel Santiago. "Walters: Top Blue Cross Execs Swayed Meridia Vote." *Crain's Cleveland Business,* 10/21/96.

80. Sullivan, Thomas A., Mayfield Heights, OH, by telephone 5/12/03.

80a. Titterington, Susan, Cleveland, by telephone 5/27/05.

81. Raquel Santiago. "QualChoice Cuts Losses, But Profit Still Just a Goal." *Crain's Cleveland Business*, 5/22/03.

82. Kastor, University of Pennsylvania: After Kelley. In: *Governance of Teaching Hospitals*, chap. 5, 134–136.

83. Nochomovitz, Michael L., M.D., Cleveland, by telephone 6/30/03, and by e-mail 5/27/05.

84. Hardy, Russell W., Jr., M.D., Cleveland, 2/12/03.

85. Menges, Hermann, Jr., M.D., South Euclid, OH, 4/17/03.

86. Abbey, Charles R., South Euclid, OH, by telephone 5/8/03.

87. Daroff, Robert B., M.D., Cleveland, by telephone 5/3/04.

88. Menges, Hermann, Jr., M.D., South Euclid, OH, by e-mail 5/12/03.

89. Menges, Hermann, Jr., M.D., South Euclid, OH, by telephone 5/8/03.

89a. Menges, Hermann, Jr., M.D., South Euclid, OH, by telephone 3/7/05.

90. Kastor, *Governance of Teaching Hospitals*, 199–201.

91. Jacobs, M. Orry, Cleveland, by telephone 4/29/03.

92. Pytte, Agnar, Ph.D., Etna, NH, by telephone 2/3/03.

93. Diane Solov. "UH to Lose Renowned Genetics Researcher: Exit Seen as Blow to Local Biotech Effort." *The Plain Dealer*, 10/24/02.

94. Pardes, Herbert, M.D., New York, by telephone 4/25/03.

95. Korn, David, M.D., Washington, DC, by e-mail 10/8/03.

96. John Mangels, Diane Solov. "University Hospitals Plans $110 Million Research Site." *The Plain Dealer*, 10/17/00.

97. Hadden, Elaine G., Cleveland Heights, OH, by telephone 12/5/03.

98. Ford, Allen H., Cleveland, 6/12/03.

99. Berger, Nathan A., M.D., Cleveland, by telephone 2/6/04.

100. Rothstein, Fred C., M.D., Cleveland, 4/15/04.

101. Joan M. Mazzolini. "Second Director Leaves University Hospitals Helm." *The Plain Dealer*, 9/12/93.

102. Gottlieb, M. *The Lives of University Hospitals of Cleveland*. Cleveland: Wilson Street Press, 1991, 128.

103. Gottlieb, *The Lives of University Hospitals of Cleveland*, 173-174.

104. Kastor, JA. *Mergers of Teaching Hospitals in Boston, New York, and Northern California*. Ann Arbor: University of Michigan Press, 2001, 74.

105. Lamm, Michael E., M.D., Cleveland, by e-mail 10/8/03.

105a. Horwitz, Ralph I., Cleveland, by e-mail 1/19/05.

106. Inkley, Scott R., M.D., 3/13/03.

107. Goldberg, Victor M., M.D., Cleveland, by telephone 4/26/04.

108. Walters, FM. A Decade of Transformation: The Growth of University Hospitals Health System, 1992–2002, Cleveland, May 2002.

109. Walters, A Decade of Transformation, 6.

110. Jeff Stacklin. "CWRU-UH Talks Wavering." *Crain's Cleveland Business*, 11/19/01.

111. Walters, A Decade of Transformation, 7.

112. NIH Awards to Independent Domestic Hospitals, Fiscal Year 2001. http://grants2.nih.gov/grants/award/trends/hospita101.htm.

113. Walters, A Decade of Transformation, 8.

114. Pogue, Richard W., Esq., Cleveland, by e-mail 5/17/04.

115. Liu, James H., M.D., Cleveland, by telephone 12/17/03.

116. Behrman, Richard E., M.D., Palo Alto, CA, by telephone 12/23/02.

117. Warden, Gail L., Detroit, by telephone 2/5/03.

118. Nilson, John H., Ph.D., Cleveland, 2/13/03.

119. Berger, Nathan A., M.D., Cleveland, by e-mail 10/16/03.

120. Hundert, Edward M., M.D., Cleveland, by e-mail 7/18/04.

121. John Funk. "New Med School Dean Sees New Focus: He Says Research Will Target Specific Diseases." *The Plain Dealer*, 8/28/96.

122. "Interim Dean for CWRU Medical School Named." *The Plain Dealer*, 7/21/95.

123. Colten, Harvey R., M.D., New York, by telephone 2/15/03.

124. Meyer, Roger E., M.D., Washington, DC, by telephone 2/21/03.

125. Meyer, Roger E., M.D., Bethesda, MD, by e-mail 10/7/03.

126. Horn, Karen, Ph.D., New York, by telephone 3/20/03.

127. Landis, Story C., Ph.D., Bethesda, MD, by e-mail 10/8/03.

128. Landis, Story C., Ph.D., Bethesda, MD, by telephone 2/11/03.

129. Walters, Farah M., Florida, by telephone 2/5/03.

130. Haaga, John R., M.D., Cleveland, 3/14/03.

131. Sholiton, David B., M.D., Cleveland, by telephone 11/14/03.

132. Watson, Richard T., Cleveland, by telephone 4/23/04.

133. Healy, Bernadine P., M.D., Washington, DC, by telephone 3/19/04.

134. Seals, Thomas L., Cleveland, 11/22/02.

135. Hundert, Edward M., M.D., Cleveland, 4/15/04.

136. Harris, John W., M.D., Cleveland, by telephone 2/21/03.

137. Mahmoud, Adel A. F., M.D., Ph.D., West Point, PA, by telephone 5/18/04.

138. Daroff, Robert B., M.D., Cleveland, by e-mail 5/18/04.

139. Baznik, Richard E., Cleveland, by telephone 12/8/03.

140. Diane Solov, John Mangels. "Secret Talks Target City's Medical Future: Clinic, University Hospitals, CWRU Negotiate Partnership." *The Plain Dealer*, 10/26/00.

141. Diane Solov. "Hopes Rise for Research Mecca Here: CWRU, Hospitals Revive Push for Elite Medical Consortium." *The Plain Dealer*, 7/25/01.

142. Diane Solov. "CWRU, University Hospitals Agree on Affiliation, Won't Tell Terms." *The Plain Dealer*, 11/21/01.

143. *Univ. Hosps. of Cleveland, Inc. v. Lynch*, 96 Ohio St.3d 118, 2002-Ohio-3748. www .sconet.state.oh.us/rod/documents/0/2002/2002-Ohio-3748.doc. 6/19/02.

144. Cooper, Kevin D., M.D., Cleveland, 3/13/03.

145. Bickers, David A., M.D., New York, by e-mail 2/5/03.

146. Utian, Wulf H., M.B., B.Ch., Ph.D., Cleveland, by e-mail 4/8/04.

147. Smith, Philip C., M.D., Cleveland, by telephone 12/10/03.

148. Resnick, Martin I., M.D., Cleveland, by telephone 12/20/02.

149. Morley, John C., Cleveland, by e-mail 10/7/03.

150. Burry, John, Jr., Scottsdale, AZ, by telephone 5/7/03.

151. Coleman, Keith T., Mayfield Heights, OH, by telephone 6/18/03.

152. Marian Uhlman, L. S. Ditzen, Susan FitzGerald. "U.S. Assesses Penn Doctors $30 Million. Abuse of Medicare Billings Amounted to Some $10 Million, Investigators Said. Fines Came to $20 Million. Further Scrutiny of Teaching Hospitals Is Planned." *Philadelphia Inquirer*, 12/13/95, A01.

153. John Caniglia. "Clinic Pays $4 Million in Medicare Settlement; U.S. Claimed Improper Billings." *The Plain Dealer*, 1/15/03.

153a. Langenderfer, Randy L., by telephone 6/6/05.

154. Landmesser, Lynn T., Ph.D., Cleveland, 3/12/03.

155. Cherniak, Neil S., M.D., Parsippany, NJ, by telephone 10/17/03.

156. Sahney, Vinod K., Ph.D., Detroit, by telephone 2/10/03.

157. Kelley, Mark A., M.D., Detroit, by telephone 1/3/03.

158. Anlyan, William G., M.D., Palm Beach, FL, by telephone 12/18/02.

159. America's Best Hospitals 2004. www.usnews.com/usnews/health/hosptl/honor roll.htm.

160. Speck, William T., M.D., Woods Hole, MA, by telephone 1/13/03.

161. Wagner, James W., Ph.D., Cleveland, 4/17/03.

162. History of the MetroHealth System. www.metrohealthresearch.org/mhmchistory.html. 2002.

163. Regina McEnery. "MetroHealth CEO to Retire in a Year." *The Plain Dealer*, 1/23/03.

164. Charles H. Rammelkamp, Jr., M.D. www.metrohealthresearch.org/drrammelkamp.html. 2002.

165. Raquel Santiago. "MetroHealth Links with Clinic Heart Program." *Crain's Cleveland Business*, 12/1/97.

166. Berger, Nathan A., M.D., Cleveland, by telephone 10/9/03.

166a. Daroff, Robert B., M.D., Cleveland, by telephone 5/31/05.

167. Balke, C. William, M.D., Baltimore, 10/21/02.

168. Affiliation agreement between the MetroHealth System, the MetroHealth Medical Center, and Case Western Reserve University. 1/11/93.

169. Bickers, David A., M.D., New York, by telephone 2/5/03.

170. Mahmoud, Adel A. F., M.D., Ph.D., West Point, PA, by telephone 2/27/03.

171. Joan M. Mazzolini. "Hospitals Have Case of Sibling Rivalry." *The Plain Dealer*, 6/13/93.

172. Joan M. Mazzolini. "Mt. Sinai Medical Center Sold to For-Profit Primary Health." *The Plain Dealer*, 12/13/95.

173. Diane Solov. "Mt. Sinai, Deaconess Facing Cutbacks: Owner of 4 Hospitals Here Seeks Bankruptcy." *The Plain Dealer*, 3/18/99.

174. "Moving On." *Crain's Cleveland Business*, 2/21/00.

175. Regina McEnery, Joan M. Mazzolini. "Anatomy of Mt. Sinai's Decline and Fall." *The Plain Dealer*, 3/20/00.

176. Bill Lubinger. "University Hospitals of Cleveland Will Add." *The Plain Dealer*, 8/12/97.

177. Diane Solov. "Staff Switching Hospitals: Mt. Sinai Losing Most of Its Neurology Department to University Hospitals." *The Plain Dealer*, 10/29/97.

178. Bank, Malvin E., Esq., Cleveland, by telephone 6/7/04.

179. Campus News. Court Approves CWRU's Purchase of Mt. Sinai Property. www.cwru.edu/pubs/cnews/2001/3-8/mt-sinai2.htm. 3/8/01.

180. Jeff Stacklin. "CWRU Hire Faces Big Task: New VP Will Lead Plans for Mt. Sinai." *Crain's Cleveland Business*, 4/16/01.

181. Hundert, Edward M., M.D., Cleveland, by telephone 7/13/04.

182. Adler, Dale S., M.D., Cleveland, by telephone 12/31/02.

183. Holland, Joel B., M.D., Cleveland, by telephone 2/23/04.

184. Joan M. Mazzolini, Diane Solov. "2 Top Clinic Transplant Surgeons to Jump to UH." *The Plain Dealer*, 1/10/98.

185. Spector, Michael L., M.D., Akron, by telephone 11/7/03.

186. Rudick, Richard A., M.D., Cleveland, by e-mail 7/15/04.

187. Diane Solov. "UH Heart Surgery Unit in Turmoil: Fighting Rocks Cardiothoracic Division." *The Plain Dealer*, 4/28/02.

188. Diane Solov. "Financial Woes, Bitter Infighting at Heart of UH Surgeons' Dispute." *The Plain Dealer*, 6/15/03.

189. Diane Solov. "Doctor Suspended from UH Fights Back: Chest Surgeon Asks Judge to Order Reinstatement." *The Plain Dealer*, 5/4/02.

190. Diane Solov. "UH Panel Upholds Surgeon's Suspension." *The Plain Dealer*, 5/10/02.

191. Farah M. Walters. "Irresponsible Reporting on University Hospitals." *The Plain Dealer*, 5/1/02.

192. Diane Solov. "UH President Blasts Critics of Hospital's Heart Program: Letter Sent to Hospital Employees Discredits Two Former Surgeons." *The Plain Dealer*, 5/1/02.

193. "Bad Outcomes: Rival Surgeons' Ugly Personal and Professional Clashes Leave a Scar on University Hospitals' Cardiothoracic Unit." *The Plain Dealer*, 5/1/02.

194. Sarah Fenske. "Silencing Dr. Kirby: He Was Worried about the Growing Body Count. They Were Worried about Shutting Him Up." *Cleveland Scene*, 7/2/03.

195. Diane Solov. "Panel Revokes UH Authority to Train Doctors in Chest Surgery." *The Plain Dealer*, 9/26/02.

196. Stewart, Robert W., M.D, Cleveland, 4/18/03.

197. Michelson, Edward A., M.D., Cleveland, 2/14/03.

FIVE: University Hospitals of Cleveland: New Leaders

1. Diane Solov, Barb Galbincea. "CWRU Names New President: Rochester Dean, 45, Hopes University Will Help Economy." *The Plain Dealer*, 1/17/02.

2. Willard, Huntington F., Ph.D., Cleveland, by telephone 11/25/02.

3. Ford, Allen H., Cleveland, 6/12/03.

4. Ford, Allen H., Cleveland, by fax 10/7/03.

5. Jeff Stacklin. "New CWRU President Placing Priority on Forging Partnerships." *Crain's Cleveland Business*, 1/21/02.

6. Kastor, JA. Johns Hopkins University and Hospital: Unified Governance. In: *Governance of Teaching Hospitals: Turmoil at Penn and Hopkins*. Baltimore: Johns Hopkins University Press, 2004, chap. 7, 234.

7. Inkley, Scott R., M.D., 3/13/03.

8. Murad, Ferid, M.D., Ph.D., Houston, by telephone 7/18/03.

9. Horwitz, Ralph I., M.D., Cleveland, 4/17/03.

10. Rothstein, Fred C., M.D., Cleveland, 4/15/04.

11. White, Terry R., Cleveland, by telephone 12/23/02.

12. Korn, David, M.D., Washington, DC, by telephone 2/10/03.

13. Daroff, Robert B., M.D., Cleveland, by telephone 12/19/02.

14. America's Best Colleges 2004. www.usnews.com/usnews/edu/college/rankings/brief/natudoc/tier1/t1natudoc_brief.php. 2004

15. Lewis, John F., Esq., Cleveland, 4/16/03.

16. Pytte, Agnar, Ph.D., Etna, NH, by telephone 2/3/03.

17. Watson, Richard T., Cleveland, by telephone 4/23/04.

18. Baznik, Richard E., Cleveland, by telephone 12/8/03.

19. Hadden, Elaine G., Cleveland Heights, OH, by telephone 12/5/03.

20. Anker, Daniel E., Ph.D., Cleveland, by telephone 12/13/02.

21. Diane Solov. "UH's Chief Suddenly Announces Retirement: Walters, 57, Seen as Casualty in Effort to Join with CWRU." *The Plain Dealer*, 4/11/02.

22. Diane Solov. "Walters' Retirement Costs UH $6 Million." *The Plain Dealer*, 1/23/04.

23. Diane Solov. "CWRU, University Hospitals Deal Hits Snag." *The Plain Dealer*, 2/26/02.

24. Hundert, Edward M., M.D., Cleveland, 4/15/04.

25. Lewis, Catharine M., Cleveland, 6/11/03.

26. Meyer, Henry L., III, Cleveland, 6/11/03.

27. Berger, Nathan A., M.D., Cleveland, 2/13/03.

28. Walters, Farah M., Shaker Heights, OH, by telephone 6/10/04.

29. Pogue, Richard W., Esq., Cleveland, by e-mail 5/17/04.

30. Walters FM. Review and rebuttal by Farah M. Walters (with background and some documentation) as to draft of chapters received from Dr. John Kastor. 5/31/04.

31. Pogue, Richard W., Esq., Cleveland, 3/13/03.

32. Regina McEnery. "Next UH Chief to Get Smaller Job." *The Plain Dealer*, 5/17/02.

33. Michael K. McIntyre. "UH Is Bargaining with Outsider." *The Plain Dealer*, 11/25/02.

34. Diane Solov. "UHHS' New Leading Man Known for Focus, Energy." *The Plain Dealer*, 2/23/03.

35. Diane Solov. "UH Names New Leader." *The Plain Dealer*, 12/19/02.

36. Zenty, Thomas F., III, Cleveland, by telephone 1/5/04.

37. Jeff Stacklin. "Zenty Ready to Take Reins at UHHS." *Crain's Cleveland Business*, 2/24/03.

38. Diane Solov. "UHHS Shakes Up Senior Leadership." *The Plain Dealer*, 7/3/03.

39. Jacobs, M. Orry, Cleveland, 4/16/03.

40. Morley, John C., Cleveland, 6/12/03.

41. Diane Solov. "Consultant to Review: UHHS Operations System to Use Analysis in Spending Plan." *The Plain Dealer*, 11/1/03.

42. Regina McEnery, Mike Tobin. "Leaders Begin to Examine Issues Surrounding St. Michael's Closing." *The Plain Dealer*, 9/18/03.

43. Kastor, JA. UCSF Stanford: Development. In: *Mergers of Teaching Hospitals in Boston, New York, and Northern California*. Ann Arbor: University of Michigan Press, 2001, chap. 7, 364.

44. Sam Fulwood III. "Health Ills Go beyond Hospital." *The Plain Dealer*, 9/20/03.

45. Diane Solov, Regina McEnery, Harlan Spector. "Sinai-East St. Michael Win New Lifer: Nine-minute Auction Ends Hospital Fight." *The Plain Dealer*, 5/2/00.

46. Ivancic, Robert, Cleveland, by telephone 12/3/03.

47. Diane Solov. "Bond Rating Company Raps UH Operations: Hospital System Suffers 2-Step Drop in Score." *The Plain Dealer*, 9/26/03.

48. Kastor, UCSF Stanford: Development. In: *Mergers of Teaching Hospitals in Boston, New York, and Northern California*, chap. 7, 378–384.

49. Kastor, University of Pennsylvania: Kelley in Trouble. In: *Governance of Teaching Hospitals*, chap. 4, 100–101.

50. Diane Solov. "University Hospitals Taps Rothstein President, CEO." *The Plain Dealer*, 2/19/03.

51. Avner, Ellis D., M.D., Cleveland, 6/13/03.

52. Shakno, Robert J., Cleveland, by telephone 2/20/04.

53. Cowen, Scott S., Ph.D., New Orleans, by telephone 7/22/03.

54. Jeff Stacklin. "Rothstein Lands Deal, Not Job." *Crain's Cleveland Business*, 12/23/02.

55. Morley, John C., Cleveland, by e-mail 10/7/03.

56. Bolton, Charles P., Cleveland, 6/13/03.

57. Diane Solov. "CWRU Picks Yale Man to Lead Medical School." *The Plain Dealer*, 1/17/03.

58. Aach, Richard D., M.D., Cleveland, 2/13/03.

59. CWRU board to consider Yale general internist, clinical epidemiologist and researcher: To be VP for medical affairs, medical school dean and director of Case Research Institute. www.cwru.edu/pubaff/univcomm/2003/1-03/horwitz.htm. 2003.

60. Landis, Dennis M. D., M.D., Cleveland, by telephone 12/23/03.

61. Linsalata, Frank N., Cleveland, 4/15/04.

62. Colten, Harvey R., M.D., New York, by telephone 2/15/03.

63. Karn, Jonathan, Ph.D., Cleveland, 4/18/03.

64. Jeff Stacklin. "Research Star Lands at CWRU." *Crain's Cleveland Business*, 2/4/02.

65. Landmesser, Lynn T., Ph.D., Cleveland, 3/12/03.

66. Kirby, Albert C., Ph.D., Cleveland, by telephone 12/8/03.

67. Mieyal, John J., Ph.D., Cleveland, by telephone 12/23/03.

68. Shuck, Jerry M., M.D., Cleveland, by telephone 12/1/03.

69. Hundert, Edward M., M.D., Cleveland, by telephone 7/13/04.

70. Horwitz, Ralph I., M.D., Cleveland, by e-mail 4/22/04.

71. Daroff, Robert B., M.D., Cleveland, by telephone 5/3/04.

72. Shannon Mortland. "Hundert Has $181M Vision." *Crain's Cleveland Business*, 10/13/03.

73. Horwitz, Ralph I., M.D., Cleveland, 4/15/04.

74. Liu, James H., M.D., Cleveland, by telephone 12/17/03.

75. University Hospitals & CWRU launch 50-year landmark partnership pact to create new model for education, research and patient care. http://cerebrum.cwru.edu/news release/Partnership.htm. 2002.

76. Diane Solov, Barb Galbincea. "UH Signs Research Pact with CWRU: Joint Institute to Recruit Top-Flight Clinical Scientists." *The Plain Dealer*, 1/18/02.

77. Wagner, James W., Ph.D., Cleveland, 4/17/03.

78. "CWRU and UHC Receive $25 Million Gift from Wolsteins." *Global News Wire*, 1/17/03.

79. $25 Million Wolstein Gift to CWRU-UHC. www.uhhs.com/article_detail.asp?id =92&GNAV=&MID=0&PageId=68. 1/17/03.

80. Hundert, Edward M., M.D., Cleveland, by telephone 7/14/04, by e-mail 7/14/04.

81. Diane Solov, Barb Galbincea. "A New Medical School for Cleveland: CWRU, Clinic Will Collaborate to Train Physician-Researchers." *The Plain Dealer*, 5/15/02.

82. Singer, Lynn T., Ph.D., Cleveland, by e-mail 12/4/03.

83. Schulak, James A., M.D., Cleveland, 3/12/03.

84. Goldberg, Jerold S., Cleveland, 3/13/03.

85. Horwitz, Ralph I., M.D., Cleveland, by telephone 3/24/05.

SIX: The New Medical School

1. Roger Mezger. "Clinic Gets $100 Million: Lerner Gift Supports New Medical School." *The Plain Dealer*, 10/20/03.
2. Topol, Eric J., M.D., Cleveland, 7/8/02.
3. Linsalata, Frank N., Cleveland, 4/15/04.
4. Licensing Committee on Medical Education. www.lcme.org/.
5. Berger, Nathan A., M.D., Cleveland, 2/13/03.
6. Kirby, Albert C., Ph.D., Cleveland, by telephone 12/8/03.
7. Berger, Nathan A., M.D., Cleveland, by telephone 12/13/02.
8. Hundert, Edward M., M.D., Cleveland, by telephone 7/14/04, by e-mail 7/14/04.
9. Henson, Lindsey C., M.D., Ph.D., Cleveland, 11/22/02.
10. Diane Solov. "Hopes Rise for Research Mecca Here: CWRU, Hospitals Revive Push for Elite Medical Consortium." *The Plain Dealer*, 7/25/01.
11. Pytte, Agnar, Ph.D., Etna, NH, by telephone 2/3/03.
12. Neuhauser, Duncan V., Ph.D., Cleveland, by telephone 2/4/04.
13. Vidt, Donald G., M.D., Cleveland, by telephone 3/1/04.
14. Bolton, Charles P., Cleveland, 6/13/03.
15. Mixon, A. Malachai, III, Cleveland, 7/10/03.
16. Loop, Floyd D., M.D., Cleveland, 7/9/03.
17. Korn, Stephen J., M.D., Sharon, MA, by telephone 11/22/03.
18. Fishleder, Andrew J., M.D., Cleveland, by e-mail 4/23/04.
19. Harvard-MIT Division of Health Sciences and Technology (HST) community. http://hst.mit.edu/public/about/. 2004.
20. Daroff, Robert B., M.D., Cleveland, by e-mail 5/31/04.
21. Nilson, John H., Ph.D., Cleveland, 2/13/03.
22. Singer, Lynn T., Ph.D., Cleveland, 7/10/03.
23. Hutzler, Jeffery C., M.D., Cleveland, by telephone 12/1/03.
24. Henson, Lindsey C., M.D., Ph.D., Cleveland, by mail 4/7/04.
25. Fishleder, Andrew J., M.D., Cleveland, 10/31/02.
26. Henson, Lindsey C., M.D., Ph.D., Cleveland, 2/12/03.
27. Loop, Floyd D., M.D., Cleveland, 7/9/02.
28. Fishleder, Andrew J., M.D., Cleveland, by e-mail 11/11/03.
29. Horwitz, Ralph I., M.D., Cleveland, 4/15/04.
30. Topol, Eric J., M.D., Cleveland, by telephone 4/23/04.
31. Henrich, William L., M.D., Baltimore, 8/16/02.
32. Anker, Daniel E., Ph.D., Cleveland, by e-mail 1/16/03.
33. Richard Goldstein. "Alfred Lerner, 69, Banker: Revived Cleveland Browns." *The New York Times*, 10/25/02.
34. Harris, C. Martin, M.D., Cleveland, 9/11/02.
35. Loop, Floyd D., M.D., Cleveland, by mail 4/12/04.
36. Blazar, James M., Cleveland, 9/9/02.
37. Ponsky, Jeffrey L., M.D., Hunting Valley, OH, by telephone 12/18/03.
38. Education. In: Clough, JD, editor. *To Act as a Unit: The Story of the Cleveland Clinic*, 3rd ed. The Cleveland Clinic Foundation, 1996, chap. 18, 211–220.
39. Healy, Bernadine P., M.D., Washington, DC, by telephone 3/19/04.

40. Eckardt, Robert E., Cleveland, by telephone 3/11/03.

41. Fishleder, Andrew J., M.D., Cleveland, by telephone 4/28/04.

42. Fishleder, Andrew J., M.D., Cleveland, by e-mail 11/26/02.

43. Rehm, Susan J., M.D., Cleveland, by telephone 11/20/03.

44. Pohl, Marc A., M.D., Cleveland, 9/10/02.

45. Francis, Gary, M.D., Cleveland, 10/30/02.

46. Ludmerer KM. Academic Health Centers under Stress: Internal Dilemmas. The Dilemmas of Graduate Education. In: *Time to Heal: American Medical Education from the Turn of the Century to the Era of Managed Care*. New York: Oxford University Press, 1999, chap. 15, 313–326.

47. Levine, Michael A., M.D., Cleveland, by telephone 1/7/04.

48. Hoogwerf, Brian, M.D., Cleveland, 11/21/02.

49. Lordeman, Frank L., Cleveland, 11/21/02.

50. Clough, John D., M.D., Cleveland, 9/11/02.

51. Novick, Andrew C., M.D., Cleveland, 7/10/03.

52. Research Institute. In: Clough, *To Act as a Unit*, chap. 19, 221-234.

53. DiCorleto, Paul E., Ph.D., Cleveland, 9/11/02.

54. Stark, George R., Ph.D., Cleveland, 9/9/02.

55. Diane Solov. "Rivals in Medical Research Explore Cooperation: 'Star' Scientists, New Treatments Possible If Clinic Works with University Hospitals." *The Plain Dealer*, 1/24/99.

56. Loop, Floyd D., M.D., Cleveland, 9/10/02.

57. Mayberg, Marc C., M.D., Cleveland, 11/1/02.

58. Lauer, Michael S., M.D., Cleveland, 7/11/03.

59. Bolwell, Brian J., M.D., Cleveland, 7/9/03.

60. Rudick, Richard A., M.D., Cleveland, 11/20/02.

61. Lüders, Hans O., M.D., Ph.D., Cleveland, 10/31/02.

62. Kay, Robert, M.D., Cleveland, 9/11/02.

63. Clough, John D., M.D., Cleveland, by telephone 11/26/03.

64. Petrovic, Frank, by email 5/27/05.

65. Petrovic, Frank, and Topol, Eric J., by e-mail 11/12/02.

66. Rudick, Richard A., M.D., Cleveland, by e-mail 7/15/04.

67. Gerson, Stanton L., M.D., Cleveland, by telephone 1/5/04.

68. Bukowski, Ronald M., M.D., Cleveland, by telephone 12/11/03.

69. Diane Solov. "UH Asks to Add Clinic to Cancer Center." *The Plain Dealer*, 6/5/03.

70. Hundert, Edward M., M.D., Cleveland, 4/15/04.

71. Horwitz, Ralph I., M.D., Cleveland, by e-mail 4/22/04.

72. Mahmoud, Adel A. F., M.D., Ph.D., West Point, PA, 1/14/03.

73. Shuck, Jerry M., M.D., Cleveland, 2/14/03.

74. Davis, Pamela B., M.D., Ph.D., Cleveland, 4/16/03.

75. Devereaux, Michael W., Ph.D., Cleveland, 4/17/03.

76. Landis, Dennis M. D., M.D., Cleveland, 4/18/03.

77. Scarpa, Antonio, M.D., Ph.D., Cleveland, 4/17/03.

78. Landmesser, Lynn T., Ph.D., Cleveland, 3/12/03.

79. Topol, Eric J., M.D., Cleveland, by e-mail 4/23/04.

80. Goldberg, Jerold S., Cleveland, 3/13/03.

81. Horwitz, Ralph I., M.D., Cleveland, 4/17/03.

82. Wagner, James W., Ph.D., Cleveland, 4/17/03.

83. Walsh, Patrick C., M.D., Baltimore, 1/16/03.

84. Topol, Eric J., M.D., Cleveland, by e-mail 3/25/04.

85. McCarthy, Patrick M., M.D., Cleveland, 10/30/02.

86. Modic, Michael T., M.D., Cleveland, by telephone 1/26/04.

87. Loop, Floyd D., M.D., Cleveland, by telephone 7/25/04.

88. Iannotti, Joseph P., M.D., Ph.D., Cleveland, 11/21/02.

89. Markman, Maurie, M.D., Cleveland, 11/1/02.

90. Hardy, Russell W., Jr., M.D., Cleveland, 2/12/03.

91. Borden, Ernest C., M.D., Cleveland, by telephone 11/17/03.

92. Cosgrove, Delos M., M.D., Cleveland, by telephone 7/7/04.

SEVEN: Conclusions

1. Lordeman, Frank L., Cleveland, 10/31/02.

2. Bronson, David L., M.D., Cleveland, 9/10/02.

3. Wade, Richard H., Washington, by e-mail 2/10/04.

4. Egan, Michele, Cleveland, by e-mail 2/10/04.

5. Kastor, JA. University of Pennsylvania: Kelley in Trouble. In: *Governance of Teaching Hospitals: Turmoil at Penn and Hopkins.* Baltimore: Johns Hopkins University Press, 2004, chap. 4, 91.

6. Neuhauser, Duncan V., Ph.D., Cleveland, by telephone 2/4/04.

7. Neuhauser, Duncan V., Ph.D., Cleveland, by e-mail 4/2/04.

8. Kastor, University of Pennsylvania: Kelley in Trouble. In: *Governance of Teaching Hospitals*, chap. 4, 91–93.

9. Longnecker, DE, Henson, DE, Wilczek, K, Wray, JL, Miller, ED. Future Directions for Academic Practice Plans: Thoughts on Organization and Management from Johns Hopkins University and the University of Pennsylvania. *Acad.Med.* 2003;78:1130–1143.

10. Diane Solov. "Clinic-UH Skirmish Moves to West Side." *The Plain Dealer*, 6/29/03.

11. Block, James A., M.D., Baltimore, 3/18/03.

12. Smith, Philip C., M.D., Cleveland, by telephone 12/10/03.

13. Goldberg, Victor M., M.D., Cleveland, by telephone 4/26/04.

14. Walters, Farah M., Cleveland, by telephone 7/8/04.

15. Kiser, William S., M.D., Cleveland, 7/10/03.

16. Lewis, John F., Esq., Cleveland, 4/16/03.

17. Lintz, Robert L., Cleveland, 7/11/03.

18. Kastor, JA. UCSF Stanford: Formation. In: *Mergers of Teaching Hospitals in Boston, New York, and Northern California.* Ann Arbor: University of Michigan Press, 2001, chap. 6, 282–288.

19. Kastor, University of Pennsylvania: Before Kelley. In: *Governance of Teaching Hospitals*, chap. 2, 8–11.

20. The Wasmuth Years, 1969–1976. In: Clough, JD, editor. *To Act as a Unit: The Story of the Cleveland Clinic*, 3rd ed. The Cleveland Clinic Foundation, 1996, chap. 7.

21. Cosgrove, Delos M., M.D., Cleveland, by telephone 7/7/04.

22. Ivancic, Robert, Cleveland, by telephone 12/3/03.

23. Coulton, Robert W., Jr., Cleveland, by telephone 11/26/03.

24. Ulreich, Shawn M., R.N., Cleveland, by telephone 11/24/03.

25. Horn, Karen, Ph.D., New York, by telephone 3/20/03.

26. Landis, Story C., Ph.D., Bethesda, MD, by telephone 2/11/03.

27. Mixon, A. Malachai, III, Cleveland, 7/10/03.

28. Jeff Stacklin. "Same Names Dot Research Boards." *Crain's Cleveland Business,* 5/14/01.

29. Diane Solov. "Can Boardroom Who's Who Snarl What's What? CWRU Chief's Departure Raises Issue of 1 Decision-Maker Serving on 2 Boards." *The Plain Dealer,* 5/19/01.

30. Hundert, Edward M., M.D., Cleveland, by e-mail 7/18/04.

31. Baznik, Richard E., Cleveland, by telephone 12/8/03.

32. Bank, Malvin E., Esq., Cleveland, 6/11/03.

33. Geha, Alexander S., M.D., Chicago, by telephone 5/17/03.

34. Scarpa, Antonio, M.D., Ph.D., Cleveland, 4/17/03.

35. Ratcheson, Robert A., M.D., Cleveland, 3/12/03.

36. Bolton, Charles P., Cleveland, 6/13/03.

37. Hadden, Elaine G., Cleveland Heights, OH, by telephone 12/5/03.

38. Murad, Ferid, M.D., Ph.D., Houston, by telephone 7/18/03.

39. Grimberg, William C., Cleveland, by telephone 11/26/03.

40. MacDonald, William E., Cleveland, 7/11/03.

41. Weimer, Gary W., Cleveland, by telephone 1/15/04.

42. "A. Malachi Mixon, III, Elected Chairman of Cleveland Clinic Foundation's Board of Trustees." *Business Wire,* 5/16/97.

43. MacDonald, William E., III, Cleveland, 7/10/03.

44. Modell, Arthur B., Baltimore, 9/23/03.

45. Cowen, Scott S., Ph.D., New Orleans, by telephone 7/24/03.

46. Gifford, Ray W., M.D., Phoenix, AZ, by telephone 12/3/03.

47. Thomas George. "For 42 Years, Modell Had Watched, and Helped, the N.F.L. Grow." *The New York Times,* 9/5/03.

48. Gregory Jordan. "N.F.L. Ownership, on the Installment Plan." *The New York Times,* 12/28/03.

49. Kovner, Anthony R., Ph.D., New York, by telephone 12/15/03.

50. Gray, Bradford H., Ph.D., New York, by telephone 12/11/03.

51. McCartan, Patrick F., Esq., Cleveland, 7/9/03.

52. Roberts, Kevin V., Cleveland, 3/14/03.

53. Daroff, Robert B., M.D., Cleveland, by e-mail 7/3/03.

54. Landis, Dennis M. D., M.D., Cleveland, by telephone 8/8/03.

55. Bank, Malvin E., Esq., Cleveland, by telephone 10/20/03.

56. Korn, David, M.D., Washington, DC, by telephone 2/10/03.

57. Bank, Malvin E., Esq., Cleveland, by telephone 5/4/04.

58. Pytte, Agnar, Ph.D., Etna, NH, by telephone 2/3/03.

59. Meyer, Henry L., III, Cleveland, 6/11/03.

60. Lewis, Catharine M., Cleveland, 6/11/03.

61. Jackson, J. Brooks, M.D., Baltimore, 4/29/03.

62. Markowitz, Alan H., M.D., Cleveland, 3/13/03.

63. Haaga, John R., M.D., Cleveland, 3/14/03.

64. Cowen, Scott S., Ph.D., New Orleans, by telephone 7/22/03.

65. NIH Awards to Medical Schools by Rank, Fiscal Year 2003. http://grants1.nih.gov/grants/award/rank/medttl03.htm. 2004.

66. NIH Support to Research Institutes, Fiscal Year 2003. http://grants.nih.gov/grants/award/trends/resins03.htm.

66a. NIH Awards to Medical Schools by Rank, Fiscal Year 2003. http://grants.nih.gov/grants/award/rank/medttl03.htm.

67. Ornt, Daniel B., M.D., by e-mail 4/23/04.

68. Ornt, Daniel B., M.D., by e-mail 5/14/04.

69. Ouriel, Kenneth, M.D., Cleveland, by e-mail 4/26/04.

70. Topol, Eric J., M.D., Cleveland, by e-mail 3/17/04.

71. Hardy, Russell W., Jr., M.D., Cleveland, 2/12/03.

72. Clough, John D., M.D., Cleveland, by telephone 11/26/03.

73. Ginzberg, E. *Teaching Hospitals and the Urban Poor.* New Haven: Yale University Press, 2000, 57.

74. Blumenthal D. New Steam from an Old Cauldron—The Physician-Supply Debate. *New England Journal of Medicine* 2004;350:1780–1787.

75. Hundert, Edward M., M.D., Cleveland, by telephone 7/14/04, by e-mail 7/14/04.

Index